A Textbook on HIV Infection and AIDS in Adolescents

A Textbook on HIV Infection and AIDS in Adolescents

M.S. Bhatia

Professor & Head
Department of Psychiatry
University College of Medical Sciences
and associated Guru Teg Bahadur Hospital
Delhi (India)

Vijay Grover

Professor
Department of Community Medicine
Maulana Medical College
Ambala (India)

Ravi Gupta

Department of Psychiatry
University College of Medical Sciences
and associated Guru Teg Bahadur Hospital
Delhi (India)

–Editors

PUBLISHING FOR ONE WORLD

NEW AGE INTERNATIONAL (P) LIMITED, PUBLISHERS

New Delhi • Bangalore • Chennai • Cochin • Guwahati • Hyderabad
Jalandhar • Kolkata • Lucknow • Mumbai • Ranchi

Visit us at **www.newagepublishers.com**

Published by New Age International (P) Ltd., Publishers
First Edition: 2009

Branches:

- 36, Malikarjuna Temple Street, Opp. ICWA, Basavanagudi, **Bangalore**. ✆ (080) 26677815
- 26, Damodaran Street, T. Nagar, **Chennai**. ✆ (044) 24353401
- Hemsen Complex, Mohd. Shah Road, Paltan Bazar, Near Starline Hotel, **Guwahati**. ✆ (0361) 2543669
- No. 105, 1st Floor, Madhiray Kaveri Tower, 3-2-19, Azam Jahi Road, Nimboliadda, **Hyderabad**. ✆ (040) 24652456
- RDB Chambers (Formerly Lotus Cinema) 106A, Ist Floor, S.N. Banerjee Road, **Kolkata**. ✆ (033) 22275247
- 18, Madan Mohan Malviya Marg, **Lucknow**. ✆ (0522) 2209578
- 142C, Victor House, Ground Floor, N.M. Joshi Marg, Lower Parel, **Mumbai**. ✆ (022) 24927869
- 22, Golden House, Daryaganj, **New Delhi**. ✆ (011) 23262368, 23262370

ISBN : 978-81-224-2245-0

Rs. 295.00

C-08-07-2702

Printed in India at Glorious Printers, Delhi.
Typeset in-house.

PUBLISHING FOR ONE WORLD

NEW AGE INTERNATIONAL (P) LIMITED, PUBLISHERS
4835/24, Ansari Road, Daryaganj, New Delhi - 110002
Visit us at **www.newagepublishers.com**

Preface

Human Immunodeficiency Virus (HIV) infection and Acquired Immunodeficiency Syndrome (AIDS) are most dreaded infectious disorders known to the world during twentieth century. This disease which was initially limited to a few areas is now widespread and according to recent statistics, has emerged as the most prevalent and deadly disorder in the developing countries.

Unfortunately, it is most common in the adolescents, since they are exposed to a number of risk factors, e.g., drug addiction, unsafe sexual practices etc. Moreover, psychological factors also play their role. Since a long time, clinicians and researchers were feeling the dearth of a dedicated book that addresses the health issues of adolescents with HIV infection. Moreover, India is now having the largest number of adolescents. Almost all factors that help in spreading the infection, e.g., illiteracy, poor economic conditions, unsafe sexual practices, intravenous drug abuse, recycling of medically used syringes, unsafe blood transfusion etc. are common in India.

Hence, this book entitled, **"A Textbook on HIV Infections and AIDS in Adolescents"** was planned. It is specially compiled by a number of renowned contributors of their field keeping the adolescent population and their need into consideration. We hope that this book will give insight into this important health problem and shall help in planning and implementing the strategies to control and prevent HIV and AIDS in a more effective manner.

Editors

Preface

Contents

CHAPTER

1 An Overview of Selected Curable Sexually Transmitted Infections in Adolescents

Vijay Grover

The transition from childhood to being health sexual adults is one of the major tasks and challenges facing young people. A successful transition implies forming intimate relationships while avoiding the acquisition of sexually transmitted infections.

The recent emergence of HIV/AIDS has added new relevance to the history of sexually transmitted diseases (STDs). In a remarkably short period of time, AIDS has become a dominant issue in both medical and social dimensions of health. The history of HIV itself reinforce ideas about the complexity of STDs both medical and cultural entities painfully reminding us of the ties between sex and disease. HIV confirms that STDs will remain as much a problem for the twenty first century as they have been for past century.

Sexually transmitted infections (STIs) are among the most common causes of illness in the world and have far reaching health, social and economic consequences. In addition to their sheer magnitude, STIs are a major public health problem for two additional reasons: their serious sequelae, and the fact that they facilitate transmission of HIV. In addition, complications from STIs are found more often in resource poor settings and, as a result, the greatest burden falls on the least well off countries, and, within countries on the poor.[1]

Sexually transmitted infections (STIs) are infections that can be transfered from one person to another through sexual contact. According to the Centers for Disease Control there are over a million cases of sexually transmitted infection reported annually. Adolescents and youth (15-24) are the age groups at the greater risk for acquiring an STI. 3 million teenagers becoming infected each year – that is 13% of all young people between the ages of 13 and 19 — contact an STI. This represents about 25% of sexually experienced adolescents.[2]

It is apparent from the current data that around the world, for a combination of reasons involving biology, psychology, ambient culture and changing moods of adolescents who have had sexual intercourse have the highest rates of STIs – including HIV/AIDS in some locale – of any age group. As stated by one researcher, "the challenge lies in getting teenagers to view their relationships in a more realistic light without destroying the positive ways in which these (relationships) may also add to their lives."[3]

The recent emergence of HIV/AIDS has added new relevance to the history of STIs. In a remarkably short period of time, AIDS has become a dominent issue in both medical and social dimension of health. HIV confirms that STIs will remain as much as the twenty first century as they have been for past centuries.

Extend of STIs

Sexually transmitted infections (STIs) are the most common causes of illness in the world. Gonorrhoea, syphilis and now AIDS are the most widely known STIs. Most population based rates of sexually transmitted underestimate of the risk of STI for sexually active adolescents because the rate is inappropriately expressed as cases of disease divided by number of individuals in this age group. For rates to reflect risk among those who are sexually experienced, appropriate denominators should include only the number of individuals in the demographic group who have had sexual intercourse, this is true of only 50% of women 15-19 years old.[4]

This underestimation of rates is greater among the youngest adolescents, since only a small proportion of them have had sex. In general when rates are corrected for the percentages in group who are sexually active, the youngest adolescents have the highest STI rates of any age group.[5]

It is seen that globally nearly half of the new HIV cases occur in the young people aged 15-29. Also a large percentage of new STIs occur in this age group reflecting 7000 young people worldwide acquire the infection every day.[6,7]

STIs take a great toll on health through their sequelae i.e. the conditions resulting from its spread to reproductive tract, such as fallopian tubes in women. Sequelae of some sexually transmitted infections, in particular gonorrhoea and chlamydial infection which cause pelvic inflammatory disease in women, impair the fertility in both men and women. Another sequela of STIs is the increased risk of ectopic pregnancy, a condition that can kill from sudden and severe internal bleeding following rupture of fallopian tube.

Some STIs attack foetus and the infant as well. In two-thirds or more of pregnant women with early spyphilis, for example, the infection spreads through the placenta and infects the foetus and because of this up to one-half of syphilis-infected pregnancies and in spontaneous abortion, stillbirth, or perenatal death. Gonorrhoea or chlamydial infection may likewise infect the eyes of babies as they pass through the cervix and vagina during birth, while chlamydial infection may spread to the lungs of newborns, resulting in chlamydial pneumonia.

Young adults between 15 and 19 years of age often have high rates of STIs on account of their frequent and multiple casual sex partners and present important problems of their lack of easy access to medical services and supply of condoms.[6,7]

Because treatments of STIs and their sequelae, have such a widespread effect on men, women, youth and newborns, the problem of curable STIs is expensive to the individual's and health care system as well as to individuals. The World Bank has estimated that STIs collectively rank second only in importance among diseases for which intervention is possible among women between 15-44 years of age worldwide.[8]

WHO estimated that in the year 1990, there were over 250 million new cases of sexually transmitted infections. The Delphi technique was chosen at that time to arrive at the estimates because of the lack of information on STIs in many regions. Recently there has been an increase in publications on STI prevalence in developing countries in Africa, Asia, Latin America and the Carribbean. Using this information, and information from other sources such as official STI prevalence estimates from industrialized countries and WHO archival information from country specific reports, prevalence rates of gonorrhoea, chlamydial infection, syphilis and trichomoniasis were estimated by sex and by (UN standard) region.[4]

In 1990 the WHO generated global estimates for the number of new cases of STDs in adults between 15 and 49 years of age using a modified Delphi approach. The expert panel estimated that in 1990 there were over 78 million new cases of the three "classes" STDs (gonorrhoea, chlambdia and syphilis) and an additional 120 million new cases of trichomoniasis in this age group. More recently, the WHO in partnership with the Rockefeller Foundation, has generated a new set of estimates of or 1995 drawing on data from the Global Data Bank of STDs established by the WHO.[9]

Because of a lack of published and archival information on chancroid, no estimates of this disease could be made. Likewise estimates were not made for the viral STIs such as herpes, human papilloma virus and hepatitis B.

Based on the probability of a symptomatic or an asymptomatic person getting treatment for his/her STI, the duration of each infection by sex and region were estimated. Regional adult STI incidence for 1995 was calculated by dividing the estimated prevalence by the estimated duration of each disease and the results are shown in Table-1, which summarises population, prevalence and incidence data by region.

Table 1. ***Estimated Prevalence and Annual Incidence of Curable STIs by Region***

Region	*Population 15-49 (Millions)*	*Prevalence (Millions)*	*Prevalence Per/1000*	*Annual Incidence*
North America	153	8	52	14
Western Europe	211	10	45	16
Australasia	11	0.6	52	1
Latin America and the Caribbean	251	24	95	36

(Contd...)

Sub-Saharan Africa	254	53	208	65
Northern Africa and Middle East	163	6.5	40	10
Eastern Europe and Central Asia	158	12	75	18
East Asia and Pacific	803	16	19	23
South and South East Asia	943	120	128	150
Total	**2946**	**250**	**85**	**333**

Source: WHO; Global Programme on AIDS

Adolescent women are much more likely to have chlamydia infection than older women and are also more likely to have repeated infection.[2]

Men aged 15 to 19 have the second highest gonorrhoea rates among men; women 15 to 19 years old have the highest gonorrhoea rates among women.[11]

Gonorrhoea and syphilis rates among adolescents while decline are disproportionately high for Afro-American youth compared to white and Hispanic youth.[12]

The consequences of STIs can be devastating: infants, infected at birth, with blinding eye infection of pneumonia, women suffering chronic abdominal pain, ectopic pregnancy or infertility; and men with infertility. Young people are specially exposed to the infection. Around 50% of the new infections worldwide are occurring in young people. Women, in addition, may suffer social consequences as well; telling a husband about an infection may lead to beatings and divorce, and husbands may abandon infertile wives.

The high incidence of STIs among women attending antenatal, family planning or gynaecological clinics indicates the extent of STI problem. For example, in studies in developing countries, up to 18% of these patients have gonorrhoea, upto 17% have syphilis and upto 30% have trichomoniasis. Sexually transmitted infections are a major public health problem in both developed and developing countries, but prevalence rates apparently are far higher in developing countries, where treatment of STIs is less accessible. Among women, syphilis prevalence rates may be 10 to 15 times higher; and chlamydia rates may be 2 to 3 times higher[13]. Incidence rates also are higher. For example, the annual rate of new gonorrhoea infections in large African cities is 3000 to 10,000 population, or as many as one in every 10 people. By comparison, in the US the annual incidence of gonorrhoea was 233 per 100,000 population in 1991 and in Sweden, about 30 per 100,000 in 1987.[14,15,16]

Among developing region STIs appear to be more common in Africa than in the Asia or Latin America. In a review by Judith Wasserheit, a median of 20% of women attending family planning, antenatal, or other clinics in Africa had trichomonasis, for example, while the median prevalence in Asia studies was 11% and in Latin American studies 12%.[17]

Youth have high rates of STIs.[18,24] In a study at Kenyatta hospital in Nairobi, for example, 23% of women ages 15 to 19 seeking antenatal care had gonorrhoea, and men ages 15 to 19 had the second highest incidence of any age group.[16]

In many countries clinic surveys are the available indicators of STI levels. The true extent of STIs in the general population remains unknown for several reasons:

- Both men and women may suffer from asymptomatic STIs, but women suffer more so than men. For example, 70% of women and 30% of men infected with chlamydia may be asymptomatic as well as 30% of women and 5% of men infected with gonorrhoea.[25,26]
- Many people with STIs do not seek care. In developing countries people are not routinely screened for STIs when they seek other health care.
- Because of stigma attached to STIs many people seek care from providers, who do not report cases.
- Some governments are reluctant to admit to a high prevalence of STIs. However, the AIDS epidemic is beginning to change this attitude.

The few studies in developing countries report mixed trends. For example, between 1987 and 1991 in 15 to 21 Latin American countries, the incidence of primary, secondary, or congenital syphilis increased.[27] Evidence from developed countries also shows mixed trends. The incidence of chlamydia is increasing in North America and some European countries.[28] Chancroid and primary syphilis are becoming common in USA.[29,30] In contrast, the incidence of gonorrhoea has been decreasing in Canada, Sweden, the UK and the US and the incidence of primary syphilis has decreased in Sweden.[14]

Sexual behaviour involves risk. The same is true of experimentation with drug usage, legal or illegal. Some young people may be infected with STIs. The behaviour that causes teenage pregnancies and STIs also causes AIDS. HIV/AIDS is no longer restricted to certain groups. It is the behaviour that puts people at risk.

According to Marx et al. (1989), nearly all 20 to 24 years old have had sexual intercourse, this was true for only 50 percent of women 15 to 19 years old. This underestimation of rates is greatest among the youngest adolescents, since only a small proportion of them have had sex.[4]

Chlamydial Infection

Chlamydia trachomatis has become the most prevalent sexually transmitted bacterial infection in North America and Europe. During 1995, it is estimated there will be approximately 89 million new adult chlamydial infections worldwide, again with the greatest number in South and South East Asia followed, as for syphilis and gonorrhoea, by Sub-Saharan Africa.

Chlamydial infection, like gonorrhoea, is a common adult disease, which has asymptomatic rates in women similar to those for gonorrhoea, but higher rates of asymptomatic infection than gonorrhoea in men. Like gonorrhoea, chlamydia has serious sequelae such as pelvic inflammatory disease and infertility. Diagnosis of chlamydial infection is costly and those diagnostic test, which are most sensitive are not generally available in developing countries. Even in industrialized countries laboratory testing is not available in all health facilities. Screening programs in women at risk of infection are therefore not consistently conducted. As many infections are neither detected nor treated, prevalence rates are high. Rates of infection among women attending family planning clinics from 1989 to 1993 in the United States of America were shown to vary from 4.5% to 8.5%.[30]

Chlamydia trahomatis is the most common of all bacterial sexually transmitted infections, which is strongly associated with adolescents, with an estimated 4 to 8 million new cases occurring each year. In both men and women, chlamydial infection may cause an abnormal genital discharge and burning with urination.

Numerous clinic based studies have demonstrated that prevalence of cervical chlamydia is greatest among sexually active individuals under 20 years of age, being approximately twice that found among older individuals.[25-28]

We, in India, are only beginning to realize the importance of this disease. It causes an estimated 4 million infections annually, primarily among adolescents and young adults. In women, untreated Chlamydia is a very dangerous STI as it usually has no symptoms; 75% of infected women and 25% of infected men, have no symptoms at all and without testing and treatment the infection may persist for as long as 15 months. Although majority of studies have been performed among females, tests performed on urine specimens, among other tests have been used recently to evaluate prevalence among males. The findings are similar to those for females. With prevalence of chlamydia being greater among those under 25 years of age, and somewhat greater among minority youth, prevalence among males is usually found between 5 to 10 percent, somewhat less than among females.[25,26]

Recurrent infections may be particularly worrisome since such infections are associated with development of significant tissue damage than in primary infection. Many recurrent infections are associated with continuing presence of a sex partner, who has remained untreated. The risk of recurrent infection is twice as high among adolescents as among older women.[27,28] However, in much of the developing world rates are still very high, as shown by the prevalence of disease (up to 22%) in antenatal or family planning clinics in a rural survey.[31,32]

When age specific data are available from other countries, chlamydia prevalence is found to be greatest among adolescents.[27,28]

Treatment: Infection can be cured with antibiotics. However, it cannot undo the damage done before the treatment.

Possible consequences for infected person: In women, untreated infections can progress to involve the upper reproductive tract and may result in serious complications with an estimated 4 to 8 million new cases occurring each year. If untreated in women, up to 20-40 percent will experience pelvic inflammatory disease (PID), which in turn often leads to entopic pregnancy, infertility, a chronic pelvic pain. In men, if untreated can cause epididymitis, an inflammation of testicles which may result in sterility. Infected individuals are at greater risk of contracting HIV, if exposed to the virus.[30]

Gonorrhoea

Gonorrhoea is one of the most frequently reported STIs. 40% of its victims contract PID if not treated and it leads to infertility. During 1995, it is estimated that there will be approximately 62 million new cases of gonorrhoea among adults worldwide, with the greatest number in South and South East Asia followed, as for syphilis, by Sub-Saharan Africa. From 1981-91 although the overall rate among males declined 46%, the rate among males 15-19 years old did not decline at all and in females decreased.[31]

Gonorrhoea is a common adult disease, though a significant proportion of those with infection (up to 80% among women, 10% among men) are asymptomatic, i.e. they do not have symptoms and therefore they are neither aware of the need for treatment nor of the risk of transmitting the disease to others. Men aged 15-19 have the second highest gonorrhoea rates, women 15-19 years old have the highest annual gonorrhoea rates.[12,15]

Infected men, who have symptoms, usually seek treatment spontaneously. Women frequently have only minor symptoms or are asymptomatic, so detection of infection depends mainly on screening by culture. This is costly and requires relatively sophisticated facilities. Few countries operate regular screening programs and gonorrhoea reporting, therefore, seldom reflects true levels of infection. Co-infection with chlamydia is very common and treatment with antibiotics is simple and highly effective.

WHO estimated that by successfully treating 100 women for gonorrhoea, among whom one-quarter are pregnant, 25 would be prevented from developing pelvic inflammatory disease and 7 of their newborns would be spared from ophthalmia neo natorum, an eye infection acquired during passage through the birth canal which, if untreated, can result in blindness. Serious sequelae such as ectopic pregnancy, chronic pelvic pain and infertility could also be averted by treatment of these women.[30]

The complications and sequelae of gonorrhoea infection clearly demonstrated in reports from Cameroon in the mid-1980s, when up to 30% of newborns to women infected with gonorrhoea at the time of delivery developed ophthalmia neonatorum, leading to an overall rate of ophthalmia neonatorum of 4% among all births. In West and Central Africa, upto 40% of women over the age of 45 years were unable to conceive, mainly due to STI induced infertility among young women, resulting from the potential of 17% rate of gonorrheal infection in the area.[31,32]

Gonorrhoea is one of the most frequently reported STIs. 40% of its victims contract pelvic inflammatory diseases (PID), if not treated and can cause sterility. It can be treated with antibiotics. While gonorrhoea rates among adults have declined, rates among adolescents have risen or remained unchanged. Adolescent females aged 15-19 have the highest rates of gonorrhoea and an estimated 50% of women with gonorrhoea have no symptoms without early screening and treatment, 10 to 40 percent of women with gonorrhoea will develop PID.[31]

Consistent and correct use of condom is very effective for reducing a variety of STIs: There is a growing difference between the rates among older females and among females 15 to 19 years of age. The rate of gonorrhoea declined least among adolescents as observed in the United States.[15] However, much of the developing world, it is still heavy high.

Possible consequences for the infected person: Untreated in women, the disease is a major cause of pelvic inflammatory disease. PID can lead to ectopic pregnancy, infertility and chronic pelvic pain. Untreated gonorrhoea can cause sterility in men. It can infect joints, heart valves and/or the brain.

Prevention: Abstaining from vaginal, anal and oral sex with an infected person is the only 100% effective means of prevention. Latex condoms can reduce but not eliminate the risk of contracting the disease during sex.

Syphilis

Syphilis fluctuates in incidence more dramatically than gonorrhoea as sexual behaviour changes. Syphilis is a chronic systemic infection caused by treponema pallidum subspecies pallidum. Following an incubation period averaging 3 weeks a primary lesion appears and is often associated with regional lymphodenopathy, a secondary bacteremic stage is associated with generalized muco cutaneous lesions and generalized lympho adenopathy, followed by a latent period of sub clinical infection lasting many years. In about one third of untreated cases, the tertiary stage is characterized by progressive destructive mucocutaneous musculoskeletal or parenchymal lesions, aortitis, or symptomatic central nervous system disease.[32]

Approximately 12 million new cases of syphilis were estimated among adults worldwide, with the greatest number of cases occurring in South and South East Asia followed by Sub-Saharan Africa.

Syphilis was first described in the sixteenth century. In industrialized countries syphilis apparently declined during the latter half of the nineteenth century. In these same countries, however, there was a sharp rise in incidence after the First World War, but following the Second World War the incidence fell rapidly, coinciding with the availability of improved diagnostic tests and antibiotics. In some industrialized countries, syphilis began to rise again in the 1960s and has been increasing steadily in some industrialized and developing countries since then. Syphilis cases increased dramatically from 1985 to 1990 among women of all ages. An analysis of 1993 data has shown that rates of syphilis were higher among females than among male adolescents; rates among females were more than twice as higher rates among males in the 15-19 age group.

Syphilis is the classic example of an STI, which can be successfully controlled by public health measures; a simple and highly sensitive diagnostic test is available. If untreated, however, syphilis may lead to nerve damage, arterial wall damage, and mental disorientation and eventually to death.

Treponema pallidum, the causative agent of syphilis, can cross the placental barrier and infect the fetus. There is evidence that in approximately two-thirds of pregnancies, infection spreads across the placental barrier, and that many of these pregnancies end in spontaneous abortion, stillbirth, or perinatal death. Congenital defects may occur in those fetuses, which go to term and are delivered. In a study in Ethiopia, for example, pregnant women with a positive serological test for syphilis were shown to have a five times greater chance of having a spontaneous abortion or stillbirth than those who were serologically negative[5] while in Zambia, 24% of stillbirths could be attributed to syphilis and congenital syphilis was implicated in 30% of all perinatal infatal mortality.[42]

Syphilis is quite prevalent in the developing world (2 to 16%) among antenatal patients, up to 30 percent in other clinic based evaluation.[35 to 42] The pattern of primary and secondary syphilis are the highest among 20 to 24 years old all over the world.[34] Rates among 15 to 19 years old are around half of those in the older group.[15]

No similar data is available for Indian adolescents. However, a population based survey in rural Nigeria found 2.6% of sexually active teenagers (under 20 years old) to have syphilis.[33]

A recent study in Houston found that not only adolescents had the highest rate of syphilis but also that the increase in the rate was associated with a sharp increase in HIV sero prevalence from 1.6 to 3.8 percent among adolescents attending STI clinic.[41]

Syphilis if untreated can lead to serious damage of the brain or heart.

Link between STIs and HIV

Genital sores (chancres) caused by syphilis make it easier to transmit HIV infection sexually. There is an estimated 2 to 5 fold increased risk of acquiring HIV infection when syphilis is present.

Ulcerative STIs that cause sores, ulcers, or breaks in skin or mucous membranes, such as syphilis, disrupts barslers that provide protection against infections. The genital ulcers caused by syphilis can bleed easily and when they come into contact with oral and rectal mucus during sex, increase the infectiousness of and susceptibility to HIV. Having other STIs is also an important predictor for becoming HIV infected because STIs on a marker for behaviour associated with HIV transmission.

By 1992 between 9 and 11 million adults and about 1 million children had been infected with the AIDS causing human immunodeficiency virus (HIV), according to WHO, two-thirds of these people live in developing countries. It was expected that by 2000, 30 to 40 million will be infected and 10 million people with HIV infection will have developed AIDS, and 90% of them will be living in developing countries.[43]

Biological factors of the curable STIs which increase the risk of HIV transmission and infection include disruption of the normal epithelial barrier by genital ulceration and/or microulceration; and by accumulation of pools of HIV-susceptible or HIV-infected cells (lymphocytes and macrophages) in semen and vaginal secretions. Epidermiological studies from Sub-Saharan Africa, Europe and North America have suggested that there is approximately, a four times greater risk of becoming HIV-infected in the presence of a genital ulcer such as caused by syphilis and/or chancroid; and a significant though lesser increased risk in the presence of STIs such as gonorrhoea, chlamydial infection and trichomoniasis which cause local accumulations of lymphocytes and macrophages.[44]

Other sexually transmitted infections make it easier for HIV to pass from one person to another. Chancroid, chlamydia, gonorrhoea, syphilis, and trichomoniasis may increase the risk of HIV transmission by two to nine times.[45-54] The link between HIV infection and other STIs may partly explain why HIV in haterosexual populations is more prevalent in Africa than in Europe and the US, where STIs are more than treated and cured.[55]

Carried in boy fluids, HIV may leave one person's body and enter another's body more easily through genital ulcers. HIV itself has been isolated from the genital ulcers of women with HIV infection. Thus the link is clearest between HIV infection and STIs that cause genital ulcers, although not all studies find an association. Six of 10 studies in Kenya and Zaire, for example, found that people with genital ulcers, caused mainly chancroid, were more likely to be infected with HIV than people without ulcers. Their risk was two to five times greater. Nine of 11 studies of syphilis and HIV infections found an association. Syphilis increased the risk of HIV infection threefold to ninefold for heterosexual men. Three of six studies of genital herpes and HIV infection found an association. Herpes doubled the risk of HIV infection for women and heterosexual men.[54]

Six studies found that chlamydia, gonorrhoea and trichomoniasis, which do not cause ulcers, increase the risk of HIV transmission to women by three to five times.[54] Several studies, however, have found no link between these STIs and HIV infection, but methodological problems may have obscured the connection. These STIs may enhance HIV transmission because they increase the number of white blood cells – which are both targets and sources of HIV in the genital tract and because genital inflammation may cause microscopic cuts than can allow HIV to enter the body. Diseases causing vaginal and urethral inflammation are far more common than genital ulcer and so may be responsible for a larger share of HIV transmission.

Infection with HIV also affects the other STIs. In people with HIV infection, other STIs may be more resistant to treatment. For example, several studies have reported that one-dose treatment for chancroid failed at least six times more often in HIV-infected patients than in patients without HIV infection.[45] Also syphilis lesions may last longer in people infected with HIV, and these people may get gonorrhoea more often.[54] Thus, HIV enhances its own transmission. With longer lasting STI symptoms, people with HIV infection are more likely to transmit HIV and increase the pace of AIDS epidemic.

Perceived susceptibility to adverse health outcome is major factor in theoriclinical models of behaviour change. Accurately accessing personal risk and making the connection between behaviour and susceptibility to infection are important first steps in preventing disease.

Inaccurate perceptions of susceptibility may be a significant barrier to preventing STIs and, ultimately, human immunodeficiency virus (HIV) infection. In order to perceive themselves as susceptible, adolescents should be able to recognize a number of factors as indicators of risk for STIs. For instance, unprotected intercourse and multiple sexual partners, the focus of most prevention programs are significant sources of STI risk. Although STIs are often asymptomatic, symptom recognition is an important aspect of diagnosis, treatment and prevention. Finally, an STI history is a strong predictor of future STI diagnosis and in terms of adolescents cognitive associations, previous experience with an STI could increase awareness of behaviour and symptoms that indicate STI risk. If adolescents appropriately understand the factors that put them at risk for STI, they should recognize that these indicators make them more susceptible to STI. Further accurate perceptions of susceptibility of STI should be related to actual infection.

Complications and Sequelae

STIs take their greatest toll through their sequelae-conditions resulting from the spread of STI pathogens (bacteria or viruses, for example) from the point of infection to another part of the reproductive tract or another part of the body. Chlamydia, gonorrhoea and syphilis can have severe sequelae. Human papilloma virus may cause cervical cancer 5 to 30 years after the initial infection.[56]

Some sexually transmitted infections threaten the fertility of both men and women. In women STI pathogens migrate up from the lower reproductive tract, causing pelvic inflammatory disease (Inflammation of the uterus, fallopian tubes, ovaries, or other pelvic structures), chronic pelvic pain and infertility. Sexually transmitted infections, mainly Chlamydia and gonorrhoea, cause most cases of pelvic inflammatory disease.[57,58] An estimated 8% to 20% of women with untreated cervical gonorrhoea develop pelvic inflammatory disease.[59-61] In a Swedish study begun in 1960, one of the largest studies of pelvic inflammatory disease, 18% of women with pelvic inflammatory disease had chronic pelvic pain compared with about 5% of women who had not had pelvic inflammatory disease.[62] Often the first symptom that women with chlamydial infection notice is the pain of pelvic inflammatory disease. At that point, any damage to the fallopian tubes is irreversible.

Pelvic inflammatory disease can cause infertility. Without treatment 55% to 85% of women with pelvic inflammatory disease may become infertile[62]. In some areas pelvic inflammatory disease is a common cause of women's infertility. In a study in Zimbabwe, 84% of 135 infertile women with abnormal fallopian tubes had a history of pelvic inflammatory disease.[63] Many women may lose their fertility without ever realizing that they had pelvic inflammatory disease. For example, in 14 studies of women with blocked fallopian tubes, 40% to 80% did not report that they had pelvic inflammatory disease.[64]

STIs also can increase a women's risk of ectopic pregnancy, a condition that can kill from sudden and severe internal bleeding when the out-of-place pregnancy ruptures the fallopian tube. Studies in the 1980s in developing countries found that ectopic pregnancy caused 1% to 15% of all maternal deaths.[65] Pelvic inflammatory disease, by permanently scarring narrowing the fallopian tubes, increases the risk that a pregnancy will be ectopic by 7 to 10 fold.[62] A US study found that genital chlamydial infection more than doubled a woman's risk of having an ectopic pregnancy.[66]

In men, infertility may follow an infection that spreads from the urethra (where it is described urethritis) to the epidimytis (epididymitis). In men under age 35, the most common cause of epididymitis is gonorrhoeal or chlamydial infection. Before antibiotics became available, 10% to 30% of men who had gonorrhoea developed epididymitis and 20% to 40% of men with epididymitis became infertile.[67]

Some STIs attack the fetus and infant. In two-thirds or more of pregnant women with syphilis, the infection spreads to the amniotic sac and infects the fetus.[68] About 40% of infected pregnancies end in spontaneous abortion, stillbirth or perenatal death.[15] Gonorrhoea or Chlamydia may spread to the eyes of babies as they pass through the cervix and vagina. Without preventive therapy 2% to 50% of infants exposed to the gonorrhoea-causing bacteria Neisseria gonorrhoea during birth develop eye infections (ophthalmia neonatorum).[69-71] In a number of developing countries ophthalmia enonatorum afflicts 5% of newborns.[72] Without treatment ophthalmia, neonatorum permanently damages the vision of 1% to 6% of affected infants.[73,74] Chlamydia also may spread to the lungs of newborns and lead to Chlamydia pneumonia.

Economic Costs

Sexually transmitted infections and their sequelae are costly to individuals and the health care system. Many people with STIs seek care from private providers, where they may pay one-quarter to one-third of their monthly earnings for drugs.[75,76] Also, STIs reduce the productivity of men and women in the prime of their lives. For example, in urban areas of sub-Saharan Africa with a high prevalence of STIs, syphilis causes the loss of an estimated 9 productive days per capita per year or the entire urban population; HIV infection leads to the loss of 48 days.[77]

Clinic and hospitals must devote their time and resources to patients with STIs. In a province of Mozambique, for example, 10% to 15% of visits to primary health clinics are for STIs treatment.78 In reports from sub-Saharan Africa pelvic inflammatory disease accounts for 17% to 40% of gynaecological admissions to hospitals; in Asia, 3% to 37%.[65]

Determinants of STI/HIV Risk Among Adolescents

Adolescence is a unique time of life, when societal, biologic, behavioural and developmental factors all act in concert to increase the likelihood of STI acquisition.

Biological factors

Several aspects of physical development may be relevant to the high risk of STIs among adolescents. The histology of the cervix and vagina undergo dramatic changes from childhood through puberty and into adulthood. Newborns show effects of exposure to maternal estrogen, which produces the squamous epithelium lining of the vagina as seen in adults. Soon after birth these squamous cells are replaced with columnar epithelium. At puberty, estrogen exposure causes the vaginal lining to thicken again which layers of squamous epithelium. Such epithelial changes may be particularly important at the cervix, since the persistence of cervical columnar epithelium in young women appears to significantly increase their vulnerability to STIs. Although cervical columnar epithelium eventually recedes completely, to be replaced with squamous epithelium, this replacement is a gradual process, continuing well into adulthood. Typically, the cervix in the adolescent still displays areas of exposed columnar epithelium,[81] a condition often referred to as ectopy. This is significant because chlamydia trachomatis infects columnar, no squamous, epithelium.

The presence of ectopy has repeatedly been associated with chlamydial infection, even after adjusting for sexual behaviour and other confounders.[82,83] Although it may be that chlamydial infection causes the appearance of columnar epithelium on the cervix, 62 longitudinal studies have demonstrated that ectopy is associated with increased risk of subsequent infection.[84,85]

The presence of ectopy also appears to increase the risk for other STIs and their adverse outcomes, Neisseria gonorrhoea attaches preferentially to columnar epithelium rather than squamous tissue. In addition, there is growing evidence that ectopy may contribute to HIV acquisition[86,87] and HIV shedding.[88] Ectopy may therefore partially account for the high incidence of HIV among adolescent women[87] by increasing both infectivity and susceptibility.[89] The vasculature found with the columnar epithelium associated with ectopy is more superficial and more easily traumatized than that of squamous epithelium, theoretically permitting HIV-infected cellular elements from the circulation to gain access to the mucosal surface, and infected monocytes and lymphocytes to reach the circulation.

The vaginal flora also changes during puberty. The appearance of Lactobacillus spp. results in reduction of the high vaginal pH levels of childhood to the more acidic pH associated with adulthood. The higher vaginal pH of early adolescence of hydrogen-peroxide producing organisms. However, casual links between these anatomic or physiologic changes and STI acquisition have not yet been demonstrated.

Changes in mucosal anatomy produce changes in mucus production, which is minimal in childhood. Mucus production is greatly increase in early puberty, but the mucus of thinner than that found in older adolescents or adult women. Thinner mucus may permit organisms to penetrate more easily and to attach to mucosal sites or gain access to the upper tract.

Unfortunately, there is very little information about how development in males affects their risk of STI acquisition or transmission.

Psychological and Cognitive Development

The stages of adolescence have been arbitrarily categorised as "early". "middle", and "late" and have been considered in terms of psychologic, physiologic and social development.

Development in each of these areas is not necessarily parallel. Individuals are often advanced in some categories but slower than their age-matched peers in others. Furthermore, growth in some of the cognitive areas is strongly influenced by the quality of teaching or role modeling they experience.[90] This is particularly relevant for STI prevention, where adults may use indirect methods of educating or reply on "scar tactics" rather than utilize skills training. Several characteristics of adolescents, particularly in early or middle stages of development may have important implications for STI risk and prevention. Younger adolescents frequently use a concrete style of reasoning, focusing on the present times, and are unable to conceptualise the long-term impact that current actions may have until they teach middle or late adolescence. Since some STIs (for example, HIV or Chlamydia) may have adverse effects that are not experienced for a decade or more, it should not be surprising that younger adolescents may not take actions needed to avoid such consequences. Furthermore, adolescents may have difficulty correctly implementing complex tasks (such as condom use) involving a series of steps that must be accomplished in a certain sequence to be effective. Finally, many parents, educators and health care workers do not teach about STI risk or even details of pubertal development until long after many adolescents are at risk for STIs. Therefore, these youths do not have even the basic information to make informed choices.

Sexual Behaviour

Over the last century, socio-cultural and behavioural changes have combined with changes in aspect if the developmental physiology of adolescents to increase the risk of STIs among these young people. Biologically, the average age at menarche has decreased (although it has been stable over the last generation). At the same time societal changes have resulted in increase in the average age in which young men and women marry. As a result, whereas 100 years ago young men in the United States spent approximately 7 years between maturation and marriage, today the interval is 13 years; for young women, the interval between menarche and marriage has increased from 8 years to 14. For this reason alone, it should be expected that premarital sex in the United States has increased.[91]

Changes in sexual behaviour have placed adolescents at increased risk of STIs, with the trend to earlier age at first intercourse occurring worldwide.[92-95] In the United States, several ongoing, population-based surveys provide information about the sexual behaviour of adolescents. They show that during the past several decades the proportion of teenagers who have experienced premarital sexual intercourse has steadily increased, and that age of first intercourse has steadily decreased, although recent data indicate that this trend has leveled off in the United States over the half-decade through 1995.[96-98] These trends have occurred despite concern about HIV infection. As a result, in the late 1980s, 56 percent of 18 years-old females and 73 percent of 18-year old males had sex. Of particular note, in 1970 only 5 per cent of women in the United States had premarital intercourse by age 15, whereas in 1988, 26 per cent had engaged in intercourse by this age.[99] At each age a greater percentage of males than females have been sexually active; in general, the percentage of males who have had sexual intercourse if approximately equal to that of females 1 year older.

In addition, younger ages of sexual "debut" is associated with a greater number of sexual partners, an important determinant of STI risk.[100] In 1988, among American women 15 to 24 years of age who were sexually active for the same length of time (less than 24 months), over 40 percent of 15 to 19 olds had two or more partners, compared with only 26 percent of women 20 years of age or older 80 younger age of sexual debut (below age 18) is also associated with ongoing sexual risk among unmarried partners. Nevertheless, partner acquisition tends to follow a pattern of serial monogamy, with fewer than 10 percent of sexually active adolescents having more than one partner within a 3-month period.[101]

Population-based data demonstrate that condom use has increased substantially, but also that use is not consistent. Surveys indicate that more adolescents are using condoms. In the United States between 1983 and 1988, 65 percent of females used contraception at first intercourse, compared with 47 percent of females in the period 1975 to 1979; this increase was entirely a result of increased use of condoms.[102] Comparison data over time are also available for adolescent males. In 1979, 21 percent of never-married urban males 17 to 19 years old reported using condoms at last intercourse, compared with 58 percent in 1988. Reported use was greatest among African American males.[103] However, follow-up data indicate that as males get older and as the duration of the existing relationship increases, condoms are less likely to be used, while forms of contraception that offer less protection against STIs are used more, particularly oral contraceptives.[104] This pattern has also been reported from other countries, such as Australia,[105] Canada,[106] and New Zealand.[107] It is noteworthy that the combined effect of serial monogamy and diminishing use of condoms over the duration of a relationship may be particularly important in exposure to and ongoing transmission of organisms such as HSV-2, Chlamydia, HPV, and HIV, which are associated with chronic and often asymptomatic infection.

Although more people are using condoms, few people, including adolescents, use them consistently. Among unmarried women in the United States 59 percent of 15 to 19 years old reported using condoms for at least 1 month during the 4 years before interview, but only 31 percent of these women's partners used condoms consistently.[108] Furthermore, the young people most at risk for STIs appear to use condoms least.[109] A survey among adolescent males indicated that those who were substance abusers or had paid for sex were among the least likely to have used condoms at last intercourse.[110] Young males were less likely than older males to use condoms at first intercourse with partners they perceived to be at higher STI risk.[104] Among young people with two or more partners, individuals with greater numbers of partners were less like to use condoms consistently with either primary or secondary partners.[110] A similar pattern has been observed in other countries.[111]

Use of condoms is a complex behaviour, but we can make some generalization about determinants of condom use upon which to base prevention strategies. Many studies,[112,113] but not all,[114,115] indicate that use is associated with perceived risk of HIV infection. Youths who think their peers use condoms are more likely to use them,[114-118] as are adolescents who feel that their partner would support their use.[109,119,120] Adolescents are often mistaken about what their partners believe, however, with females overestimating the resistance and negative attitudes that males have about condom use.[121]

Studies have noted that self-efficacy, perceived risk, and partner support are important factors in increased condom use.[117-122] For example, many young females who feel confident that they could get their partner to use condoms or could discuss condom use with them are not using condoms.[123] An important factor appears to be the extent to which young people underestimate their partners' risk of infection. Young homosexual males[124] believe that they are safe if they have sex with younger partners. Heterosexual females often feel that they have little or no risk of acquiring HIV from their male partners and believe in their boy friends' statements of fidelity, often despite having a history of STI themselves.[3] A major concern, however, is the belief that their partners, particularly their steady partners, would view the request to use a condom as indicating a lack of trust. Conversely, if the request for use is made by the male, the female may assume he is dating outside the relationship, approaches to reconciling these issues are complex and require skillful and practiced communication, as well as interventions suitable for sexually active adolescents who are in the formative phases of social skill development. Other barriers to condom use that are unique to adolescents include lack of ready availability.[113]

Embarrassment about purchasing condoms may be a particular obstacle for girls.[123]

Legal and Ethical Issues

Adolescents have unique legal status with regard to the provision of health care. Legally they are accorded more rights than children, but in some matters they may have rights that differ from those of adults. However, in all states of the United States, adolescents can be diagnosed and treated for STIs without parental consent or knowledge, and some states have specific provisions regarding testing for and treating HIV infection. Beyond STI diagnosis and treatment, they are three basic issues providers confront in dealing with adolescents.[124]

1. Does the adolescent have the authority to consent to care without parental involvement?
2. Does the adolescent have the authority to release or prevent release of confidential information (particularly to parents)?
3. Is the adolescents or another source responsible for payment for services rendered? Can adolescents insist that parents not be contacted?

Parents usually have the responsibility for medical care for their minor children and are liable for the costs of their care. However, as stated, all states, either have specific status or otherwise permit the diagnosis and treatment of "venereal disease" (the usual terminology) without parental consent.

Consent

Although all states permit a minor to consent to STI care without parental consent, some states identify an age criterion. As of 1994, in five states (Alabama, California, Delaware, Illinois, and Vermount) minors must be at least 12 years old to consent to STI related care, and in five states (Hawaii, Idaho, New Hamsphire, North Dakota and Washington), they must be 14 years old.

Health Care Utilization

Till to-date very few studies have been conducted on the felt needs of adolescents regarding health care utilization and compliance. However, data from ICMR study in 1998 suggest that adolescents in Delhi do not obtain health group they do not need health services. In the focus group discussion they came out that they need health care, they should be regarded for seeking health services as a separate group (ICMR, 1998).

Reducing the Toll of STIs

Timely and effective care for STIs can reduce their toll by preventing transmission and sequelae. To provide care for the most people, STI services need to be widely available. Several steps are necessary:

- Adopting a quick, simple, and effective way to diagnose and treat STIs. Microscopes and laboratory tests permit specific diagnosis. Many health care providers lack equipment or time to await test results, however. They manage STI patients by relying on symptoms (what the patient notices) and easily observable signs (what the provider notices). Often STIs can be identified by syndromes (groups of symptoms). The syndromic approach to case management, now begin prompted by the World Health Organization (WHO), gives providers a systematic way to use this information and NACO has already recommended for Indian situation.
- Making effective services accessible. Most important is offering STI services in primary health centres, which serve the most people. The syndromic approach can help primary health care providers to diagnose STI patients. At the same time, primary health care providers need help and support from STI experts in district and medical college level hospitals and in apex hospitals. Such support includes ensuring a steady supply of drugs, training, managing difficult cases referred by the primary health system, that means a good support of referral system and surveillance must be established.
- Getting people with STIs to treatment. There are a variety of approaches: mass – media communication to alert people and inform them about STIs, screening people for STIs when they seek health care for other reasons, notifying the sexual

partners of STI patients that they should seek treatment, and setting up special programs for high risk populations.

- Encouraging people to avoid STIs by following, what Philipine health secretary Juan Flavier calls the ABCs of safe sex: "A for abstinence. If you can't abstain, B for be faithful, and if you can't be faithful, then use C for condom's".

Managing STIs

Effective managements of STIs as of most infections, requires that patients and health care providers cooperate in a series of steps leading to cure:

1. Obtaining information: Providers question about patient's health and sexual activity; patients answer questions completely and truthfully.
2. Performing a physical examination: Patients are willing to be examined; providers check patients for signs of STIs.
3. Diagnosing and treating patients: Providers know the signs and symptoms of STIs and have the right drugs to treat them; patients can obtain the drugs, and they take the full course as directed.
4. Counseling: Providers counsel patients to cure the current infection and prevent re-infection; patients follow the counseling advice and help get their sexual partners treated.

Effective STIs prevention for adolescents require involvement by numerous individuals and institutions that have contact with young people, and it should include activities implemented in several different settings. Despite the many challenges facing prevention of STIs among adolescents, there are encouraging findings from interventions based in schools, colleges, and hospitals.

There are effective strategies, if coordinated and implemented broadly, should result in healthier behaviour and lower rates of STIs among adolescents. Health education messages found to be effective can be provided with consistency across the different levels of social context of adolescents' lives, and educational and health service activities can be systematically linked across schools, media, community organizations, and health care delivery systems.

References

1. Rowley J, Berkley S: Sexually Transmitted Diseases in Murray, CJ I, Lopez, A D eds. Health Dimension of Sexual Reproduction; The Global Burden of STD and HIV, Maternal Conditions, Perenatal and Congenital Anamalies; Cambridge Harvard University Press, 1993.
2. Centers for Disease Control, Division of Sexually Transmitted Disease Prevention, STD, Surveillance, 1994, CDC, Atlanta, US 1995. Department of Health Sciences, Public Health Service, 1996.
3. Overby KJ, Kegeles SM: The Impact of AIDS in an Urban Population of High Risk Female Minority Adolescents: Implications for Intervention. *J Adolesc Health* 15:216, 1994.
4. Marx R, Aral: Gonorrhoea Rates: What Denominator is Most Appropriate? *Am J Public Health* 79: 1057, 1989.
5. Ball TA, Holmes KK: Age Specific Risks of Syphilis, Gonorrhoea and Hospitalized Pelvic Inflammatory Disease in Sexually Experienced US Women Sex Trans. Dis. 11:291.
6. http//www/niard.nih.gov/factsheets/STI info.htm
7. http//statie./highbead.com r/reporodti.
8. Weinstock HS, Bolan GA, *et al.*: Challenges for International Health Policy, Programs and Research In: Germain, A Holmes, *et al.:* eds. Reproductive Tract Infections: Global Impact and Priorities for Women's Reproductive Health, New York, Plenum Press, 1992, p. 7-32.
9. WHO, Feature No. 152, Geneva, WHO 1990.
10. Gerbase AC, JT Rowley, DHL, Heymann, SFB *et al.*: 1998. Global Prevalence and Incidence Estimates of Selected Curable STD, Sexually Transmitted Disease, 74 Supply (1) 512-516.

10a. WHO Global Prevalence on AIDS, 1992.

11. 11 *Ibid.*
12. 12 *Ibid.*
13. Wasserheit JN, Holmes KK: Reproductive Tract Infections; Challenges for International Health Policy, Programs and Research, In; Germain, A Holmes, KK, Piot, P, and Wasserheit, JN, eds. Reproductive Tract Infections; Global Impact and Priorities for Women's Reproductive Health, New York, Plenum Press, 1992, p. 7-33.
14. Aral SO and Holmes KK: Sexually Transmitted Diseases in the AIDS era, *Sci Am* 1991, 264, 62-69.
15. Schryver DA, Meheus A: Epidemiology of STI, The Global Picture, Bull, WHO, 68:629, 1990.

16. United States Department of Health and Human Services Centres for Disease Control (CDC), Division of STD/HIV Prevention; 1991 Annual Report (Atlanta, Georgia) CDC, 1992, p. 12 (Unpublished).
17. Wasserheit JN: The Significance and Scope of Reproductive Tract Infections Among Third World Women, International Journal of Gynaecology and Obstetrics (Suppl. 3); 145-168, 1989.
18. Bernal JN, Martinez MA, Triantafro VI, Suarez M, Dabancens A, Hurtado C, Montaldo G: Diagnosis of Sexually Transmitted Diseases in Pregnant Chilean Adolescents, Revista Chilena de Obstricia Ginec Logia 54 (2); 66-70, 1989.
19. Donovan, P: Testing Positive; Sexully Transmitted Disease and The Public Health Response, New York, Asia Guttmacher Institute, 1993, p. 47.
20. Goicochea, P, Peru: Reaching Boys Who Sell Sex? AIDS Watch; 11; 2-3, 1990.
21. Maggwa ABN and Ngugi EN: Reproductive Tract Infections in Kenya; Insights for Action from Research. In Germain, A Holmes, KK, Piot, P and Wasserheit, JN eds. Reproductive Tract Infections; Global Impact and Priorities for Women's Reproductive Health, New York, Plennum Press, 1992, p. 275-295.
22. OH, MK, Feinstein RA and Pass, RF: Sexually Transmitted Diseases and Sexual Behaviour in Urban Adolescent Females Attending a Family Planning Clinic; *Journal of Adolescent Health Care* 9 (1); 67-71, Jan. 1988.
23. Urmil AC, Dutta PK, Sharma KK and Ganguly SS: Medico-social Profile of Male Teenagers STD Patients Attending A Clinic in Pune, Indian Journal of Public Health 33 (40); 176-182, Oct-Dec, 1989.
24. World Health Organization, Global Program (WHO) The Health of Youth. Facts for Action. Youth and Sexually Transmitted Diseases, Geneva, WHO, 1989 (A 42/Technical Discussion/10) p. 6.
25. Werner M J, Biro FM: Urinary Leukocytes Esterase Screening for Asymptomatic Sexually Transmitted Disease in Adolescents Male, *J Adolesc Health* 12, 326, 1991.
26. Leonardi, GP *et al.*: Evaluation of Areas Immunoassay for Detection of Chlamydia Trachomitis in Urine Specimen from Asymptomatic Males. *J Clin Microbio* 30; 2793, 1992.
27. Hills SD *et al.*: Risk Factors for Recurrent Chlamydia Trachomitis Infection in Women. *FM J Obstet & Gynaecol*, 170: 801, 1994.
28. Brabin L *et al.*: Reproductive Tract Infection and Abortion among Adolescent Girls in Rural Neigeria Lancet 345: 300, 1995.
29. Gershman KA and Rolfs RT: Diverging Gonorrhoea and Syphilis Trends in the 1980s: Are They Real? *Am J Public Health* 81(10): 1263-1267, Oct. 1991.
30. Schmid GP, Sanders LI, Jr, Blount JH and Alexander ER: Chancroid in the United States. Re-establishment of an old disease. Journal of the American Medical Association 258 (22); 3265-3268.
31. Ellen JM *et al.*: Socio Economic Differences in Sexually Transmitted Disease Cases among Black and White Adolescents, San Francisco, 1990 to 1992. *Am J Public Health*, 85; 1546, 1995.
32. Sheila A, Lukehart King K, Holmes: Spirochetal Diseases Harrison Principles of Internal Medicine, Vol. I, International Edition, p. 651.

33. Meheus A *et al.*: General Infections in Prenatal and Family Planning Attendants in Switzerland, *East Afr Med* J 57:212, 1980.

34. Adolescents Health Program: Sexually Transmitted Diseases Amongst Adolescents in the Developing World. WHO/ADH/93, 1, 1993.

35. Howard M, Mc Cabe JB: Helping Teenagers Postpone Sexual Involvement, *Fam Plann Perspect* 22: 21, 1990.

36. Mulder D, *et al.*: Decreasing HIV-1 Sero Prevalence in Young Adults in a Rural Ugandan Cohort. BMJ 311; 833, 1995.

37. Piot P, Islam MQ: Sexually Transmitted Diseases in the 1990s. Global Epidemiology and Challenges for Control. Sex Tranm Dis (suppl) 21:S7, 1994.

38. Kohl PK: Epidemiology of Sexually Transmitted Diseases. What does it tell us? *Sex Trans Dis* (suppl) 21: S81, 1994.

39. Berkley S: The Public Health Significance of Sexually Transmitted Diseases for HIV Infection in Africa, in ADIS and Women's Reproduction Health, LC Chen, JS Amor (Eds), New York, Plenum Press, 1990, p. 73-84.

40. Daly, CC *et al.*: Risk Factors for Gonorrhoea, Syphilis, and Trichomonas Infections among Women Attending Family Planning Clinics in Nairobi, Kenya, Genitour Med, 70: 155, 1994.

41. Levine WD, *et al.*: Dual Epidemics of Syphilis and HIV Infection among Adolelscent African – American Women in Houston, 1938-1993. The 11th Meeting of the International Society for STD. Research, abstr 051, 1995.

42. Malotte CK *et al.*: Screening for Chlamydial Cervicitis in a Sexually Active University Population. *Am J P Health* 80; 469; 1990.

43. World Health Organization (WHO), Global Programme on AIDS, Current and Future Dimensions of the HIV/AIDS Pandemic; A Capsule Summary, Geneva, WHO, Jan, 1992, p. 12.

44. Adexunle AO and Ladipo OA: Reproductive Tract Infections in Holmes KK, Piot P and Wasserheit JN eds. Reproductive Tract Infections; Global Impact and Priorities for Women's Reproductive Health, New York, Plenum Press, 1992, p. 297-315.

45. Cameron DW, Plummer FA, D'Costa L J, Ndinya Achola JO, and Ronald AR: Prediction of HIV Infection by Treatment Failure for Chancroid, A Genital Ulcer Disease. In 4th International Conference on AIDS, Book 2, Stockholm, Jan, 12-16, 1988, p. 334.

46. Cleghorn F, Jack N, Edwards J, Murphy I: STD Clinic Clients in Trinidad (Abstract), In 9th International Conference on AIDS/4th STD World Congress, Vol. 2, Berlin, Germany, Jaun 6-11, 1993, p. 653.

47. Greenblatt RM, Lukehart SA, Plummer FA, *et al.*: Genital Ulceration As A Risk Factor for HIV. AIDS 210; 47-50, Feb, 1988.

48. Kreiss JK, Koech D, Plummer FA, *et al.*: AIDS Virus Infection in Nairobi Prostitutes, New England Journal of Medicine 314(7); 414-418, Feb, 13, 1986.

49. Laga M: HIV Prevention, The Need for Complementary STD Control. In Germain, A Holmes KK, Piot P and Wasserheit, J N, Eds. Reproductive Tract Infections; Global Impact and Priorities for Women's Reproductive Health, New York, Plenum Press, 1992, p. 131-144.

50. Laga M, Nzila N, Manoka A T, Malele M, Bush TJ, Behets F, Heyward WL, Piot P and Ryder R: Non-ulcerative Sexually Transmitted Diseases (STD) as Risk Factors for HIV Infection (Abstract). In 6th International Conference on AIDS, Vol. 1, San Francisco, Jun 20-21, 1990 p. 158.

51. Plummer FA, Simonsen JN, Cameron DW, Ndinya Achola JO, Kreiss JK, Gakinya MN, Waiyaki P, Cheang M, Piot P, Ronald AR and Ngugi EN: Co-factors in male-female Sexual Transmission of HIV Type 1. Journal of Infection Diseases 163: 20; 233-239, Feb, 1991.

52. Ryder R, Hassig S, Ndilu M, Behets F, Nanlcle K, Malele B, Bishagara U and Kashamuka M: Extramarital/Prostitutes Sex and Genital Ulcer Disease (GUD) are Important HIV Risk Factors in 5th International Conference on AIDS; The Scientific and Social Challenges, Montreal, Quebec, Jun 4-9, 1989, p. 51.

53. Simonsen JN, Cameron DW, Gakinya MN, Ndinya Achola JO, d'Costa L J, Karasira P, Cheang M, Ronald AR, Piot P and Plummer LA: HIV among Men with Sexually Transmitted Diseases; Experiences from a Center in Africa. New England Journal of Medicine 319 (5); 274-278, Aug 4, 1988.

54. Wasserheit JN: The Significance and Scope of Reproductive Tract Infections Among Third World Women, International Journal of Gynaecology and Obst (Suppl. 30) 145-168, 1989.

55. Cameron W, Ngugi E, Ndinya Achola JO and Corey L: Isolation of HIV from Genital Ulcers in Nairobi Prostitutes. Journal of Infectious Diseases 160 (3); 380-384, Sep 1989.

56. Shah KV: Biology of Human Genital Tract Papilloma Viruses. In: Holmes KV, Mardh PA, Sparling PF, Wiesner PJ, Cates W, Jr. Lemon SM, and Stamm WE, eds. Sexually Transmitted Diseases, 2nd ed. New York, McGraw Hill, 1990, p. 425-432.

57. Rice PA, and Schachter J: Pathogenesis of Pelvic Inflammatory Disease, Journal of the American Medical Association 266 (18): 2587-2593, Nov 13, 1991.

58. Westrom L and Mardh PA, Sparling PF: A Acute Pelvic Inflammatory Disease (PID). In Holmes KK, Holmes K, Mardh PA, Sparling PF, Wiesner PJ, Cates W, Jr. Lemon SM and Stamm WE eds. Sexually Transmitted Disease 2nd ed. New York, McGraw Hill, 1990, p. 593-614.

59. Eschenbach DA, Buchanan TM, Pollock HM, Forstyth PS, Alexander ER, Lin JS, Wang SP, Wentworth BB, Mccormock WM and Holmes KK: Polymicrobial Etiology of Acute Pelvic Inflammatory Disease, New England Journal of Medicine 293(4); 166-171, July 24, 1975.

60. Kramer DG and Brown ST: Sexually Transmitted Disease and Infertility, (1982) p. 22 (Unpublished).

61. Estrom L, Svensson L, Wolnner-Hanssen P and Mrdh PA: Chlamydial and Gonococcal Infections in a Defined Population of Women, Scandinavian Journal of Infectious Disease (Suppl. 32); 157-162, 1982.

62. Westrom I, Mardh PA: Acute Pelvic Inflammatory Disease (PID) In: Holmes KK, Mardh PA, Sparling PF, Weiner PJ, Cates W, Jr, Lemon SM and Stamm WE eds. Sexually Transmitted Diseases.

63. De Muylder X, Laga M, Tennsted C, Van Dyck E, Aelbers GNM and Piot P: The Role of Neisseria Gonorrhoea and Chlamydia Trachomitis in Pelvic Inflammatory Disease and its Sequelae in Zimbabwe. Jr of Infectious Diseases 162 (2); 501-505, Aug, 1990.

64. Bernal JN, Martinez M A, *et al.*: Dragnostico de enfermedades de Transmission Sexual in Adolescents Embarazades, Summaog in Eng. Revista Chilena: 54 (2): 66-70, 1989.
65. Meheus A, Women's Health: Importance of Reproductive Tract Infections, Pelvic Inflammatory Diseases and Cervical Cancer in Germain A Holmes KK, Piot P and Wasserheit JN, eds. Reproductive Tract Infections; Global Impact and Priorities for Women's Reproductive Health. New York, Plenum Press, 1992, p. 61-91.
66. JM Yonekura, ML Richwald, GA Greenland, S Sweet, RL and Schaachter J: The Association between Chlamydia Trachomatis and Ectopic Pregnancy, Journal of the American Medical Association 263(23): 3164-3167, June, 20, 1990.
67. Pelouze PS: Gonorrhoea in the Male and Female; A Book for Practitioners, Philadelphia, WB Sounders, 1941, p. 489.
68. Zenker PN and Rolfs RT: Treatment of Syphilis, 1989, Reviews of Infectious Discases 12 (Suppl. 6); 5590-5609, July, Aug, 1990.
69. Gutman LT and Wilfert CM: Gonococcal Diseases in Infants and Children In; Holmes KK, Mardh PA, Sparling PF, Wiesner PJ, Cates W, Jr Lemon SM and Stamm WE eds. Sexually Transmitted Diseases 2nd ed. New York, McGraw Hill, 1990, p. 803-810.
70. Laga M, Meheus A and Piot P: Epidemiology and Control of Gonococcal Ophthalmia Neonatorum, Bulletin of the World Health Organization 67 (5): 471-478, 1989.
71. Ronald A, Plummer F, Ngugi E, Ndinya-Achola JO, Piot P, Kreiss J and Brunham R: The Nairobi STI Program: An International Partnership. Infectious Disease Clinics of North America S(2): 337-352, Jun 1991.
72. Knox SR, Mandel B and Lazarowicz R: Profile of Callers to the V.D. National Hotlines: Sexually Transmitted Diseases 8 (4): 245-254, Oct-Dec 1981.
73. Fransen L, Nsanze H, Klauss V, Van Der Stuyft P, D'Costa L, Burnham RC, and Piot P: Ophthalmia Neonatorum in Nairobi, Kenya: The Roles of Neissaria Gonorrhoea and Chlamydia. Journal of Infectious Diseases 153 (5): 862-869, May 1986.
74. Piot P and Rowley J: Economic Impact of Reproductive Tract Infections and Resources for Their Control. In: Germain A, Holmens KK, Piot P and Wasserheit JN eds. Reproductive Tract Infections: Global Impact and Priorities for Women's Reproductive Health. New York, Plenum Press, 1992, p. 227-249.
75. Centers for Disease Control and Prevention: Health Risk Behaviour among Adolescents who do and do not attend school – US, 1992, MMWR 43 : 129, 1994.
76. Moran J: Centre for Disease Control, STD Programs in Developing Countries. Personal Communication, Mar. 10, 1992.
77. Over M and Piot P: HIV Infection and Sexually Transmitted Diseases, In Jamison DT and Mosley WH, eds. Disease Control Priorities in Developing Countries. New York, Oxford University Press, June, 1991, p. 130 (to be published).
78. Latif AS: WHO STD Services in Zimbabwe. Personal Communication, Apr 13, 1992.
79. Moran S: (CDC) STD programs in developing countries. Personal communication, Mar 10, 1992.

80. Bastosdos Santos R, Folgosa E and Fransen I: Reproductive Tract Infection in Mozambique: A Case of Integrated Services. In: Germain A, Holmes KK, Piot P and Wasserheit JN, eds. Reproductive Tract Infections; Global Impact and Priorities for women's Reproductive Health, New York, Plenum Press, 1992, p. 343-160.
81. Critchlow CW, *et al.*: Determinants of Cervical Ectopia and of Cervicitis – Age, Oral Contraception, Specific Cervical Infection, Smoking and Douching. *Am J Obstets Gynaecol* 173; 534, 1995.
82. Stergachis A, *et al.*: Selective Screening for Chlamydia Trachomitis Infection in a Primary Care Population of Women. *Am J Epidemiol* 138: 143, 1993.
83. Johnson BA, *et al.*: Derivation and Validation of a Clinical Diagnostic Model for Chlamydial Cervical Infection in University Women. *JAMA* 265: 3161, 1990.
84. Louv WC, *et al.*: Oral Contraceptive Use and the Risk of Chlamydial and Gonococcal Infections. *Am J Obstet Gynaecol* 160: 369, 1989.
85. Rahn VA, *et al.*: Chlamydia Trachomitis in Sexually Active Teenage Girls. Factors Related to Genital Chlamydial Infection: A Prospective Study, *Genito Ur Med* 67: 317, 1991.
86. Moss GB, *et al.*: Association of Cervical Ectopy with Heterosexual Transmission of Human Immunodeficiency Virus; Results of A Study of Couples in Nairobi, Kenya. *J Infec Dis* 164; 588, 1991.
87. Plourde PJ, *et al.*: Human Immunodeficiency Virus Type 1 Sero Conversion in Women with Genital Ulcers. *J Infec Dis* 170: 313, 1994.
88. Clemetson DB, *et al.*: Detection of HIV, DNA in Cervical and Vaginal Secretions: Prevalence and Correlates among Women in Nairobi, Kenya. *JAMA* 269: 2860, 1993.
89. Bultrerys M, *et al.*: Incidence HIV-1 Infection in a Cohort of Young Women in Butare, Rwanda. AIDS 8: 1585, 1994.
90. Forrest JD: Timing of Reproductive Life Stages. *Obstetr and Gynaecol* 82: 105, 1993.
91. Friedman HL: Changing Pattern of Adolescent Sexual Behaviour, Consequences for Health and Development. *J Adolesc Health* 13: 345, 1994.
92. Graham CA: AIDS and the Adolescent. Internet J STD AIDS 5:305, 1994.
93. Haffner DW: Facing Facts: Sexual Health for Americans' Adolescents. Report of the National Commission on Adolescent Sexual Health, 1995.
94. Oakley A, *et al.*: Sexual Health Education Interventions for Young People: A Methodological Review, *BM J* 310:158, 1995.
95. Carael M, *et al.*: Overview and Selected Findings of Sexual Behaviour Surveys, AIDS 5:565, 1991.
96. Centers for Disease Control and Prevention: Trends in Sexual Risk Behaviour among High School Students – US, 1990, 1991 and 1993. *MMWR* 44: 124, 1995.
97. Sonnenstein FL: Preliminary Data from National Survey of Adolescent Males, Personal Communication, 1996.
98. Centers for Disease Control and Prevention: CDC Surveillance Summaries. *MMWR* 44: 124, 1995.
99. Centers for Disease Control and Prevention: Premarital Sexual Experience among Adolescent Women – US, 1970-1988, *MMWR* 39: 929, 1991.

100. Kost K, Forrest JD: American Women's Sexual Behaviour and Exposure to Risk of Sexually Transmitted Disease. *Fam Plann Perspect* 24: 244, 1992.

101. Seidman SN, *et al.*: Predictors of High Risk in Unmarried American Women Adolescent Environment at Risk Factor. *J Adolesc Health* 15: 126, 1994.

102. Mosher WD, Mc Nally JW: Contraceptive Use at First Premarital Intercourse: US, 1965-1988. *Fam Plann Perspect* 23: 1108, 1991.

103. Sonnenstein FL *et al.*: Sexual Activity, Condom and AIDS Awareness among Adolescents males, *Fam Plann Perspect* 21: 152, 1989.

104. Ku L, *et al*: The Dynamics of Young Men's Condom Use During and Across Relationships. *Fam Plann Perspect* 26; 246, 1994.

105. Dunne MP, *et al.*: Age Related Increase in Sexual Behaviours and Decrease in Regular Condom Use Among Adolescent in Australia. International J STI AIDS 5:41, 1994.

106. Ngyur NT, *et al.*: Sexual Behaviour and Condom Use: A Study of Suburban Male Adolescents. *Adolescence* 29:37, 1994.

107. Furgusson DM, *et al.*: AIDS Knowledge and Condom Use Birth Cohort of 16-year olds. *NZ Med J* 107:480, 1994.

108. Potter LB, Anderson JE: Patterns of Condom Use and Sexual Behaviour Among Never Married Women. *Sex Transm Dis* 20: 201, 1993.

109. Weisman CS, *et al.*: Consistency of Condom Use for Disease Prevention among Adolescent Users of Oral Contraceptives. *Fam Plann Perspect* 23: 71, 1991.

110. Binson D, *et al.*: Data from National AIDS Behavioural Surveys: IV. Multiple Sexual Partners among Young Adults in High risk Cities. *Fam Plann Perspect* 25:268, 1993.

111. Mac Donald NE, *et al.*: High Risk STI/HIV Behaviour among College Students. *JAMA* 263: 3155, 1990.

112. Hingson RW *et al.*: Beliefs about AIDS, Use of Alcohol and Drugs, and Unprotected Sex among Massachusetts Adolescents. *Am J Public Health* 80: 295, 1990.

113. Donald M: Determinants of Condom Use by Australian Secondary School Students. *J Adolesc Health* 15: 503, 1993.

114. Brown LK, *et al.*: Predictors of Condom Use in Sexually Active Adolescents. *J Adolesc Health* 13: 6513, 1992.

115. Weisman CS *et al.*: AIDS Knowledge, Perceived Risk, and Prevention among Adolescent Clients of a Family Planning Clinic. *Fam Plann Perspect* 21: 213, 1989.

116. Romer D *et al.*: Social influences on the Sexual Behaviour of Youth at Risk for HIV Exposure. *Am J Public Health* 84: 977, 1994.

117. Shafer MA, Boyer CB: Psychosocial and Behavioural Youth at Risk of Sexually Transmitted Diseases, Including Human Immunodeficiency Virus Infection, among Urban High School Students. *J Pediatr* 119: 826-833, 1991.

118. Di Clementre RJ *et al.*: African Adolescents Residing in High Risk Urban Environments do use condoms – Correlates and Predictors of Condom Use Among Adolescents in Public Housing Developments. *Pediatrics* 98: 269, 1996.

119. Pendergrast RA, Jr, *et al.*: Attitudinal and Behavioural Correlates of Condom Use in Urban Adolescents Males, *J Adolesc Health* 13: 133, 1992.

120. Plichta SB *et al.*: Partner specific Condom Use Among Adolescent Women Clients of a Family Planning Clinic. J Adolesc Health 13: 506, 1992.

121. Kegeles SM *et al.*: Sexually Active Adolescents and Condoms: Changes over one year in Knowledge, Attitudes, and Use. *Am J Public Health* 78: 460, 1988.

122. Joffe A, Adolescents and Condom Use. *Am J Dis Children* 147: 746, 1993.

123. Guttmacher S, *et al.*: Gender Differences in Attitudes and Use of Condom Availability Programs among Sexually Active Students in New York City Public High Schools. *J Am Med Wom Assoc* 50:99, 1995.

CHAPTER

2 Epidemiology of STDs

Parvathy Nair* and *Vijay Grover

Sexually transmitted diseases, or STDs, are infections that can be transferred from one person to another through sexual contact. According to the Centers for Disease Control there are over 15 million cases of sexually transmitted disease reported annually. Adolescents and young adults (15-24) are the age groups at the greatest risk for acquiring an STD, 3 million becoming infected each year. These diseases can be classified on the basis of either their etiologies or their clinical manifestations. They can be classified according to the causative agent in the following manner:

Agent	*Disease or Syndrome*
Bacteria	
Neisseria gonorrhoea	Gonorrhoea
Chlamydia trachomatis	Chlamydia, Lymphogranuloma Venerium
Mycoplasma hominis	Postpartum fever, salpingitis
Ureaplasma urealyticum	Nongonococcal urethritis, chorioamnionitis, premature delivery
Treponema pallidum	Syphilis
Hemophilus ducreyi	Chancroid
Calymmatobacterium granulomatis	Donovanosis (granuloma inguinale)
Gardenerella vaginalis	Gardenerella associated ("nonspecific") vaginosis
Shigetta sp.	Shigellosis in homosexual men
Campylobacter sp.	Enteritis, proctocolitis
Group B streptococcus	Neonatal sepsis, neonatal meningitis
Viruses	
Herpes simplex virus	Genital Herpes

(Contd...)

Hepatitis B virus	Acute hepatitis B, chronic active hepatitis, hepatocellular carcinoma
Cytomegalovirus	Infectious mononucleosis, congenital infection, gross birth defects and infant mortality
Human papillomavirus	Condylomata acuminata, cervical dysplasia
Molluscum contagiosum virus	Genital molluscum contagiosum
Protozoa	
Trichomonas vaginalis	Trichomonal vaginits
Entamoeba histolytica	Amebiasis in homosexual men
Giardia lambia	Giardiasis in homosexual men
Fungi	
Candida albicans	Vulvogaginitis, balanitis
Ectoparasites	
Phthirius pubis	Pubic lice infestation
Sarcoptes scabiei	Scabies

Social Factors in STDs

There are numerous social factors that aid in the spread of STDs. They include changing behavioural patterns among youth, sexual disharmony, broken marriages and urbanization that has increased the sexual permissiveness and hence incidence of STDs in the society. Prostitution and sexual promiscuity remain the single major factor in the spread of the disease. Social stigma associated with STDs is a major road block in the detection of cases. The prevalence of STDs is higher amongst those indulging in substance abuse.

Gonorrhoea

The Problem: An estimated 62 million cases of gonorrhoea occurred in 1999; globally affecting more women than men. Out of 62.35 million cases reported worldwide in 1999, 27.2 million were from India.

Agent: Gonorrhoea, also known as "the clap", is a curable infection caused by the bacteria Neisseria gonorrhoea, a gram negative bacteria. Symptoms of infection may show up at anytime between 1 and 14 days after exposure. It is possible to be infected with gonorrhoea and have no symptoms. Men are far more likely to notice symptoms than women.

Host: It is an exclusively human disease. The highest rates of infection are usually found in 15 to 19 years old women and 20 to 24 years old men. The incidence of gonorrhoea is highest in high-density urban areas among persons under 24 years of age who have multiple sex partners and engage in unprotected sexual intercourse. Increases in gonorrhoea prevalence have been noted recently among men who have sex with men. A higher incidence has been observed in persons belonging to Blood Group B. Antimicrobial resistance in N. gonorrhoea has been noted. Antimicrobial resistance in N. gonorrhoea occurs as plasmid mediated resistance to penicillin and tetracycline, and chromosomally mediated resistance to penicillins, tetracyclines, spectinomycin, and recently to fluoroquinolones.

Mode of Transmission: It is sexually transmitted and can infect the cervix, fallopian tubes, urethra, rectum, anus and throat. Gonorrhoea is spread during sexual intercourse. Infected women also can pass gonorrhoea to their newborn infants during delivery, causing eye infections, ophthalmia neonatorum, in their babies. When the infection occurs in the genital tract, mouth, or rectum of a child, it is due most commonly to sexual abuse.

Syphilis

Agent: It is a curable bacterial infection caused by treponema pallidum, a spirochete.

The Problem: An estimated 12.22 million cases of Syphilis occurred worldwide in 1999, similar to the estimated rates of 1995 (11.76 million), however between these years individual country rates increased and decreased rapidly. Studies of pregnant women in Africa revealed rates of infection as high as 17.4. Most cases of primary and secondary syphilis occurred in persons between 20 to 39 years of age. The incidence of infectious syphilis was highest in women 20 to 24 years of age and in men 35 to 39 years of age. Rates in women have continued to decrease over the years while, the rate in men in about 3.5 times higher especially in homosexuals. Syphilis rates usually increase and decrease in seven-to-ten years cycles.

Mode of Transmission: It is spread by close sexual contact with an infected person, an infected mother to the child during birth and blood transfusions from infected person. Syphilis is passed from person to person through direct contact with a syphilis sore that occur mainly on the external genitals, vagina, anus, or in the rectum and rarely on the lips and in the mouth. Genital sores (chancres) caused by syphilis make it easier to transmit and acquire HIV infection sexually and there is an estimated 2 to 5 fold increased risk of acquiring HIV infection when syphilis is present.

Chlamydia

It is the most common treatable bacterial STD.

The Problem: Chlamydial prevalence rates across the world vary enormously. Prevalence rates in Latin America and the Caribbean are often lower than that of countries in Europe though in Asia rates tend to be much higher. The WHO quotes a rate of up to 17% in India. Out of 91.98 million people suffering from Chlamydia world-wide in 1999, 85 million were reported from South Asia, South East Asia and Sub-Saharan Africa alone (WHO 1999).

The Agent : There are two types of chlamydia: (a) C. trachomatis (biovar: trachoma) is the most common sexually transmitted bacterial disease in the United States (4 million new cases each year) and 50 million new cases occur yearly worldwide. In the United States, the highest infection rates occur in Native and African Americans with a peak incidence in the late teens/early twenties. (b) C. trachomatis (biovar: LGV) is a sexually transmitted disease that occurs sporadically in the United States but is more prevalent in Africa, Asia and South America. Humans are the only natural host. It can cause serious problems later in life if it is not treated. Incubation period is 5 to 20 days.

The Host : Because the cervix of teenage girls and young women is not fully matured, they are at particularly high risk for infection if sexually active. The women under 25 and sexually active, have a 1 in 10 chance of having chlamydia while risk is even higher for adolescents are under 20 having unprotected sex. About 75% of infected women and 25% of infected men have no symptoms at all.

Mode of Transmission : One can get genital chlamydial infection during oral, vaginal, or anal sexual contact with an infected partner. It can cause serious problems in men and women as well as in newborn babies of infected mothers. The primary risk factors for chlamydia include: unsafe sex and having multiple sexual partners. The infection can be passed when the mucous membrane, the soft skin covering all the openings of the body, comes into contact with the secretions or semen of an infected person. Chlamydia infects the cervix in women. The urethra, rectum and eyes can be infected in both sexes. It can also be passed from mother to newborn as the baby passes through the infected birth canal. This can result in eye infections, pneumonia or other complications.

Chancroid

Chancroid is characterized by one or more genital ulcer and painful inguinal lymphadenopathy.

Agent: The causative agent is Heamophilis ducreyi which is a Gram negative coccobacillus that on Gram stain, has a "school of fish" appearance. Culture is difficult, requiring blood factors and is often negative. Incubation period is 2-5 days.

The Problem: Chancroid is common in parts of Africa, Asia and Latin America where its incidence is more than syphilis as a cause of genital ulceration. Chancroid is endemic in tropical and subtropical countries, but it is sporadic in temperate countries. It is common in Africa and parts of Asia. Recently, there have been outbreaks in the United States, Canada and some European countries.

Host Factors : Number of sexual partners is known to be a critical factor in the spread of chancroid. It may explain the association of the disease with other risk factors; like drug addiction and alcohol as substance abuse leads to high risk sexual behaviour. Majority of cases occur in males. STDs especially those presenting with genital ulcers are risk factors in transmission of HIV in two ways it increasing the shedding of virus through ulcer and increases the susceptibility to HIV infection by disrupting the epithelial barrier and increasing HIV susceptible cells at the point of entry. The disease is also more common in the uncircumcised men, and in unhygienic and low socio-economic conditions, asymptomatic carriers exist.

Mode of Transmission: Chancroid is transmitted in two ways, sexual transmission through skin-to-skin contact with open sore(s) and non-sexual transmission by means of auto inoculation when contact is made with the pus-like fluid from the ulcer. A person is considered to be infectious when ulcers are present. There has been no reported disease in infants born to women with active chancroid at time of delivery.

Genital Herpes

The Problem: According to the U.S. Center for Disease Control and Prevention, 1 out of 5 of the total adolescent and adult population, are infected with HSV-2.

Agent: Genital herpes is an infection caused by the herpes simplex virus or HSV. There are two types of HSV, and both can cause genital herpes. HSV type 1 most commonly infects the lips, causing sores known as fever blisters or cold sores, but it also can infect the genital area and produce sores. HSV type 2 is the usual cause of genital herpes, but it also can infect the mouth. A person who has genital herpes infection can easily pass or transmit the virus to an uninfected person during sex. Both HSV 1 and 2 can produce sores (also called lesions) in and around the vaginal area, on the penis, around the anal opening, and on the buttocks or thighs. Occasionally, sores also appear on other parts of the body where the virus has entered through broken skin. HSV remains in certain nerve cells of the body for life, and can produce symptoms off and on in some infected people.

The Host: The largest increase is occurring in young teens. HSV-2 infection is more common in three of the youngest age groups which include people aged 12 to 39 years. Genital HSV-2 infection is more common in women (approximately one out of four women) than in men (almost one out of five). This may be due to male-to-female transmissions being more likely than female-to-male transmission. While some people realize that they have genital herpes, but as many as 90% are unaware that they have the virus. This is because many people have very mild symptoms or no symptoms at all. Once the first outbreak of herpes is over, the virus hides away in the nerve fibres, where it remains totally undetected and causes no symptoms.

Mode of Transmission: Herpes is transmitted through direct skin-to-skin contact. This occurs when a contagious area comes into contact with a mucous membrane, primarily the mouth and genitals. As the skin on the body is too thick for the virus to go through most people get genital herpes by having sex with someone who is having a herpes "outbreak". This outbreak means that HSV is active. When active, the virus usually causes visible lesions in the genital area. Herpes can be transmitted when there are no symptoms present i.e. there are several days throughout the year (called asymptomatic reactivation, asymptomatic shedding or subclinical shedding) when a person can be contagious without having a symptom.

Bacterial Vaginosis (BV)

Bacterial Vaginosis (BV) is the most common vaginal infection in women of childbearing age. It is the name of a condition in women where the normal balance of bacteria in the vagina is disrupted and replaced by an overgrowth of certain bacteria. It is sometimes accompanied by discharge, odor, pain, itching, of burning.

Host: It is seen in sexually active women. Vaginal symptoms may be caused by vaginal or cervical infections resulting in abnormal discharge. After puberty under the influence of esterogen, the Ph of vagina decreases to less than 4.5. Though not proved, it is suggested that the alkaline nature of semen that upsets the acidic nature of the vaginal bacteria after sexual intercourse.

Agent: Bacterial Vaginosis is also thought to be a result of a complex interaction of many species of bacteria. The development of the disease is due to the result of shift in vaginal ecosystem from one predominated by acid producing lactobacilli to Gardenella Vaginalis and anaerobic bacteria. G. Vaginilis produces amino acids, which act as substrates for production of amines by anaerobic bacteria, that are responsible for the foul smelling discharge associated with this condition. This disease is more prevalent in women with multiple sex partners. Use of intra utereine device and history of trichomoniasis have been associated with bacterial vaginosis.

Vaginal Syndrome and Etiology/Causative Agents

Type	*Etiology*
Infectious causes Bacterial vaginosis	Mixed Gardnerella Vaginalis, anaerobes and genital mycoplasma
Yeast Vulvovaginitis	Candida albicans
Trichomoniasis	Trichomonas Vaginalis
Desquamative inflammatory Vaginitis	Group B Streptococci, Other unknown Causes
Non Infectious Causes	
Post-Partum Atrophic Vaginitis	Lack of esterogen especially during lactation
Allergic Vaginitis	Systemic allergy, Passive transfer of IgE in semen, Local response to chemical irritants.
Atrophic Vaginitis	Lack of estrogen during or after menopause

Genital Warts

They are small fleshy growths which may appear anywhere on a man or woman's genital area. They are caused by a virus called the Human Papilloma Virus (HPV). More than 80 types of HPV are known to exist and quite a few of these types cause genital warts, e.g. HPV types 6 and 11. Other HPV types cause common warts on the hands, feet, or elsewhere on the body. Other types (HPV types 16 and 18) can cause cancer of the cervix, the external genital skin, or the anus. Warts can grow on the genitals, or on different parts of the body, such as the hands. After you have been infected with the genital wart virus it usually takes between 1 and 3 months for warts to appear on your genitals.

Hepatitis

Hepatitis causes the liver to become inflamed. There are various different types of hepatitis, the most common being hepatitis A, B and C. Each of these viruses acts differently. Hepatitis can be caused by alcohol and some drugs, but usually it is the result of viral infection.

Molluscum

It is a skin disease caused by the Molluscum Contagiosum Virus. It appears as small bumps on the skin, and can last from a couple of weeks to a few years. Molluscum cause small, pearl-shaped bumps the size of a freckle on the thighs, buttocks, genitalia and sometimes the face. They are passed on through body contact during sex and through skin-to-skin contact. Transmission can help to be prevented by using condoms, by avoiding skin-to-skin contact with someone who is infected and by not having sex until they have been treated. In most cases molluscum do not need treatment and will disappear over time.

Non-specific Urethritis (NSU)

Non-specific Urethritis is an inflammation of a man's urethra. This inflammation can be caused by several different types of infection, the most common being Chlamydia. NSU may be experienced months or even in some cases years into a relationship. The symptoms of NSU may include pain or a burning sensation when passing urine, a white/cloudy fluid from the tip of the penis that may be more noticeable first thing in the morning, feeling that you need to pass urine frequently. Often there may be no symptoms, but the infection is transmitted on to the partner(s).

Thrush

It also known as candiasis, is yeast, which lives on the skin, normally kept in check by harmless bacteria. If this yeast multiplies however, it can cause itching, swelling, soreness and discharge in both men and women. Women may experience a thick white discharge and pain when passing urine. Men may experience the same discharge in the penis and difficulty pulling back the foreskin. Thrush can be passed on when having sex with someone who is infected, but also if you wear too tight nylon or lycra clothes or if you are taking certain antibiotics. Transmission can be prevented by using condoms during sex and maintenance of proper hygiene. Treatment for thrush involves taking or applying anti fungal treatments. Thrush can reoccur, especially in women.

Trichomonas Vaginosis

It is caused by a parasite that is found in women's vagina and men's urethra. Often there are not any symptoms. If symptoms are present, they can include pain when urinating and discharge in men and discharge, soreness when having sex and when urinating and inflammation of the vulva in women. Transmission normally occurs through having oral, anal or vaginal sex with an infected person. Treatment consists of taking antibiotics, and the infection should not reoccur.

HIV and STDs

The Agent : Human immunodeficiency virus, measures 1/10000th of a millimeter in diameter belongs to the lentivirus subgroup of family Retroviridae. It is an enveloped virus, 90-120 nm in diameter with a nucleoprotein core containing single stranded RNA genome and proteins. In association with Viral RNA is reverse transcriptase enzyme. The virus core is surrounded by a nucleocapsid shell composed of protein. The virus replicates in actively dividing T_4 lymphocytes and like other retroviruses can remain in lymphoid cells in a latent state that can be activated. The virus has a unique ability to destroy T4 helper cells and can spread through out the body, even crossing the blood brain barrier. The virus mutates radidly, and new strains are continuously developing. Two types of HIV are known – HIV1 is most common while HIV2 is found mostly in West Africa. The virus is susceptible to heat, either, acetone, ethanol (20%) and beta-propiono lactone (1:400 dilution), but is relatively resistant to ionizing radiation and ultra violet light.

Transmission of HIV

The Human Immunodeficiency Virus has been isolated from a variety of body fluids. The risk of transmission through contact with a given fluid is related to

(a) the amount of virus present in the fluid, and
(b) the type of exposure to it.

HIV is found in such small concentrations in tears, saliva, and urine that though transmission through casual contact with these fluids is possible it is highly unlikely but sexual behaviours that lead to exposure to blood, semen, vaginal secretions, and breast milk-all fluids with higher HIV concentations can cause HIV infection. HIV is spread primarily by unprotected sexual intercourse, irrespective of gender or sexual orientation, and sharing of unsterilized needles and syringes. It can be transmitted from an infected mother to an infant in uterus during pregnancy, parentally, or through breast-feeding.

(a) Sexual, Sexual behaviours with exchange of body fluids can transmit HIV. Man to man and heterosexual intercourse are considered the high risk behaviours, with transmission more likely in the presence of other sexually transmitted diseases or genital lesions or during sexual activities that cause a rupture of tissue or bleeding. Studies have shown that male to female transmission is twice more likely than female to male transmission. Women are more vulnerable due to larger surface area exposed and due to higher concentration of HIV virus in semen compared to vaginal secretions.

Anal intercourse carries higher risk of transmission of HIV than vaginal intercourse as there is a greater chance of tissue injury to the receptive partner. A menstruating woman is at a higher risk for containing infection.

Adolescent girls and post menopausal woman are more prone to infection because their cervix would not have been well developed to protect them from HIV and due to thinning of mucosa with age respectively. Also production of mucous is deficient in these age groups.

Two patterns of sexual transmission has been observed First sexual transmission amongst those with multiple partners and Homosexuals (MSM), which is widely recognized. Second pattern which is being recognized now as a major threat is sexual transmission between the infected person and his/her regular partner (WHO).

(b) Injection drug use: Sharing the equipment used to prepare and inject drugs with an HIV-infected person is a very efficient means of transmitting HIV and essentially amounts to a direct inoculation of viral particles from one person to another. The risk of transmission is directly related to the concentration of virus present in the blood and the volume of blood exchanged. Extensive episodes of HIV epidemics among IDUs have occurred in 100 areas throughout the world (WHO).

(c) Blood transfusion: Blood transfusion with infected whole blood cells, platelets and factors VIII and IX remains a significant risk for acquiring HIV. The risk of contacting HIV infection from transfusion of a unit of infected blood is more than 95%. The instance of transmission of infection due to blood transfusion has become low after strict legislation on screening of donated blood/donors for HIV before transfusion. Before the use of lyophilized factor VIII, recurrent inoculation with pooled donated factor VIII was a major source of HIV transmission in hemophilia patients. Transmission due to blood transfusion has been reported from Russia, Libya and Romania account for 2-3% of HIV infection in Africa (WHO).

(d) Perinatal: Infection from mother to infant can occur during gestation, delivery, or breast-feeding. The risk is higher if mother is newly infected or has full blown AIDS. About one third of children born to HIV positive mothers can be infected in this manner. Without intervention, overall risk of transmission is 25-45% in developing countries and 16-20% in Europe (De cock). The absolute risk in utero (antepartum) transmission is 5-10% and intra-partum i.e. approximately 13-18% (Fowler). Meta analysis shows that the transmission via breast milk in women with established infection is 14% (Dunn DT). A study by Miaotiin Malawi demonstrated that the incidence of transmission of infection to child through breast milk among HIV1 infected mothers was 0.7% during 1-5 months, 0.6% during 6-11 months and 0.3% during 12-17 months.

(e) Co-factors for transmission: Co-factors can enhance but do not cause the transmission of HIV. Physical co-factors include the presence of sexually transmitted diseases (such as gonorrhoea, syphilis, and chlamydia, which may cause genital lesions) or genital/mucous membrane bleeding during sexual activity. The use of mood or mind-altering substances may serve as a behavioural co-factor because they can lower sexual inhibitions, impair judgment, or increase impulsivity. Data are inconclusive regarding the effect of mind altering substances on immunocompetence and HIV subsceptibility or progression.

Socio-demographic Variables

1. **Race/ethnicity**: In 1998, African Americans in United States accounted for 45% of AIDS cases reported that year while constituting only 12% of the total

population. The same year, the rate of reported AIDS cases for Hispanics in the United States was 20%, although Hispanics constituted only 13% of the general population. African American and Hispanic women are disproportionately affected, with AIDS rates 17 and 6 times higher, respectively, than for Caucasian women. Three inter- related issues seem to account for the high rates of HIV/AIDS in minority communities: (1) inequities in the general health status in economically disadvantaged minorities, (2) problems controlling substance abuse in minority communities, and (3) the role of substance abuse in the spread of HIV sexually and perinatally.

2. **Gender:** The percentage of women with both HIV infection and AIDS has been steadily rising over the past decade. AIDS cases in USA among women and adolescent girls rose 364% between 1991 and 1997. Trends in HIV diagnoses showed a slight decrease in men but a increase in women. There are issues that are unique to women and HIV/AIDS. Male-to-female transmission is estimated to be eight times more likely than female-to-male transmission. Sex differences in HIV measurements such as viral load, side effects of anti-retroviral medications, and access to quality health care have all been documented.
3. **Age:** AIDS has always had the greatest impact on ages 25-44. Because of the impact associated with new medical therapies, many people's lives have significantly lengthened, which has led to older generations of persons living with HIV/AIDS.
4. **Economic Factors:** The majority of HIV + patients are socially and economically disadvantaged.
5. **Urban versus Rural:** Although HIV has historically disproportionately affected urban areas, rural populations are increasingly at risk. When compared to urban dwellers living with HIV/AIDS, rural inhabitants report significantly lower life satisfaction, lower perceptions of social support from family and friends, reduced access to medical and mental health care, elevated levels of loneliness, more community stigma, heightened personal feal that their HIV status might be disclosed by others, and more maladaptive coping strategies.

Incidence and Prevalence of HIV

The incidence of new HIV infections among adolescents can give a more accurate picture of the trends in the epidemic compared to the overall prevelance of HIV infection.

Among the 5 million new infections in the year 2003, 7 lakh were amongst children less than 15 years of age. Out of them more than 3 million were from the African subcontinent. This bring the total number of people suffering from HIV to 40 million around the world. There were 3 million deaths due to AIDS in the year 2003, while 21.8 million deaths due to AIDS have been recorded till 2001.

Africa

Sub-Saharan Africa is the region of the world that is most affected by HIV/AIDS with an estimated 26.6 million infected people while 3.2 million were newly infected in 2003. Nearly 8% of adults aged 15-49 are infected with HIV/AIDS (UNAIDS and WHO, 2003). Approximately 2.3 millon Africans lost their lives to the disease last year. There were ten million young people (aged 15-24) and almost 3 million children under 15 are living with HIV. An estimated eleven million children have been orphaned by AIDS in Sub-Saharan Africa. Mwaluko *et al* reports and increase of HIV prevalence among adults aged 15-44 years in Tanzania from 5.9% to 8.1% from 1994-1995 to 1999-2000.

In about 16 countries in Africa more than 10% of the adult population aged 15-49 are infected with HIV. In four southern African countries, the national adult HIV prevalence exceeds 30%. These countries are Botswana (37.5%), Lesotho (31.5%), Switzerland (38.6%) and Zimbabwe (33.7%). In South Africa, 20% are now infected compared to 13% three years age. West Africa is relatively less affected by HIV infection, the prevalence rates in some large countries are increasing. Cote d'Ivoire is already among the 15 worst affected countries in the world. East Africa was once the highest on the continent, but now the prevalence in Southern Africa has exceeded the East African countries. Significant Africa has exceeded the East African countries. Significant declines have been noted in Kenya, Ethiopia, Zambia and Zimbabwe. Heterosexual route is the commonest mode of transmission in Africa.

Asia and the Pacific

There are an estimated 7.4 million people living with HIV in Asia and Pacific. Further AIDS has claimed half a million lives in 2003 while one million were newly infection with the virus in the same year.

China accounts for two thirds of the HIV infections in the Western Pacific region.

The prevalence is still under 1% in most of this region's countries. But it may be an underestimation as many Asian countries are quite large and populous and the focus is concentrated on urban areas, without taking into account epidemics in smaller districts and states. Although national adult HIV prevalence in India, for example, is below 1%, five states have an estimated prevalence of over 1% among adults.

However, due to the mushrooming sex trade, drug trafficking and abuse as well as transmigration among porous borders of countries in East and South East Asia like India, Thailand, Burma and China there is a fear of a steep increase in HIV infection rates in near future in this part of the world.

Eastern Europe and Central Asia

The AIDS epidemic in Eastern Europe and Central Asia shows no signs of declining. There were 230,000 new HIV infections in 2003 that brought up the total number patients to 1.5 million. Approximately 30,000 deaths were attributed to AIDS in 2003. It is now estimated that around 1 million people aged 15-49 are living with HIV in the Russian Federation with Ukraine, Estonia, Latvia, and Lithuania being worst affected.

Caribbean & Latin America

It is the worst affected region in the world after Sub-Saharan Africa. While in Haiti, over 6% of adults are living with HIV, in the Bahamas the adult prevalence rate is over 3.5%. In the Dominican Republic 2.5% adults are infected and in Trinidad and Tobago the rate exceeds 1%.

Unprotected heterosexual intercourse is the major route of spread of virus in these countries though injectable drug abuse is a major risk factor in some countries, such as Puerto Rico.

The most vulnerable section of the population are young girls between 15-19 years of age, about one third of whom had sex with older men. HIV rates are five times higher in girls than boys aged 15-19 in Trinidad and Tobago, and at one surveillance centre for pregnant women in Jamaica, girls in their late teens had almost twice the prevalence rate of older women.

There is a lot of diversity in HIV epidemic data obtained from Latin America. Most common risk factor for HIV transmission is hetrosexual sex. In addition very high rates of infection among men who have sexer with men and injecting drug users has been observed in Brazil. In Mexico, Argentina, and Colombia, HIV infection is restricted largely to these high-risk groups. Columbian and Peruvian studies have observed a prevalence rate of 18-22% among men who have sex with men (WHO).

Europe and America

HIV infections in these nations are confined mainly among injecting drug users and gay men. However, heterosexual transmission is the predominant route of spread of infection in several western European countries.

North Africa and Middle East

HIV prevalence is still very low in the region with Sudan remaining most affected with an national adult prevalence of 2%. There has been an increase in incidence of infection amongst IDU users in Libya, Iran and Bahrain (WHO).

HIV/AIDS in India

After the first diagnosis of HIV/AIDS amongst commercial sex workers in Chennai, Tamil Nadu in 1986, the focus has shifted from screening foreigners initially to blood banks and finally setting up of national network of HIV screening centres in major urban areas (Dakar). The National AIDS Control Program was launched in 1987 followed by establishment of National AIDS Control Organization or NACO in 1992 (Bhupesh).

The States were categorised as high, moderate or low, based on following definitions:

High Prevalent States: States where HIV prevalence in antenatal women is 1% or more.

Moderate Prevalent States: States where the HIV prevalence in antenatal women is less than 1% and prevalence in STD and other high risk groups is 5% or more.

Low Prevalent States : States where the HIV prevalence in antenatal women is less than 1% and HIV prevalence among STD and other high-risk group is less than 5%.

HIV prevalence in antenatal women provide a reasonable estimate of HIV prevalence within the general population in each state.

There are a total of 69559 cases of AIDS in India as on April 2004, of whom 26.8% are females. In 2004, it was estimated that 22% of HIV cases in India were house wife with a single partner (Heffman). The increasing HIV prevalence among women can consequently be seen in the increase of mother to child transmission of HIV and paediatric HIV cases.

With 29782 cases Tamil Nadu has approximately 42.8% of total AIDS patients in India followed by Maharashtra and Andhra Pradesh with 23.1% and 10.3% of cases respectively. The prevalence amongst ANC women was more than 1% in Karnataka (1.75%), Tamil Nadu (1.25%), Goa (1.38%), Manipur (1.13%), Maharashtra (1.25%), Mizoram (1.50%) and Nagaland (1.25%).

HIV prevalence among injecting drug users was 10.28% in Nagaland, 39.06% in Manipur.

Out of them 34% were in the age group of 15-29 years and 55% between 30-44 years. In 86.7% the route of transmission was sexual. The prevalence of HIV in India is about 0.8%. The UN Population Division projects that India's adult HIV prevalence will peak at 1.9% in 2019. A 2002 report by the CIA's National Intelligence Council predicted 20 million to 25 million AIDS cases in India by 2010, more than any other country in the world.[10]

India's prevalence rate could be an underestimation as they are based solely on sentinel surveillance conducted at public sites and there is no national information system to collect HIV testing information from the private sector, which provides 80% of health care in the country. Also there are other weaknesses in the surveillance system like there aren't enough testing centers in many parts of the country and bias while targeting specific groups for testing.

Although HIV/AIDS is still largely confined to the high risk populations the recent data suggests that the epidemic is spreading into the general population in some regions. It is also moving from urban to rural districts.

High Risk Groups

Migrants

Populational Reference Bureau had projected that 264 million Indians would be mobile by 2003. Most of them are migrant workers who usually reside in urban slums. The hard nature of their job and the isolation from family may lead to casual unprotected sexual relationships outside wedlock that makes them highly vulnerable to STDs and HIV/AIDS. Moreover they tend to have little access to HIV/STD information, voluntary counseling and testing and health services. Later they end up spreading the infection to their wives and other sexual partners at home leading to a spill over of infection in the general population.

Sex Workers

Mumbai has over 15,000 sex workers. A study in Surat found that HIV prevalence among sex workers had increased from 17% in 1992 to 43% in 2000. When the project of educating sex workers about prevention through condom promotion in Sonagachi, Kolkota was launched in 1992, 27% of sex workers reported condom use. By 1995, this had risen to 82% and in 2001, it was 86%. This proves the effectiveness of such campaigns if implemented properly. In northern Karnataka's "Devadasi" women has been pushed into sanctioned prostitution – as a result many women from this part of the country are supplied to the sex trade in big cities such as Mumbai.

According to the behavioural survey conducted on female sex workers (Female Sex Workers) in India, 94% of FSW had heard of HIV/AIDS. Among all respondents nearly 66% had correct knowledge of the two important prevention methods, i.e. consistent condom use and having one, uninfected and faithful partner.

About 83% of the respondents reported that they had heard of STD in most states, a majority of the respondents (above 80%) could describe symptoms of STD among women and 76% among men. 46% of the respondents reported that they suffered from any one of the symptoms of STD in the last 12 months. Overall, around 35% of the FSWs reported that they had genital discharge or genital ulcer or burning pain during urination. About 35% of the respondents went to a private hospital/clinic for treatment while 28% visited a government hospital and 12% went to the clinic run by NGOs.

The age at first sex was less than 15 years for 27% of the FSWs. The median age at first sex was about 17 years (Range: 7-31 years). Three out of four respondents used a condom at last sex with paying clients.

Injecting Drug Users (IDUs)

HIV infections among IDUs first appeared in Manipur. In Manipur city, the level of HIV infection increased from 61% in 1994 to 85% in 1997 and 1998 it was 80.7%. Injecting drug use is also a major problem in urban areas such as Mumbai, Kolkata, Delhi and Chennai.

The majority of drug users in India are male. According to a study in the capital of Manipur, the prevalence of HIV infection in female IDUs was 57% compared to 20% among female non IDUs. However, use of drug treatment data may underestimate the number of female drug users, with women addicts being predominately a hidden population. There is also an increasing no. of wives of infected IDU contacting HIV through their husbands.

At the national level a total of 1355 interviews were taken during a **behavioural** survey conducted by NACO. Approximately 41% respondents reported using previously used needles/syringes while 4% respondents reported sharing every time they injected. While 97% were aware of HIV/AIDS, 55% among them were aware that switching to non-injecting drugs could prevent infection. Nearly 12% of all respondents had suffered from more than one symptom and a fourth of all respondents had suffered from at least one STD symptom in the past 12 months (26%). While 37% did not take any treatment, only 18% and 17% visited any private hospital/clinic and government hospital/clinic.

Truck Drivers

Truck drivers are crucial in spreading STDs and HIV infection throughout the country. A study published in 1999 showed that 87% of the drivers had frequent and indiscriminate change of sexual partners, and only 11% of them used condoms although their AIDS knowledge was fairly good.

There have been a number of major HIV/STI prevention projects aimed at truckers. Some of these projects include not just truckers, but also other stakeholders such as gas station owners and employees.

Men Who Have Sex with Men

According to the NACO behavioural survey out of the 1387 men who had sex (manual/oral/anal) with other men surveyed in five Indian cities, 97% were aware of HIV/AIDS and 83% reported that the correct and consistent use of condoms could protect from HIV.

Overall about 16% of the respondents reported that they suffered from genital discharge while 24% of the respondents reported genital ulcer/sore and around 30% had burning pain during urination in last 12 months. Around 44% and 28% of the respondents reportedly visited private hospital/clinic and government hospital/clinic respectively during the last episode.

The mean age at first sex with any male partner was 17 years. Around 32% of the respondents reported their age at first sex with any male partner was less than 15 years. Overall, 39% of the respondents reported using condoms last time they had sex with any commercial male partner. 53% of the respondents reported using condoms last time they had sex with non-commercial male partners.

Thus, spread of HIV in India has been diverse, with most of the states reporting a low rate of infection. The HIV epidemic is affecting the Southern Indian States and Maharashtra.

REFERENCES

1. NACO (2003) 'HIV/AIDS Surveillance in India' www.naco.nic.in/indianscene/esthiv.htm
2. Ritherford GW and Werdegar D: Epidemiology of Acquired Immunodeficiency Syndrome 1-29.
3. Gorbach PM, Ryan C, Saphonn V and Detels R: Impact of Social, Economic and Political Forces on Emerging HIV Epidemics, AIDS 2002, 16 (suppl 4): s35-s43.
4. Curran JW *et al*: The Epidemiology of AIDS: Current Status and Future Prospects, Science, 1985, 229:1352-7.
5. NACO 'National AIDS Control Programme Phase-I (1992-1999)', www.naco.nic.in/nacp/phase1.htm accessed 21/8/03.
6. The Lancet (2003) 'Spreading the Word about HIV/AIDS in India', Vol. 361, May 3.
7. Dakar DN and Dakar SN (2001): 'Combating AIDS in the 21st Century Issues and Challenges', Sterling Publishers Private Limited, p. 33.
8. Mwaluko G, *et al*: Trends in HIV and Sexual Behaviour in a Longitudinal Study in a Rural Population in Tanzania, 1994-2000, AIDS 2003, Vol. 17 No. 18: 2645-2651.
9. Bhupesh M, (1992): 'India Disquiet About AIDS Control', *The Lancet*, Vol. 240, No. 8834/8835.
10. You and AIDS (2001), 'South and North-East Asia at a Glance: India.
11. World Health Organization (2004), 'Fight Stigma and Discrimination' USAID (2003) 'HIV/AIDS Country Profile India', March.
12. Hefferman G, (2004): 'Housewives Account for One Fifth of India's HIV cases, expert says', India Post and NCM, April 16.
13. Sivaram S, (2002): 'Integrating Income Generation and AIDS Prevention Efforts—Lessons from Working with Devadasi Women in Rural Karnataka, India', Abstract.
14. Population Reference Bureau (2003) '2003 Data Sheet Highlights: Using Global Population Projections', Data Sheet.
15. UNAIDS (2001) 'Population Mobility and AIDS', Technical Update, February, p. 5.
16. Dutta *et al.:* (2002): 'Strategizing Peer Pressure in Enhancing After Safer Sex Practices in Brothel Setting', Abstract TuPeF5332, The XIV International AIDS Conference.
17. Panda S, *et al.*: (2000): "Transmission of HIV from Injecting Drug Users to Their Wives in India', International Journal of STD and AIDS, July 11(7): 468-473.
18. Kootikuppala SR *et al.:* (1999): 'Sexual Lifestyle of Long Distance Lorry Drivers in India—A Questionnaire Survey', British Medical Journal, January 16.

CHAPTER

3 HIV and AIDS in Adolescents

Vijay Grover

AIDS is posing one of the biggest global challenges in the history of public health. Three decades into the epidemic, there is still no vaccine and 'cure' for AIDS, the Acquired Immunodeficiency Syndrome. The social and economic conditions that facilitate the spread of HIV are also well understood. Despite all we know, risk behaviour and risk environment persist and HIV continues to spread among individuals and across national and regional border, the latest frontier being Asia.

With nearly six million people already infected in WHO's South-East Asia Region, the potential health and socio-economic impacts of AIDS in the new millennium is a cause for serious concern (WHO, 1997). More than half of all new infection globally are in the young people below 25 years. During 1999, more than 5,70,000 children under 15 got infected with HIV.

The HIV/AIDS epidemic is deeply entrenched in several Asian countries in numbers that are escalating fast (UNAIDS, 1997). While Africa remains the worst hit region in the world, the rate of increase in the numbers of HIV infections is even higher in Asia. With more than 60 percent of the world's population, the Asian region needs prompt concerted action to avert the potential social and economic consequences of a more widespread epidemic (UNFPA, 1997).

The World Bank has predicted that there will be 35 million infected with HIV/AIDS by 2005. If these are not prevented, it will be witnessing in Africa, with 25 million infected which is hard to imagine.

The Asian epidemic is highly dynamic and evolving cultural taboos that surround sexual behaviour and talking about sex in many Asian cultures make information. Exchange and negotiating safer sexual practices a significant challenge. Poverty and low levels of education also contribute to a lack of awareness about HIV. Finally, highly mobile populations are more likely to engage in risk behaviour and can act as "bridges" transmitting HIV from one population to another (Mills, Stephen, 1994).

HIV/AIDS ranks as sixth leading cause of death among those aged 15-24 in the United States, with the number of AIDS cases reported each year in that age group increasing by 417 percent from 1981 through 1994. Additionally, since then 5 reported AIDS cases diagnosed among these age 20-29, and as the asymptomatic period may last 10 years, many of those diganosed in their 20s as having AIDS more than likely became infected with HIV in thier teens. The Centers for Disease Control and Prevention (CDC), Public Service Announcement (PSA) Campaign "Respect Yourself" launched on Nov. 30, 1995, has placed a new emphasis on the importance of educating young adults aged 18-25 about the risk they face HIV/AIDS and other sexually transmitted diseases. There are several studies, that support the perception of increased risks (CDC, Dec. 1998). Over 50 percent of all new HIV infections are occurring in young people between 15-24 years old. This is partly because a large part of the world population is young. Secondly, since AIDS is essentially a STI, it affects the young sexually active people the most. The fundamental risk for young people is their ignorance about issues on sexuality, HIV/AIDS/STIs and the dangers of unprotected sex.

Young men having sex with men constitute another marginalized group whose vulnerability is heightened by the lack of information and services available to them and directed to their concerns. Young women are more vulnerable than young men, for both physiological and socio-cultural reasons. Young people are a priority group for HIV prevention. The majority of boys and girls will be free of HIV at puberty and Family Planning Association workers, teachers and those working with young people can help them to stay that way. They will then form a reservoir of healthy parents and an insurance for future generations.

Nearly 50 percent of the developing world populations consists of young people in their sexually active 'prime'. The sexual health services are critical to their health and wellbeing.

Adolescents contribute nearly one billion in number to world population and approximately 200 million of these are in India alone. Adolescents, especially girls are very important resources of the nation. If they suffer from deadly disease, our country will suffer.

With a population of over one billion, and half of the population between ages 15-49, HIV/AIDS in India has a strong impact on the pandemic, both in Asia and globally, India is home to the largest number of people living with HIV/AIDS second only to South Africa. In India current available data, limited as they are, indicate that youth will increasingly be at the centre of the epidemic both in terms of transmission and infect over 50% of all new infection in India take place among young adults below 25 years. Every year, nearly 22,837 newborn children are infected and about 11,434 die due to HIV/AIDS. It is estimated that total of 1,80,000 children are living with AIDS in India (htpp://www.sdnpbd.org/sdi/2004/women-aids.htm).

80% of reported AIDS cases occur in the southern States of Maharashtra, Tamil Nadu, Andhra Pradesh, and Karnataka, and in the north-eastern States of Nagaland and Manipur.

In the southern States, HIV transmission through men having unprotected sex with men is also a cause for concern, as many men who have sex with men also have sex with women. In the north-eastern States of Manipur and Nagaland, transmission is mainly through intravenous drug use. In the six States with generalized epidemic, prevalence among pregnant women has remained stable at just above 1%, which some experts suggest indicates that the epidemic may have stabilized. High rates of tuberculosis in India exacerbate the growing number of HIV infections.

Adult HIV prevalence rate (2003) is 0.9%. Estimated number of adults and children living with HIV/AIDS (2003) is 3.1 million (NACO, UNAIDS, 2004).

AIDS (Acquired Immunodeficiency Syndrome) is not one disease, but a set of diseases. Not all people who develop AIDS suffer from the same diseases, but there are certain unusual illnesses that occur very frequently in AIDS. That is why it is called a "syndrome". This syndrome is caused by a virus which affects the body's immune system, making it liable to infections and cancers to which it would normally be resistant. The virus is "Human Immunodeficiency Virus" (HIV), it is one virus, in fact it seems to have changed its structure over time and in different places. Now a family of viruses, some of which are more closely related them other. Many people either shows no immediate symptoms at the time, they are infected with HIV, or else have such transient and mild symptoms that they are passed off as a "cold" or a "flu". Sometimes they have a short term illness similar to glandular fever; aching muscles, fever and a general feeling of illnesses which are much more common than AIDS. Whether or not there are symptoms, the infected person can carry the virus and infect others. It is perfectly possible to be infected with HIV from someone who appears fit and healthy, or to carry the virus on self without being aware of it.

The adolescents should be able to understand the consequences (personal and social) on a person infected with HIV/AIDS (Bureau of the Census, United States, 1987). The United Nations believes public ignorance is encouraging the spread of HIV/AIDS in India, and that the government has been slow to tackle the problem due to conservativeness of the people who oppose prevention methods that could be interpreted as promoting promiscuity. Attitudes are changing as the epidemic spread like wild fire through India's vast population. A staggering 85% of intercourses are heterosexual.

In many cultures, shame, fear and denial cloud discussion of the issue and adults to whom young people might naturally turn parents, teachers, school.

Nurses, community leaders find it difficult to speak openly about STIs. Unfortunately, when youth finally approach the formal STI care system, they often encounter an obstacle course (Kabatesi, 1996).

Adolescents, both boys and girls, have very little information on sex and HIV/AIDS prevention. Girls have almost no information, and boys have misinformation (http://www.indianngos.com/issue/hiv/children.htm).

Most young people start experimenting with sex earlier than believed and without understanding concepts like safe sex, contraception and other health issues. Many of the adolescents knew something about AIDS but it was not useful information as they had no context to place it in. This has serious implications for reproductive health because lack of information can result in unintended pregnancies, STDs or HIV.

Sex education is not widely available to children and is still an issue despite findings to the contrary that sex education delays onset of sexual activity and promotes safe sex.

Existing reproductive health services do not serve adolescents and there is an under utilization of services by adolescents for gynaecological conditions such as RTIs.

Data from a recent study in Maharashtra showed that 82% of married adolescent women did not use health services for postnatal care, and 51% did not use services for gynaecological problems.

Findings of research study by the NGO Butterflies revealed that a large number of street children had genital lesions, suggestions of secondary syphilis. One out of ten tested positive on VDRL test. None went for proper medical treatment (NACO, 2004).

Which Adolescents are at Risk?

Which groups of adolescents are at high risk of HIV? At what age do boys become sexually active? What about girls? At what age do girls marry and/or have their first baby?

In some groups girls may marry at puberty and have their first child a year later. Their husbands are likely to have other sexual partners. At this age girls usually have low status in the household and will not be able to even discuss safer sex. If bride wealth or dowry is paid, the man and his family will 'own' the girl's sexuality.

The other groups or societies, boys and girls usually later, perhaps in their early twenties. Some, if not all of them, will have sexual partners before marriage. In some societies, girls will have their first child in their teens several years before they get married.

A high incidence of pregnancy, abortions and STIs in unmarried adolescents means that they are at high risk of HIV/AIDS in areas with HIV. These problems already threaten the lives and fertility of girls and a programme to help them to have safer relationships is urgently needed.

Tragically, 50% of global HIV/AIDS infections are amongst women (most of them 'set up' to acquire the virus through no fault of their own), mainly in the developing nations. Mothers can transmit the virus to their new born children through breast milk, the food of choice for the poor, as cost is a factor (Ethener et al., 2003).

AIDS increases the urgency of extending this knowledge and skills to all children before they become sexually active. The age at which adolescents become sexually active will vary with ethnic group, religious, domestic situation, schooling etc.

Sexually transmitted infections have significant implications for the vulnerability of young people' to HIV. High rates of STIs among young people reveal the high levels of unprotected sex, which put them at high risk for contracting HIV and STIs. These are most frequent in young people aged 15-24, and 50 percent of all HIV infections are among young people, most of whom contract HIV before they are 20 years old (UNFPA, 1997).

Street children and child labourers are particularly vulnerable due to high incidence of sexual abuse and exploitation. All these children have little or no family support, no access to services without the welfare and social safety nets of the organized sector:

There are an estimated 1,00,000 street children in the metropolitan citis like Mumbai, Delhi and Kolkata, and the number are increasing due to rapid urbanization.

Street children are especially vulnerable to HIV infection due to lack of awareness and an absence of safety nets. Many of them, as young as 8, report having sex for companionship or as being victims of regular sexual abuse. Some are forced into prostitution as a means of survival.

It is estimated that 60-90% street children in Mumbai are sexually active. About 20% of street boys in the 16-20 age group visit commercial sex workers regularly and 80% periodically. A study conducted in the slums in Chennai found that 80% of youth engaged in pre marital sex; 85% of the same group reported never using condoms (http://www.inianngos.com/issue/hiv/resources/children.htm).

Government of India admits to 17.5 million children in the 5-14 age group as being in the labour force. Some live in conditions of extreme marginalization and fall prey to sexual exploitation increasing their vulnerability to HIV/AIDS. In this context, the situation of the girl child labourer calls for particular attention.

Life on the street for girl child is twice as oppressive and exploitative than that of a boy. Girl children as young as nine and ten are forced into consuming drugs and then sexually abused.

Among those at greatest risk are street children. Some estimates suggest that there are as many as 100 million children and adolescents in the world who are working or living on the street, often in violent and dangerous conditions. These groups are some of the most vulnerable to HIV infection and, of course, to many dangers. Adolescents are even more reluctant than adults to seek treatment for sexually trasmitted infections. Many are embarrassed and fearful that their parents will find out that they are sexually active. Even if treatment for STIs is sought, young people, particularly in developing countries, are less likely to be able to pay for their treatment. Some go to traditional healers or obtain antibiotics from pharmacies without proper diagnosis. Incomplete treatment may alleviate the symptoms, while not curing an STI, which can still transmit to others and lead to complications such as infertility and increased vulnerability to HIV infection.

When Sex Starts?

Boys and girls in boarding schools have a freedom and lack of family guidance which may result in sexual activity by around 13 years. Girls may be eager to get pregnant soon after primary school education as a passport to adulthood and proof of fertility for potential partners.

Unemployed young people in urban areas may sell sex for cash at an early age. Girls have sex with 'sugar daddies', older elite men who may have many partners. Adolescents may inject drugs and sell sex to pay for their habits (Gill & Tony, 1989).

What Does the Risk of HIV Infection Mean?

Talking about HIV transmission means talking about risk. No definite statement can be made that are true for everyone. People may or may not realize or admit to themselves that they are at risk of HIV infection. People with HIV may not know they have it or that they are partly others at risk. Many people who know they have HIV try to protect others, though there may be limit on how much they can do so. Getting exposed to HIV does not necessarily mean being infected, as shown in following table:

Likelihood of infection per exposure	*Exposure*
Blood Transfusion	>90%
Pregnancy-related	20% - 40%
Sexual intercourse	0.1% - 1.0%
Injection, drug use	0.5% - 1.5%
Other needle type	< 0.5%

The vast majority of people at risk through these main routes of transmission with all forms of exposure, although the relative risk differs, are exposure can lead to infection and each repeated exposure carries the same risk. In general, the more virus per exposure and the more times a person is exposed, the more likely it is that infection will occur, multiple exposure increases the risk. Re-infection through continuing exposure after infection also occurs and may contribute to disease progression.

The dimension of sexual behaviour that increases the risk of infection include individual sexual characterization, early age at sexual intercourse, large number of life time and current sex partners, high risk characterization of sex partners and specific sexual practices and frequency along with the socio-cultural beliefs of the individuals.

Studies have shown that young parents are unable to teach their children well and on growing up, these children exhibit high risk sexual behaviour (Garg, 1986; Klerman, 1993; Trad, 1993; Holder, 1993).

With this kind of global patterns it would be important to note here that due to poverty, lack of knowledge and counseling and greater numbers of people in urban areas, the spread of AIDS in the developing countries would be expected to be quick and disastrous (Anderson and Roy, 1992, 1993; NACO, 1993; Branham and Robert, 1992).

Sex and HIV/AIDS

Unprotected sexual practices, within males with males or females with males, is the most common way of transmitting HIV. Between 85-90 percent of new infections are transmitted through sexual intercourse.

Understanding sexual behaviour of different sectors of population is key to designing an effective response to the epidemic. While the commercial sex industry is often thought of as the highest risk area for contracting HIV through sex, a critical place for interventions is in the 'bridging' population the clients of sex workers who are the link or 'bridge' for HIV transmission between the sex workers and the general population.

What is Risky Behaviour?

Behaviour increasing the risk of contracting an STI includes:

- Having sexual intercourse with many partners, without using a condom.
- Having a partner who has many sex partners.
- Having sex with commercial sex workers, without using a condom.
- Continuing to have sexual contact with symptoms of an STI and without using a condom.
- Not getting any treatment for an STI; or
- Not taking the medication prescribed for an STI correctly, or not finishing the treatment.

Child prostitution, child trafficking and sexual abuse leading to forced and coerced sex increase the vulnerability of children to HIV:

A 1990 study conducted by the Central Social Welfare Board in six metros reported that roughly 40% of the total commercial sex worker population is below 18 years of age, many of them as young as 8 or 9 years.

Every year, about 50,000 more forced into prostitution. The average age of children in brothels is as low as 13. Commercial child prostitutes increase at the rate of 8-10% a year. At least 4,00,000 are minors and 20,000 are annually trafficked into India from Nepal.

The children of sex workers numbering about 53 lakhs nationwide are especially vulnerable group since they fall easy victims to the sex trade.

Recent studies indicate that incidence of rape in the under 10 age group has increased by 84% between 1990 and 1994, while the general incidence of reported rape in all age groups has increased from 20,194 in 1990 to 2,15,000 as of October 1995. These figures represent only the tip of iceberg.

Across Asia, commercial sex workers are largely young. A survey in three urban areas in Thailand found 40 per cent of low priced sex workers to be under 18. In two rural villages in northern Thailand 46 percent and 71 percent of the sex workers started before they were 18 and 29 years old respectively.

Young sex workers are at particular risk of contracting HIV as their social status makes them less able to negotiate the use of condoms, and biologically they are more vulnerable to infection. Despite this, young female sex workers are often perceived by clients as being safer than the older sex workers who are more risky (ibid). According to the figure reported at the 1996 World Congress Against Commercial Sexual Exploitation of Children, one million children enter the sex trade every year (Ahlburg, et al. 1998). In 1992, The Royal Government of Nepal estimated that there were close to 2,00,000 Nepali girls and women in Indian brothels. Many young women are abducted or sold by parent, relative or family friends in whom they had placed their trust (O'Dea, Pauline, 1993).

While poverty is a key factor driving the commercial sex trade and trafficking of young women, it is not the sole cause of prostitution in Nepal or in Mumbai. Links between the social status of girls and women, growing consumerism, violence and crime and the erosion of trditional values are well recognized (ibdi., p20, 29).

These reasons are even more compelling when social systems are inadequate and do not provide needed support to individuals and families. Sex workers even more vulnerable to HIV due to inadequate social welfare systems, vulnerable individuals, and economic needs of families.

Studies in 1993 estimates that 15% of secondary school girls have been sexually abused. The Social Welfare Board reports increased molestation, rape, sexual abuse of progressively younger children more within the family than outside.

Increasingly, adult males are targeting younger children for sex in the belief that they are free from HIV and STDs or that sex with virgin will increase their virility, or cure them of STIs.

STIs and HIV/AIDS

One of the key factors precipitating the spread of HIV is sexually transmitted infections. STIs rates not only indicate the extent of unprotected sex, it is now known that an individual with an STI is more vulnerable to contracting HIV than an individual who has no other STI. Aggressive STI prevention campaigns as well as prompt treatment of STIs are key to preventing the spread of HIV infection. The Bangladesh, for instance, a recent study revealed that 95 percent of the sex workers had contracted genital herpes and 60 percent had syphilis.[37] Fertile ground for rapid HIV infection if, such levels of STIs are not treated.

The Correlation between HIV and STIs

- The predominant mode of transmission of both HIV and other STI agents is sexual. Although other routes of transmission include blood, blood products, donated organs of tissues, and from an infected woman to her fetus or new born infant.

  STI, which causes genital ulcerations, such as syphilis, chancroid and herpes simplex, may facilitate the transmission of HIV infection to 2-9 folds more times. This is because the infected semen or vaginal secretions come into direct contact with the open sores of the mucous membrane.
- Many of the measures taken for preventing the sexual transmission of HIV and other STIs agent are the same, as are the target audience for these interventions.

- Access to STIs clinical services are important for people at high risk of contracting STIs and HIV, not only for diagnosis and treatment but also for education and counseling.
- There is a strong association between the occurrence of HIV infection, and the presence of certain STIs, making early diagnosis and effective treatment of such STIs an important strategy for the prevention of HIV transmission.
- Trend in STI incidence and prevalence can be useful early indication of changes in sexual behaviour and are easier to monitor than trends in HIV surveillance.

In view of the strong association between HIV/AIDS and STIs programmes to control HIV/AIDS now also focuses on STIs through combined HIV/AIDS and STIs programmes (WHO, 1997).

The changing nature of marital and sexual relationships in many countries, has profoundly influenced patterns of transmission of not only AIDS, but other STIs as well, STD, which causes genital ulcerations, such as syphilis, chancroid and herpes simplex, may facilitate the transmission of HIV infection. This is because the infected semen or vaginal secretions come into direct contact with the open sores of the mucous membrane.

Popular ideas about STDs suggest that little stigma is attached to male infection. Having an STI is almost a right of passage into manhood, in many countries proof of sexual activity; 'A bull is not a bull without his scars'. Consistent with both data and belief, a study on HIV infection among male factory workers found that a history of, prior STI was common among both seropositive and seronegative men 100 and 75 percent respectively. Other risk factors, now documented in numerous studies of AIDS in Africa were also more common in the HIV positive group e.g. multiple partners, a history of payment for sex. What was unexpected was the high prevalence of high risk activities among seronegative men; 40 percent reported STI in the previous year and 67 percent had paid money for sex. Seropositive men were more likely than seronegative men to report a history of genital ulcer. In the light of these data, one can hardly characterize the seronegative comparison group as 'low risk'.

The focus on genital ulcer as an important co-factor for HIV transmission has both positive and negative features while, it offers new approaches for intervention programmes, it also shifts emphasis from the broader social context of STI occurrence to more narrow medical concerns. Certainly any intervention that results in reduced rates of STIs, such as increasing public awareness about the availability of treatment for STIs. Will also mean a diminution of HIV transmission. It is said that, some women now inspect men for sex, a strategy that may be particularly useful for women engaged in commercial sex. The focus on genital ulcer is also appealing because it seems to eliminate all of the value laden issues. That accompany interpretation of other risk factors, such as multiple partners and prostitute contact. Early detection and prompt treatment of STI can reduce the risk of sexual transmission of HIV infection. However, the diagnosis of STI in women can be difficult as obvious symptoms do not always occur. Once diagnosed, however, treatment for most STIs are available.

Why Need Safer Sex?

Should everyone having intercourse be advised to practice safer sex, or only people most at risk of HIV/AIDS?

Of 17,655 women attending family planning clinic in the Philadelphia area in US from mid 1988 to mid 1989, 14 percent were at high risk of HIV infection, 31 percent at moderate risk and 55 percent at low risk. Risk was measured according to the number of STDs acquired in the previous five years, number of sexual partners in the previous year and sex with an injection drug user 3. Even on this relatively crude measure, at least half the women would have benefited from counseling about HIV/AIDS and safer sex. However, determination of risk is not fool proof. It is not always possible to recognize, who is at risk. Many mistakenly believe or realize that they are at risk. And women who are at high or low risk today do not necessarily remain that way indefinitely.

A major disadvantage of encouraging safer sex and condom use only among those with identified risk behaviour is that everyone else is helped to believe they are not vulnerable (Susan Robbin, *et al.*, 1990).

This can contribute to double standards of 'good' and 'bad' sex and discrimination against people with identified risks. Most importantly, in the long run, it may be the only effective way for safer sex to become the social norm at a global level.

Drug Use and HIV/AIDS

In many countries children resort to drug use for recreational purposes.

According to the UNDCP report, majority of the drug users are in the age group of 16-30 years. Drug use increases the potential of engaging in risk taking behaviour and consequently increases their vulnerability to HIV infection. There is little or no use of condoms among drug users.

The UNDCP reports of a close relationship between living on the street and use of drugs.

As noted earlier, adolescence is a time of experimentation with a variety of behaviour that may include sex and the use of drugs. Much drug use, even though it is considered to be a significant health threat to the individual as well as to society at large, does not constitute a direct risk factors for AIDS. IV drug use, 56 on the other hand, can play a direct role in HIV transmission, if drug injection equipment is shared. Moreover, the use of drugs that are not injected may pose an indirect threat. Even alcohol, for example, can play an indirect role in transmission by lowering inhibitions and perhaps clouding the judgement of those who are drinking, thereby facilitating unsafe sexual practices (Stall, et al, 1986 & Madoove, 1987). Another drug that has the potential to affect transmission of virus is a crack, a smokable and potent form of cocaine that is believed to heightened sensations of sexual arousal among males. Ethinographics studies indicate that some women exchange sex for crack (or for cash to by crack) (Turner et al 1989). In a study of 13-19 years old black male and female crack users in San Francisco area (n=222), virtually all (96%) were found to be sexually active, slightly more than half (52%) reported that they had combined sex with drug use and one quarter of both boys (25%) and girls (24%) had exchanged sexual favour for drugs or money (Fulli, Love et al, 1989).

Needle sharing among injecting drug users is a high risk activity that has fueled the spread of HIV and AIDS in a number of Asian countries. Since drug use is illegal and covert, these risk populations are particularly difficult to reach with interventions such as safe needle exchange and prevention education. It is also difficult to make accurate assessment of the extent of HIV (Brown, et al., 1994). It is clear, however, that injecting drug use and the related risk of HIV transmission is prevalent in all countries in the region, although varying in scope from one country to the next.

Adolescent Women Underestimate Their Susceptibility to HIV/AIDS

Adolescent females are at significant risk for HIV/AIDS and may not accurately incorporate indicators of risk into their perception of susceptibility. Perceived susceptibility to adverse health outcome is a major factor in theoretical models of behaviour change. Accurate assessing personal risk and making the connection between behaviour and susceptibility to infection are important first steps in preventing disease. In order to perceive themselves as susceptible, adolescents should be able to recognize a number of factors as indicators of risk for HIV/STIs. For instance, unprotected intercourse and multiple sexual partners, the focus of most prevention programme are significant sources of HIV/AIDS risk. Although STIs are often asymptomatic, symptomatic recognition is an important aspect of diagnosis, treatment and prevention. Finally, STI history is a strong predictor of future STI/HIV/AIDS diagnosis and interns of adolescents cognitive associations, previous experiences with an STI could increase awareness of behaviour and symptoms that indicate STI risk. If adolescents appropriately understand the factors that put them at risk for STIs they should recognise that these indicators make them more susceptible to STI. Further, accurate perception of susceptibility of STI should be related to actual infection (Holden, G.M. *et al.,* 1993).

Variation of AIDS and HIV Prevalence by Gender

Just as more AIDS cases are seen among adult males than adult females, so too there are more cases of AIDS among teenage boys than among teenage girls (Bureau of Census, US, 1987). Of all AIDS as of December 31, 1989, males outnumbered females by a 9:1 ratio (Dec. 31, 1989). The ratio of male to female by a 9:1 ratio (Dec. 31, 1989). The ratio of male to female cases is much lower among teenagers than among adults in United States. It is seen that male-female ratio, which is roughly 1:1 among cases diagnosed in infants increases to 4:1 among teenagers, to 6:1 among 20 to 24 years old, and ultimately 16:1 for cases diagnosed among persons in their forties. In India, we do not have age wise break up of data from childood to adulthood.

In addition to variations by age, the ratio of male to female cases of AIDS and HIV infection varies substantially among populations. Eleven percent of AIDS cases among teenagers have been diagnosed in the New York metropolitan areas, and the male to female, ratio for those cases is approximately 2:1. The size of this ratio indicates that girls in the New York area are supporting a greater burden of disease than girls nationally (US Bureau of the Census, 1985). Overall the number of infected men is approximately equal to the number of infected women among 17-19 year old military applicants (1.09:1), but 17 and 18 year old applicants fewer than women found to be seropositive (0.1:1) (Burks et al., 1990). Survey of clinic populations have found roughly equivalent rates of infection among teenage males and females (Project AWAKE, 1989).

The Impact of HIV/AIDS on Children

By the end of year 2000, over 13 million children globally will have lost their mothers or both parents to AIDS, and 10.4 million of them will still be under the age of 15 (UNICEF & UNAIDS, 1999).

Orphans especially disadvantaged in terms of school enrollment due to reduced ability of families to pay fees; are withdrawn from school to earn, help in family chores or care for ailing family members as indicated in data from seven African countries, Haiti and Brazil.

Child malnutrition is one of the most severe and lasting consequences of death of the adult earner through reduced household income, resulting in reduced food expenditure and consequently a drop in food consumption.

In addition to the risks of children contracting HIV from mother either at birth or through breast feeding, or due to sexual exploitation during adolescence, the impact of HIV on uninfected children is also significant. This increases the number of dependent orphans in families and communities already stressed by limited resources, compounded by the fact that those with HIV/AIDS are often the family members in their most productive years.

All children under the age of 18 living in to-day's world whether they are themselves infected with HIV, affected by AIDS in their households or communities, or living in the shadow of HIV risk are recognised by the United Nations Convention on the Rights of the child (UNAIDS, 1997).

The fear, discrimination, ignorance and social stigma associated with AIDS leave affected children completely isolated.

Beyond 2000, Responding to HIV/AIDS in the New Millennium

As we enter a new millennium, we are still faced with ever growing AIDS pandemic. HIV infection continues to spread, especially among those with high risk behaviour and among those that are vulnerable, such as women and young people. Bold steps must be taken to honesty acknowledge and address the status of epidemic, ensure adequate resources and establish needed policies and programmes (Larson & Narain, 2001).

There are many borders that need to be crossed to truly address HIV and AIDS. National plans must consider the impact of rural urban and intraregional movement of people across geographical borders and provide relevant, understandable information and services.

Young people should also be recognized as key advocates of healthy behaviour and not merely the recipients of information traditionally sanctioned gener borders limiting women's access to education and information as well as opportunities to express their views need also to be re negotiated in light of epidemic. Gender inequalities fuelling the epidemic must be explicity addressed. Prevention methods, life saving treatments and the results of scientific breakthrough in prevention and care must be made broadly available on an equitable and affordable basis to all.

That people living with and affected HIV/AIDS must be actively engaged and supported in their efforts to address the epidemic in communities around the world. Successful responses are linked to respect for human rights.

One of our greater challenges is to honour the right to health. We can do this by mobilizing political will and commitment not merely words of enthusiasm, but true commitments of financial and human resources to public awareness and action at all levels; and by catalyzing legislation ensures non-discrimination of those affected by HIV and AIDS beyond all borders (Larson & Narain, 2001).

Indian Adolescents Virtually in the Dark about AIDS, New Delhi

There is woefully inadequate knowledge among Delhi adolescents and specially among the 15-24 age group on how the AIDS virus is transmitted. A behavioural surveillance survey carried out by the Delhi State AIDS Control Society of the Government of Delhi and conducted by the Operation Research Group (ORG) covered 3,832 respondents in the 15-49 age group of which the adolescents formed a part. This survey revealed that 88.2% had never heard of HIV/AIDS. Interestingly, low awareness rates were recorded for both men and women. While, 86% of the people surveyed were aware that HIV/AIDS can be transmitted through blood transfusion; only 23.5% had correct knowledge of HIV transmission. A majority of them were aware of the benefits of consistent use of condom. The adolescents as a group were found to be not aware of sexual aspects of HIV/AIDS, says the study report (Newindpress.com, 2004).

Interestingly, the results of behaviour surveillance survey are in accordance with International trends as a recent UNICEF report has found that those who belong to 15-24 group in different countries 9 in 1 World lack knowledge of HIV transmission and prevention. It is argued in favour of reopening the entire AIDS intervention strategy in terms of empowering the 15-29 age group calling it as an "Opportunity Crisis".

Based on Delhi survey, The State AIDS Control Society has considered that there exists a definite need of information education and communication among the adolescents on an urgent basis. Though they constitute a low risk group, they are unaware of AIDS and in fact, want to know more details". This report points out "once this group is informed and motivated they can act as change agent for their own family, peer group as well as community at large" (Hindu; 2002).

Condom sales have actually dropped in India in last one year according to a BBC World Report (http://news.bbc.co.uk/2/hisouthasia/3067325.stm). It will continue to fall one of the hotspot for transmission of the disease in Mumbai, where nearly 6,000 prostitutes and sex workers live in just one red light area Many are struggling to survive and do not consider the condom a priority. "Young people are especially vulnerable and we must help them to make the right decisions in life."

We have learned in last two decades that people, particularly young people, change their behaviour and behave responsibly when they are given choices and no singly lessons based on morality said, Ex-secretary General UNAIDS, Kofi Annan, supported this view.

The Rights of the Child in a World with AIDS

The United Nations Convention on the Rights of the Child (CRC) drafted in 1989 is a global convenant on the rights of children. It holds countries morally and ethically bound to honour the rights of children as outlined by the Convention including protection from HIV/AIDS and to take concrete steps to ensure their implementation. All but two countries in the world are signatories in this landmark convenant. The Government of India accepted to this Convention in 1992.

In this context of HIV/AIDS, CRC has spelt out principles for reducing children's vulnerability to infection and protect them from discrimination because of their real or perceived HIV/AIDS status.

Children should have access to HIV/AIDS prevention, education, information and to the means of prevention. Measures should be taken to remove social, cultural, political or religious barriers that block children's access to these.

Children's right to confidentiality and privacy in regard to their HIV status should be recognized. This includes the recognition that HIV testing should be voluntary and done with the informed consent of pre-testing counseling. If the child's legal guardians are involved, they should pay due regard to child's view, if the child is of an age or maturity to have such views.

All children should receive adequate care and treatment for HIV/AIDs, including those children for whom this may require additinal costs because of their circumstances, such as orphans.

Children should suffer no discrimination in leisure, recreational sport and cultural activities because of their HIV/AIDS status.

Challenges ahead for the reduction of children's and young people's vulnerability to HIV

1. The most important challenge in India would be to reach the large majority of young people outside the school system who are part of the unorganized and informal labour force.
2. To implement youth centred programmes for the prevention of not only HIV/AIDS but to promote general development of young people through the total participation of young people themselves in every stage of programming.
3. Upscale current best practices e.g. School based HIV/AIDS education already implemented in several schools, UTA programme in colleges. These need to be scaled up to increase the extent of coverage.
4. Reorientation and strengthening of existing services to become youth friendly services to ensure accessibility and acceptability to young people.
5. Promotion and development of policies that ensure that the rights of young people are respected, protected and fulfilled.
6. Ensuring care and support of orphans and young people living with HIV/AIDS.

REFERENCES

1. http://www.indiananngos.com/issue/hiv/children.htm
2. http://news.bbc.co.uk/2/hissouthasia/3067325.htm and http://www.sdnpbd.org/sdi/2004/women-aids.htm and newindpress.com,2004.
3. Ahlburg, Dennis, A, and Eric, R Jensen, 1998: The Economics of the Commercial Sex Industry and Its Implications for HIV/AIDS Prevention Policies in Confronting AIDS: Evidence from the Developing World, M Ainsworth, L Fransen, and M Over, (eds) Brussels: European company.
4. AIDS in India: Newsletter of the NACO (National AIDS Controlling Organization), Ministry of Health and Family Welfare, New Delhi, June, 1993; 1-6.
5. Anderson and Roy, N, 1992: Some Aspects of Sexual Behaviour and the Potential Demographic Impacts of AIDS in Developing Countries. Social Sciences and Medicine, Vol. 34, No. 3: 27-280.
6. Brown, Tim and Peter Xenos, 1994, p. 10.
7. Chin and James, 1995: Scenarios for the AIDS Epidemic in Asia. Asia-Pacific Population Research reports No. 2, Hawai: East West Center Program on Population, p. 12.
8. Ethener KA, Kershaw T, Niccolas L, *et al.*: 2003: Adolescent Women Underestimates their Susceptibility to Sexually Transmitted Infections, *Sex Trans Infec* 2003; 79: 408-411.
9. Godwin, Peter *et al.*: 1997: Evaluation of Asia and Near East (ANE) Regional HIV/AIDS Activities, Prepared for the USAID Strategic Planning and Analysis Division, Office of Strategic and Economic Analysis Bureau for Asia and the Near East, p. xiv.
10. Hindu: 2002 <http://www.reuse.com>
11. HIV/AIDS Surveillance Report, mid year 1998, edition Vol. 10-11, Center of Disease Control and Prevention, National Centre for HIV, STD and TB Prevention, Atlanta, Georgia, 38333, Dec. 1998.
12. Holden G W, Nelson P W, Veleisquez J, *et al.*: 1993. Cognitive Psychological and Reported Sexual Behaviour Difference between Pregnant and Non-pregnant Adoleslcents. Adolescence, Fall 28 (111): 557-572.
13. *Ibid.*, p. 20.
14. *Ibid.*, p. 20.

15. *Ibid.*, p. 29.
16. *Ibid.*, p. 29.
17. Kabatesi, Donna, 1996: Young People and STIs—A Prescription for Change, AIDS Captions, Vol. III, i. pp. 21-22.
18. Klerman L V, 1993: Adolescent Pregnancy and Parenting Controversies of the Past and Lessons for the Future, *J Adolescent Health*, Nov, 14(7) 553-561.
19. Kofi Annan, Secretary General, UNAIDS, http://www.thecityreview .com/aids3.htm
20. Larson, Heidi J. and Narain, JP, 2001: Beyond 2000 Responding to HIV/AIDS in the New Millenium, WHO/SEA/AIDS122, Regional Office for South East Asia, New Delhi, India.
21. Many T, Bassett and Marnellous Mbloyi: Women AIDS and STDs—An Important Connation—Women and HIV/AIDS 1995; Written and Edited by Marge Berer with Sunanda Ray.
22. Mills Stephen, 1994: AIDS in Asia Facing The Epidemic AIDS Caption, p. 6.
23. National AIDS Control Program (NACO), Ministry of Health & Family Welfare, Govt. of India, New Delhi, 2004.
24. O'dea Pauline, 1993: Gender Exploitation and Violence—The Market in Women, Girls and Sex in Nepal, Report Prepared for UNICEF.
25. Preventing a Crisis, AIDS and Family Planning Work, International Planned Parenthood Federation Produced by Gill Gordon & Tony Kionda, Feb. 1989, McMillan Publishers. p. 39-40.
26. Project AWAKE, San Francisco General Hospital, Women at risk of AIDS more likely to switch Partners than Sex Practices, Press Release at 5th International Conference on AIDS Montreal, 7 June 1989.
27. Susan Robbins *et al*: A Description of HIV Risk Factors Among 17,655 Women 6th International Conference on AIDS San Francisco, 1990, Abstract No. FC 746.
28. Trad PV, 1993: Adolescents Pregnancy—An International Challenge in Child Psychiatry, *Human Dev. Winter*, 24(2): 99-113.
29. UNAIDS, 1997, Children Living in a World with AIDS, World AIDS Campaign Media Briefing, p. 5.
30. UNFPA, 1997 State of the World's Population Report.
31. UNICEF & UNAIDS, 1999, Children Orphaned by AIDS, p. 2.
32. US Bureau of the Census, 1985 Appendix 2.
33. US Bureau of the Census, 1987, 17.
34. WHO, 1997, AIDS: No Time for Complacency, New Delhi; WHO/SEARO, p. 27.
35. World Health Organization, Global Programme on AIDS. Current and Future Dimensions of HIV/AIDS Pandemic: A Capsule Summary, Sept. 1990, No. WHO/GPA/SFI/90.2 Rev.

CHAPTER

4 Adolescents' Reproductive Health

Vijay Grover

Reproductive health is of growing concern these days particularly of adolescents in the light of early gain in sexual maturity coupled with their relative ignorance of its various aspects and hazards in this population.

What is 'Reproductive Health'?

Reproductive health is defined as, "the aspect of health which addresses reproductive process, functions and systems, at all stages of life and the associated freedom and a capability to reproduce and to decide if, when and how often to do so."

Reproductive health is not merely the abuses of disease or disorders of the reproductive processes, functions, or systems among the individuals of different age groups but is a condition in which the reproductive function and process can be accomplished in a stage of physical, mental and social wellbeing. People are capable to have a responsible, satisfying and safe sex. They should have the right ability, and opportunity to regulate their fertility according to their choice without any risk to women's health, and they are able to go through pregnancy and childbirth safely and with successful outcome that would ensure survival and proper growth and development of the child (WHO, Biennial Report 1990-92).

It also encompasses information and services to improve reproductive and sexual health through disease control and increasing gender equity.

The concept of reproductive health has widened since the rapid spread of AIDS pandemic during the last two decades. It has led family planning program to reassess the type, quality and the reach of the services being provided, creating greater awareness of the choice of methods. A major problem known is that sexuality is often surrounded by strict social, moral, and religious beliefs, which makes an objective study by the subject difficult. Such knowledge is essential not only in developing social advice for people but also in dealing which type contraceptive will suit and peoples' need.

The reproductive health received worldwide endorsement at the International Conference on Population and Development (ICPD) in Cairo in 1994. It represented a move to a holistic and coherent framework encompassing a broad range of needs. Building on WHO's vision of health as a state of complete physical, mental and social well-being, and not just the absence of disease, it applies this vision to all aspects of sexual and reproductive life.

Reproductive health care thus includes family planning, maternal and newborn care, and prevention and treatment of sexually transmitted and reproductive tract infections (RTIs), as well as actions to improve sexual health and gender equality within a broad developmental framework. Reproductive Health Program aims to reduce the adverse outcomes of pregnancy ensuring that people have a satisfying and safe sex life, and to decide for themselves if and when to have children. The integrated provision of these services offers a practical and efficient approach to identifying and solving health problems related to sexuality and reproduction (UNDP/UNFPA/WHO/World Bank, 2004). Reproductive health is the centre-stage of health and development and needs support and strenthening at all levels.

Adolescence is a process of somatic, psychological, and cognitive growth, which transforms a dependent child to self sufficient adult. The adolescent period spans the ages of ten to nineteen years, which include times from onset of puberty to the attainment of legal age at majority. The World Health Organization defines adolescence as the period of biological development from the onset of puberty to full sexual and reproductive maturity, psychological development from emotional pattern of childhood to that of adulthood and the emergence from a state of total socio-economic dependence to one of relative independence (WHO, 1996). Adolescence health is one of the elements of reproductive health and is a matter of utmost importance these days. The high prevalence of tract infections in youth are seen as the direct consequences of irresponsible and risky sexual activity. Overall, sexual and reproductive ill health accounts for at least one fifth of global burden of diseases among women, and one-seventh among men (UNDP/UNFPA/WHO world Bank, 2004).

The highest rate of STDs is reported in young people aged 15-24 years (WHO, 1997). Majority of newly infected HIV cases were under 25 years of age and 50% of the new infections occur in women. Presently there are 11.3 million women, who are HIV positive and 2.8 million, who suffer from AIDS, in fact 44% of AIDS cases in India are in the age group of 15 to 29 years. Hence, it is imperative to provide proper education to adolescents, the most vulnerable age group, to reduce transmission of AIDS (NACO, 1996).

The World Health Organization (WHO) defines "young people as those between the ages of 10 to 24 years." This age group is composed of two overlapping sub-groups, namely 'adolescents' aged 10-19 years and 'youth' aged 15-24 years (WHO, 1986). The Planning Commission estimates that as of March 2000, adolescents aged 10-19 comprised 23% of the Indian population i.e. almost 230 million. Such a large group represents a major human resource that can and must contribute to the overall development of the country. Addressing their needs will contribute not only to social and economic development, but also to social harmony, gender parity, population stabilization and improved quality of life for all India.

Adolescence being a period of exploration and experimentation, young people often lack knowledge, experience and maturity to avoid grave risks that confront them. In both developed and developing countries adolescents can face overwhelming problems, among them early pregnancy, high school dropout rates, substance abuse and violence, making them more vulnerable to life threatening disease and conditions.

Adolescents comprise 20% of the total world population, 85% of whom live in developing countries, low education and high unemployment often compound the problems of developing world adolescents. Furthermore, the adolescent population in developing countries is burgeoning, with the number of urban youth growing a projected 600% between 1970-2025. (WHO Fact Sheet # 186, 12/97).

Adolescence is a period of tremendous opportunity as well as of risks. Various studies suggest that adolescents have limited knowledge of sexual and reproductive health. Even most of the adolescents do not understand the correct meaning of reproductive health. ICMR study conducted in Delhi revealed that almost three-fourth (73%) of the adolescent boys and 70% of girl adolescents had just heard of the term 'Reproductive Health'. The knowledge of urban adolescent was observed to better than their counterpart slum adolescent. A significant difference existed in the awareness level of male students, which was better than females in the group, mainly on topics such as impotency, homosexuality and genital hygiene. As expected, urban girl had a higher level of awareness (90%) than the slum girls (665). Similarly half of urban adolescent boys and a quarter of slum boys were knowledgeable about the menstruation (ICMR, Grover, 1998). Schools have to device strategies to open up more effective communication with students in relation to education on sex, STDs and AIDS. The students have no reliable means of obtaining correct information about these subjects. It is the time to face up this responsibility.

Francis et al (1994) pointed out in their South Delhi study of student adolescents that the sources of knowledge about sex was mostly obtained from books, friends or media, parents (14%) and from teachers (2%). However, in ICMR study it was mainly through mothers.

There is need to learn this young group before sexual practices are established. Schools and colleges, given their unique access to youth can provide an ideal setting for learning large number of adolescents.

Pubertal Changes

During adolescence, growth is rapid, disorganized and confusing compared to the relatively stable period earlier of childhood. Adolescence is a turbulent period of development when the changes of puberty occur significantly, the growth and maturation of the sex organs and the emergence of the powerful sex drive. Adolescents require time to get used to their changing bodies and the new body image. Moreover since emotional maturity does not occur until two or three years after the reproduction system is fully developed, therefore, becomes very important for adolescents to understand themselves and the function of their body so that their can cope with the changes that are taking place within them and develop attitudes towards sex, marriage, parenthood and the family. Awareness of all the physical changes during puberty is low in most of the Indian studies. A highly significant correlation was present between age of awareness of pubertal changes (Gandhi, 1993, Ahuja, 1995 and Nair & Grover, 1999). There is an urgent need to educate adolescents on all aspects of growing up including marriage, child bearing and family planning.

Sexual Maturation

Sexual orientation is relevant to the understanding of reproductive health as it may eliminate the risk of pregnancy. Broadly speaking, two types of services can meet the needs of adolescence at puberty information and guidance presented to them at a level, in a manner and from sources best matched to their needs and health services geared to determine, the presence of any abnormality and treat it. This may involve the families, classmates or peers and teachers as well as the adolescents themselves.

Menarche

Menarche is the beginning of a new stage in the life of a girl. It denotes the attainment of reproductive maturity and entry into womanhood. Girls these days enter into puberty at younger ages than previous generations (Population Reports, 1996). The age at menarche in America has decreased by 3-4 months each decade after 1850 till it leveled at 12.5 years in 1998. Though the reasons behind these trends are not fully understood, factors like better nutrition and improved socio-economic conditions may have a role to play in them (WHO, 1996). In many cultures the first menstrual cycle denotes the day when a girl grows up to attain adulthood. It is also considered as a marker of her fertility and fecundity. Menarche usually occurs in adolescents. From various studies it can be concluded that menarche usually occurs between 12-14 years of age. Most girls are ignorant about the physiology of reproductive system and pubertal changes. Many of them become aware of menses when they start menstruating. Hence, they react to it with shock and surprise. Their lack of proper knowledge is highlighted in many studies (Gandhi, 1993, Ahuja, 1995 & Gover, 1998).

Taboos and restrictions are very commonly placed when they are menstruating. In Indian communities girls having menses are taken as impure (Ahuja, 1995). Nearly half (45.7%) of the rural adolescent girls had prior knowledge of menarche before attaining it. Only one third (29.1%) of girls who had not attained menarche knew about menstruation (Nair and Grover, 1999).

The development of normal menstrual function is an indication that the general and anatomic components of reproductive system are intact and functioning well. Menstrual abnormalities and irregularities are common during adolescent period. The following studies were conducted to study the prevalence of menstrual complaints in adolescent girls. Klien (1981) reported 59.7% prevalence of dysmenorrhoea among Finnish adolescents. Arora (1992) study revealed that 25.4% of girls suffered from menstrual disorders. Gandhi observed that girls mainly complained of abdominal pain (57%), backache (27%), leg cramps (15%) (Gandhi, 1993). Scanty periods, menorrhagia, amenorrhoea were the common complaints which are self limiting (Nair and Grover, 1999).

There is paucity of research data on the knowledge of conception among adolescents. However, existing data reveal that majority of the young girls had poor awareness of various aspects of conception (Bali, 1972, Verma, 1994, Grover, 1998).

Marriage

In India, marriage is considered a life long partnership. It is the rock on which the family is built and which, in turn, is the foundation of society. Basically, marriage is a social and legal contract. However, under the influence of widespread education and the mass media, young people in urban areas appear to be seeking greater freedom and independence to express their feelings and to make their own decisions. Attitude towards marriage and sex among adolescents by and large, continue to be conservative and acceptance of traditional norms, which oppose late marriage, social relation between adolescent boys and girls and pre-marital sex. Those in the forefront of changing attitude are boys and girls urban and educated adolescents. A number of students access the attitudes of adolescents to the ideal age at marriage.

In many parts of India, early marriage for girls is a religious and social imperative. Despite laws that specify the legal age of marriage for girls as 18 years, cultural pressures often force parents to marry off their daughters at a younger age. In 1996, an average of 38% of girls aged 15-19 were married (Jejeebhoy, 1998). This rate was significantly higher in rural areas where 46% of girls in this age group were married, compared with 22% of girls aged 15-19 in urban areas. Age at marriage varies from state to state, however, early marriages are common in Madhya Pradesh, Andhra Pradesh, Rajasthan and Bihar, where more than 50% of young women aged 15-19 are married. In Haryana and Uttar Pradesh, 40-44% of young women aged 15-19 are married. Women in Kerala, Punjab, Goa, Manipur, Mizoram and Nagaland tend to marry later, and in those states fewer than 15% of girls aged 15-19 are married.

Because of early marriage, adolescent fertility in India is relatively high. This should be a cause for concern since many younger adolescents are physiologically immature for reproduction. Compared to adult women, childbearing during adolescence poses greater health risks to both the mother and the newborn. Fertility during this period contributes to maternal morbidity and mortality, high incidence of low birth weight babies and neonatal morbidity and mortality (Jejeebhoy, 1998). Not surprisingly 1997 age-specific fertility rates (ASFR) among 15-19 years old reveal a major urban rural differential. At 20.3 per thousand, the rural ASFR was more than double the urban ASFR of 9.8 per thousand (International Institute for Population Sciences, 1995).

Age at Marriage

For most women in India, sexually activity starts in adolescence and within marriages (UNICEF, 1990; IIPS, 1995). Early marriage was perpetuated in the past by tradition, beliefs about preservation of a girl's chastity, family honour and the need to reduce expenditure. Present laws prohibit early marriages; the minimum legal age for girls is 18 years and 21 for boys. Regardless, many girls continue to be married off at an early age and are expected prove their fertility well before they attain full biological and emotional maturity (Masuma, 1999).

Data from the 1992-93 National Family Health Survey provides some insight into marriage patterns and fertility behaviour of adolescent girls. There are some evidence of a modest increase in the average age for marriage; the singular mean age at marriage for females has gone up by 4.1 years, from 15.9 years in 1961 to 20 years in 1992-93. In all, as many as 6 percent of 10-14 years old and 38 percent of 15-19 years old are currently married. Further, 58 percent of ever married adolescent. girls between the ages of 13 and 19 years have begun childbearing. This corresponds to 17 percent of all females begun childbearing. This corresponds to 17 percent of all females aged 13-19 years. The situation appears to be particularly acute in rural India.

In Delhi study, almost half (48.6%) of adolescents agreed that ideal period of marriage for boys should be between 18 and 21 years and majority of adolescents (82.9%) were sure that ideal time of marriage for girls should be almost same as that of boys between 18 and 21 years, while 14.4% agreed that the age for marriage in boys should be around 22-25 years (Grover 1998). Hence, adolescents are well aware regarding the correct age for marriage.

In many parts of India, early marriage for girls is a religious and social imperative. Despite laws that specify the legal age of marriage for girls as 18 years and above, cultural pressures often force parents to marry off their daughters at a younger age. Adolescent marriages are prevalent due to age-old customs, traditions and the lack of awareness of the legal aspects of marriage. In the Hissar (Malhotra, 1984) and Mumbai (Gandhi, 1993) study on school students 70% and 55% of the girls was aware of the legal age of marriage responsible. Singh (1998) states that 92.3% of the study subjects knew the legal age of marriage for girls and 88.5% of boys. The awareness of legal age of marriage is high as it is evident from these studies. Yet the average age at marriage for girls in our country remain 19.4 years.[12,13]

In 1996, an average of 38% of girls aged 15-19 were married (Jejeebhoy, 1998). This rate was significantly higher in rural areas where 46% of girls in this age group were married, compared with 22% of girls in urban areas. In Madhya Pradesh, Andhra Pradesh, Rajasthan and Bihar, where 50% young women are married in the ages 15-19 years is common. In Haryana and Uttar Pradesh, 40-44% of young women aged 15-19 are married. Women tend to marry later in Kerala, Punjab, Goa, Manipur, Mizoram and Nagaland, where fewer than 15% of girls aged 15-19 are married.

Pre-marital Sex

In India, although traditional norms oppose pre-marital sex, some studies indicate growing trends towards pre-marital sexual activities among adolescents (Sharma, 2000). It is important to recognize the growing incidence of pre-marital sexual activities among adolescents owing to the widening gap between pre-marital sex age and age at marriage. Adolescents are becoming sexually active at young ages, reflecting difference in the cultural and social values, both between and within countries. There is variation in the age at which young boys and girls begin sexual relation. Studies on adolescents' sexual behaviour in different parts of the world show that premarital sexual encounters in young people are generally unplanned, infrequent, and unprotected. A much higher percentage of men reported having had pre-marital sex than women. In India, 60 to 65% of males of 15 to 20 years reported having first sexual intercourse before marriage as against 19.5% of women in the same age group. According to Delhi study, the most common age at first sexual intercourse was 16 to 20 years for both boys and girls. One-fourth of the boys who admitted having had sexual intercourse, started earlier i.e. in the age of 11 to 15 years whereas only 6.3% of the girls had first sexual intercourse in the age of 11 to 15 years (Grover, 1998). Countrywide information on adolescents' sexual behaviour is not available. However, contrary to general expectations, small scale studies suggest that sexual activities begin at relatively early age. As reported in a review of adolescents' sexual and reproductive behaviour in India, a 1993-94 study conducted by the Family Planning Association of India among educated urban youth revealed that the average age of first sexual experience among 15-19 years old was 14.8 for males and age 16.1 for females, another 1995 study found that only 38% of young men and 63% of young women disapproved of pre-marital sexual relationships (Jejeebhoy, 1998). While these studies are not representative of the entire country, they do suggest that a substantial proportion of adolescents are sexually active. The need of the hour is to obtain more culturally and context specific data for formulating interventions that address sexual decision making, gender roles and power relations between the sexes (Nanda, 1999).

Sarin (1986) in his study on unmarried pregnant girls almost 90% between the ages of 15 to 20 years mentioned that they were forced to have sex in more than 62.5% of the cases and none of them were aware of contraceptives.

Patterns of Contraceptives Use Among Adolescents

The study of the use of contraceptives among adolescents reveals an issue of key importance to this particular group that 'adolescent girls may know about contraceptives, but also not necessarily use them'.

Large scale studies as the National Family Health Survey suggests that at least half of all young women in India are sexually active by age 18 mostly within marriage and almost one in five are pregnant by age 15. Well over half of all married women aged 15-19 have experienced a pregnancy or given birth (United Population Fund, 1998). Nevertheless, the

1995 National Survey on Fertility and Family Planning Practices (International Institute of Population Sciences, 1995) found that adolescents had relatively low levels of knowledge about reversible contraceptive methods. The study revealed that while 89% of adolescents were aware of oral contraception, but only 39% knew about IUDs.

It is often seen that ignorance is the main factor behind the limited use of contraceptives by young married women of India. In 1988, All India Survey of Family Planning Practices revealed that only 8.6% of the girls between 15-19 years were using contraceptives (Pathak, 1993). Inaccessibility is another main factor as even young girls aware of contraceptives may not know where to obtain them. Malhotra (Hissar, 1984) observed that 33% of the girls were aware of condoms, 60% of oral pills, 40% of vasectomy and 38% of tubectomy. The level of awareness about contraceptives in middle and late adolescent groups of boys in Delhi study was quite significant (58.2%) for condoms and significantly girls were aware of Mala-D than boys. Vasectomy was more popular method of sterlization in both sexes in adolescents than about tubectomy. Majority of adolescents (77.4%) were aware of the availability of these birth control methods at Family Planning clinics.

Studies of attitudes towards the marital sex suggest once again that while the large majority of adolescents hold conservative attitude to pre-marital sex, there are clear indication of change.

Consequences of Adolescent Sexuality and Childbearing

Child bearing during adolescence poses greater health risk to both the mother and the new born. Fertility during this period contributes to maternal morbidity and morality, high incidence of low birth weight babies and neonatal morbidity and mortality (Jejeebhoy 1998). Not surprising, 1997 average specific fertility rate (ASFR) among 15-19 years of age reveal a major urban-rural differential. At 20.3 per 1000, the rural ASTR was more than double the urban of 9.8 per 1000 (International Institute of Population Sciences 1995). Studies have invariably shown that infant mortality rates are generally higher for babies born to adolescent mothers than for babies born to women in their twenties or thirties (United Nations, 1989).

Because adolescents are physiologically and socially immature, health risks associated with their pregnancies and childbearing are more pronounced than those among older women (United Nations, 1989). Studies reviewed by Population Reference Bureau found that adolescent women are especially vulnerable to reproductive health problems, and they are more likely than older women to die from problems related to pregnancy and childbirth. Most important, adolescent women face increased risks during pregnancy and childbirth because they have less information and access to prenatal, delivery and postpartum care as compared with older women (Ashford, 2001).

An elevated risk of dying among births occurring to adolescent women can be observed from data tabulated from the demographic and health surveys carried out in Asia. It is evident from it that in Bangladesh, India, Nepal and Pakistan, over 1 in 10 babies born to adolescent women die before reaching the age of one year. The risk of dying during infancy is at least 1.3 times higher among births occurring to adolescent women as compared with women 20-29 in countries like Bangladesh, India, Nepal and Pakistan. Although the infant mortality rate is much lower in Vietnam the risk of dying during infancy is between 1.4 and 1.6 times higher among births to adolescent women as compared with women aged 20-29. These data reaffirm the fact that in virtually all societies adolescent childbearing is detrimental to both mothers and their offspring.

The risk of early childbearing to the health of mother and child is focused mainly on married adolescents, as in many Asian countries sexual activity and childbearing begin within marriage and data on childbearing are typically gathered from married women. However, in several countries of Asia there is evidence of pre-marital sexual relationships leading to pre-marital births, although such births vary greatly across societies. Young unmarried women who have children are socially as well as economically disadvantaged.

This is partly because of the traditional values that strongly oppose sexual relationships, pregnancy and child bearing among the unmarried. Most importantly, births to unmarried adolescents are likely to be unplanned or unwanted and, above all, single mother may be living in poverty.

Age at First Sexual Intercourse

The first thing in sexual behaviour is access age at first intercourse, whether pre-marital or post-marital. In a WHO study conducted in STD clinic of Medical College Hospital (1995), reported that a majority of male had their first sexual intercourse before marriage (66.6%) and in the case of females, it was post-marital (76%). This could be inferred that while men (92.2%) could have acquired STDs outside marriage, the women (88.1%) acquired from their marriage. However, the most common age group for men at first pre-marital intercourse was 15 to 24 years and 20 to 24 years at post-marital sex. In case of females, the most common age at first intercourse was 15 to 19 years for pre-marital sex and 15 to 24 years for post-marital sex (Grover, 1995).

There is growing evidence that sexual activity among unmarried adolescents is increasing, especially in the urban areas. In an excellent review of reproductive behaviour of adolescents in India, Jejeebhoy (1996) suggests that around 20-30 percent of all males and upto 10 percent of all females, many from the urban areas, are sexually active during adolescence before marriage.

Early Pregnancy

Worldwide, one in every ten is a teenage mother (Youth Coalition for ICPD). Early pregnancy adversely affects a girl's education, economic well-being and health. Adolescent mothers often fail to complete their education, which, in turn, affects their future job perspectives and their economic well being and health of their child. Pregnancies before the age of 18 is also caused greater medical risk for the mother. The risk of dying from complications related to pregnancy or childbirth is 2.5 times higher for girls under 15 and two times higher for those aged 15-19 (UNFPA Med. St.). The UNFPA (2001) estimates that raising the mother's age at first birth from 18 to 23 could reduce population growth by 40 per cent.

The young adolescent mother faces greater hazards, both to the mother as well as their babies. Adolescent mothers often fail to use antenatal services, partly because they are unwilling to inform their parents or other adults who can help them.

A major consequences of adolescent sexual activity is adolescent pregnancy with the risk of sexual activity in youngsters the rates of adolescent pregnancy is also increasing. Both the adolescent mothers and adolescent fathers have fewer years of education, poor paying jobs and greater medical problem than older parents. Once a adolescent is pregnant, few choices are available. The practitioners must provide unbiased information about all options including for adoption and abortion. Although ideally the adolescents will involve a parent in making her decision, this is not always possible. Fortunately, in India, such cases are not commonly seen. Early pregnancies in the age of 12 to 19 years are associated with greater health risks. Maternal mortality rate (MMR) was 3.8/1000 live births in the age group with the average birth weight 1.9 kg.

Pregnancies in adolescents are risky as they are more prone to complications both physical as well as psychological (Reddy Rani, 1992, Das 1993). A pregnant adolescent can be literally viewed as a 'child carrying a child', has to meet the growing demands of the fetus when her own physical growth experience premature labour, spontaneous abortion and stillbirth; the corresponding figure for 20-24 years old is 8% (IIPS, 1995). Maternal mortality is around one and half to two times higher for adolescents than for older women. Complications of pregnancy, such as anaemia, spontaneous abortion and eclampsia are also significantly higher among adolescent mothers.

The results also indicate that babies of adolescent mothers are more likely to have low weight, run a higher risk of being premature and have higher perinatal mortality.

The poor nutritional status of adolescent girls in India is well documented (Gopalan, 1990; Kanani and Consul, 1990; Ramachandran, 1989).

Adolescence, malnutrition, anaemia and the extra nutritional demands exacerbate health risks during pregnancy. These risks may be further heightened due to lack of antenatal care. The Family Health Servey shows that 35% of pregnant women under 20 years did not receive any antenatal care (IIPS, 1995). In all, 15 percent of all deaths of rural women aged 15-24 years are attributed to diseases of childbirth and pregnancy; the second largest cause of death following accidents and violence, which account for 34 percent of all deaths and which may often be associated with marriage or pregnancy (Sundari Ravindran, 1996).

Though adolescents pregnancy rates in India have come down from 10% in 1971 to 8.8% in 1987, the absolute number of pregnant adolescent women has increased due to increasing population in that age group in India. There were 2.2 million adolescents mother in 1961, 2.7 million in 1971, 3.3 million in 1998. In most North Indian States, the practice of gauna is prevalent in which girls marry early and makes frequent visits between her natal and nuptial places. It can lead to early pregnancy, childhood adolescent mothers experience a 16% to 24% higher mortality risk as compared to children of mother in 20-24 years age group. Out of 300, 200 children of older mothers are during infancy (Pathak, 1993). Other studies conducted on adolescent pregnancy reflect higher maternal and prenatal mortality and morbidity (Das, 1993; Morris, 1993).

Induced Abortion

It would be possible to provide a relatively safe and simple service to enable young adolescent to procure an induced abortion. Generally, abortion presents a gender risk to the health and life of an adolescent than to an adult woman. It is estimated that roughly only half a million abortions are performed under the medical services network while another 4-5 million occur illegally in India.

Adolescents seems to be not different and indeed one much more vulnerable than adult. Although a number of studies have documented the prevalence of abortion among adolescents, they do not present an adequate profile of current studies in the country. In Solapur Hospital setting, as many as 30% (499 of 1684) were adolescents (Solapurkar, 1985).

Data on level of induced abortion in developing countries are notoriously difficult either because abortion is restricted or because the issue is too delicate. Even so, among young females reporting a pregnancy, the overwhelming majority in almost every case, induced abortion is widely used by pregnant young women.

Estimates from National Family Health Survey for married women reveal that induced abortion is somewhat more likely among adolescents aged 15-19 than among 20-24 year olds: 1.7 percent and 1.2 percent of pregnancies, respectively (IIPS, 1995). For example, adolescents accounted for 27 percent of the 2,755 abortions conducted in a rural hospital (Chhabra et al, 1988). And 30 percent of the 1,684 abortions conducted in an urban hospital (Solapurkar and Sangam, 1985), with a disproportionately large number of them being unmarried in both instances. Adolescents are also considerably more likely to delay seeking abortion services and undergo second trimester abortions which are not safe; 90,81 and 66 percent of adolescent abortion seekers in Baroda (Bhatt, 1978), Mumbai (Purandare and Krishna, 1974) and Sevagram (Chhabra, 1992) respectively. Unmarried adolescents in particular, are more inclined to delay seeking an abortion until late pregnancy mainly due to the lack of awareness as well as ignorance of services, and fear of social stigmatization (Chowdhury and Mukherjee, 1979; UNICEF, 1990).

Unwanted Pregnancies, Illness and Death from Complications of Pregnancies

A minority of sexually active unmarried young women experience pregnancy, which is typically unplanned and unwanted. Between 10% and 40% of young females reported having experienced an unwanted pregnancy.

Illness and death from unwanted pregnancies are very high. Frequent pregnancies are correlated in the world with poor health and poverty. One in five births is unwanted, in part because safe and effective methods, and fertility regulations are not available. About half of the 45-60 million abortions performed each year are unsafe, and over 65,000 deaths occur from unsafe abortions annually, most in developing countries.

At least forty percent of the 200 million women who become pregnant each year, experience complications that require treatment from a trained provider, and one in ten require hospitalization. But most women in developing countries lack access to basic prenatal and delivery care. As a result, countless millions suffer from preventable or treatable conditions. 15-20 million develop long term disabilities and 6,00,000 die.

Health consequences of unsafe abortions are acute, ranging from complications such as a perforated uterus, cervical lacerations or haemorrhage in the short term to an increased risk of ectopic pregnancy, chronic pelvic infection and possible infertility in the long term. The existing health services are ill equipped to address the needs of these young girls, including emergency and timely evacuations, post abortion care, counseling and contraceptives services (Masuma, 1999).

Media has the strongest influence on adolescent for the promotion of a small family norm and birth control measures. Young girls with access to moderate means of communication are more aware of contraceptives than their counterparts (Punia and Kaur, 1986). Media can be effectively used to impart education about population dynamic and reproductive physiology to the adolescents. It is not only necessary to be aware of family planning method but also about maternal and child health services that can be availed there to ensure safe delivery and health of their children.

Contraceptive Patterns among Adolescents

In Delhi ICMR study, 48.6% were not aware that certain oral pills were used a method of contraceptive; only 34.9% were aware of this fact, 59.6% were aware of condom while 26.8% were not, 67.8% were not aware of the intra utrine devices, while 20.5% claim that they did not know. Tubecomaties were known by 29% while 51.9% did not know of it. Vasectomies were known by 20.7%, while 59.6% mentioned unaware of it. Only 0.8% were aware of any other method of contraceptive.

Regarding the adolescents' awareness of birth control methods, 42.2% of urban males and 32.8% urban females and 31.1% of slum males and 27.4% of slum females know of oral pills. Knowledge on condoms was available to 61.7% of urban male and 56% urban female and by 68.4% slum males and 53.6% of slum females. 12.6% urban males and 11.1% urban females, and 8.4% slum males and 7.4% slum females were aware of the copper T, 28.1% of urban male and 27.4% urban female and 28.9% of slum males and 34.2% slum females were aware of tubectomy, 19.3% of urban male and 19.7% urban females and 26.8% urban male and 19.5% slum female were aware of the vasectomy. The higher awareness of condom were probably due to advertisement in the media regarding birth control and AIDS.

Illness and Death from STDs

Sexually transmitted diseases are a major cause of serious illness and death. They usually affect people in the 15-44 age group, the most economically production years. In some countries, congenital syphilis is one of the principal causes of illness and death of newborns. The presence of STDs –especially those associated with genital ulceration – speeds the rate of transmission of HIV, substantially increasing both the susceptibility to HIV and AIDS and the infectiousness of an HIV infected individual. Some 23 million people are infected with HIV worldwide and nearly two-third of them live in sub-Saharan Africa.

Early and unprotected sexual activity is likely to expose adolescents to an increased risk of contracting STIs including HIV/AIDS. In general, female sex workers are reported to be an important source of STIs for majority of adolescent and pre-adolescent boys seen at STD clinics (Bansal, 1992; Kanbargi and Kanbargi, 1996; Pandhi et al, 1995; Grover, 1995).

Despite this frightening scenario, both unmarried and married adolescent girls continue to be vulnerable to early, and often, unprotected sexual activity. Adolescent girls are least likely to seek assistance, especially if they are unmarried. Why is this the case?

Traditional Practices Harmful to Health

Two million young girls are subjected to circumcision and other from genital mutilation every year. These practices can lead to death, acute pain, recurrent urinary tract infection, mental trauma, painful intercourse, and complications during childbirth. Discrimination in the way girls are treated can damage their reproductive health – for example, inadequate feeding childhood may stunt growth, bringing hire risk of complication during childbirth. Early marriage and adolescent pregnancy are serious problems because of greater health risk of pregnancy for adolescence than for women in their 20s and early 30s, the adverse effect on education and employment opportunities, poor nutrition is also harmful to women's health. In sufficient nourishment and inadequate iron not only reduce productivity and well being, but also increase the likelihood of pregnancy related complications and poor infant outcome.

Reproductive Health of Youth and the UN Support

At the UN special session on children, the world's nations have an opportunity – and a responsibility to reaffirm and strengthen existing commitments to meeting young people's developmental needs, including those relating to reproductive health. The international community has repeatedly agreed to take a comprehensive approval to meeting these challenges that reflects young peoples right to reproductive health. Yet young people are too often denied the information and services they need to make healthful, informed decisions about their sexual and reproductive lives.

The social and developmental consequences of reproductive decisions are far-reaching. Health, education and preparation for the world of work are closely connected. An unintended pregnancy can irrevocably disrupt a young girl's life, precluding further schooling and training. Contracting HIV in an unprotected sexual encounter can bring a young person's prospects for a healthy and productive future to an end.

Young people have a right to the information and services they need to make healthful decisions about their lives. Since the International Conference on Population and Development (ICPD) in 1994, the International Community has consistently reaffirmed the right of young people to age-appropriate reproductive health information and services that safeguard their rights to privacy, confidentiality, respect and informed consent. The International community has also reaffirmed that the rights and responsibilities of parents to provide guidance in such matters should not prevent young people from having access to the information and services they need to enjoy good reproductive health.

Good reproductive health is crucial to national development. The challenges of preparing the next generation for adult roles are remarkably similar across both developed and developing country settings. Half of the world's 6.1 billion people are under age 25; more than one billion are between the ages of 10 and 19. Within 15 years, all 3 billion will have reach reproductive ages. Countries that fail to provide boys and girls with the means to remain healthy and in school will not benefit as fully from other investments they make in young people and globalization sharpens this reality. In addition to the impact on individual health and welfare, the decisions these young people make about the timing and number of their children will have long-lasting consequences for population growth (WHO).

Status of Young People's Reproductive Lives

Most young people everywhere becomes sexually active during their adolescent years. Expectations that girls will marry and have children while very young, may lead them to have sex early in some places, in others, later marriage is often preceded by sexual activity. Young people's sexual experience is often gained under circumstances that make them vulnerable to coercion, sexually transmitted infections (STIs) and unintended pregnancy—factors that undermine their health and can complicate their lives in the longer term.

Because young people tend to be denied explicit information about sexuality and reproduction, they are often ill-prepared for sexual relations or unable to protect themselves from unintended pregnancy and STIs. The young and the unmarried are often rebuffed or treated with little respect by reproductive health care providers. Surveys in Mozambique found that three-quarters of girls and close to two-thirds of boys aged 15 to 19 did not know how to protect themselves from HIV infection. Prevention-oriented programs should make a special effort to reach young people, both in school and out of school, with sexual and reproductive health information and services.

Worldwide, over ten million young people aged 15 to 24 have HIV or AIDS. Every year almost half of all new HIV infections and at least one-third of all new sexually transmitted infections occur to people under 25. Young people tend to consider themselves invulnerable to risk, even in countries where HIV is widespread, unplanned and sometimes secretive nature of their sexual encounters make protecting themselves difficult even when they are aware. The immature reproductive tracts of young people make them more susceptible than adults to acquiring HIV/AIDS and other STIs. In the United States, young people 15 to 19 years old have higher rates of STIs than any other age group.

Girls are more vulnerable to reproductive health problems than boys for both biological and social reasons, and often have little say over the conditions of sexual relations and childbearing. Young women who become pregnant outside of marriage may have to decide whether to obtain abortions or try to support their children on their own. Faced with an unintended pregnancy, an adolescent will often resort to self-induced abortion or take the services of an untrained provider. A recent study estimated that about 700 adolescents resorted to abortion each day in Kenya – all of them illegal and almost all unsafe.

Schooling and reproductive behaviour are closely linked. Education is associated with differences in adolescent childbearing throughout the world. The proportion of women who have their first child by age 18 ranges from 1 percent in Japan to 53 percent in Nigeria. Women with primary education are, on average, about half as likely as women with less schooling to have a child before age 18. Girls who give birth are far less likely to complete high school than their childless peers. And around the world, young women, even at cost of their lives, seek unsafe or illegal abortions.

Adults who are traditional sources of information on sexual and reproductive matters are increasingly unavailable to young people or are unfamiliar with current threats to reproductive health. Urbanization, evaluation of family structures away from the extended family and towards the nuclear family, and other social and economic changes have all had an effect on traditional systems that, in the past, prepared young people for their future reproductive roles. The epidemic of STIs, including HIV/AIDS, adds to the challenge of providing sufficient information to young people about threats to their sexual and reproductive health.

Strategies Needed to Ensure Good Reproductive Health

Leadership from the very top is key to addressing young people's reproductive health needs. In places as diverse as Uganda and the Netherlands, the government has waded fearlessly into the territory of youth reproductive health because it has so clearly understood the public health mandate for doing so. In Uganda, where HIV infection rates peaked in the 1990s, the president's outspokenness made it possible for information about the causes of AIDS and how to prevent it to be communicated through a broad range of channels—television, political leaders, religious centers, schools and others. In the Netherlands, ongoing collaboration between the government and the media has educated the population and dramatically reduced pregnancy abortion and STIs.

Successful reproductive health policies and programs cut across sectors such as education and public health. While useful policies and programs exist in various sectors, they are often undermined by a lack of coordination. In many countries, unintended pregnancy abruptly ends girls' schooling. To change this pattern, the government should support a program that provides them schooling, job training, childcare and nutrition for pregnant girls and young mothers.

All couples wishing to obtain a marriage licence must attend compulsory sex education counselling program.

Sex education and services in schools reach millions of students; they work best when they start with parents. Since a large share of young people attend school in most parts of the world, integrating sex education into school curricula is an important strategy. Studies have shown that fears that sex education will contribute to earlier and less thoughtful sexual activity are misplaced. Providing parents with basic health information and educating them about the importance of sex education can help them become comfortable with and supportive of such efforts.

In the country, sex education should be universal, public message about sexuality should be widespread, and access to services should be viewed as a basic human right. Adequate teacher training and the development of educational materials that are consistent with regards to the information they seek to communicate is key to the success of sexually education programs.

Because young people often do not seek medical care and treatment they need, school based health centres. These school-based health centres should nationwide provide affordable, convenient and confidential services, through most side-step contraceptives and abortion counselling as a result of school policy.

Sex education and services through the public health system can also reach out-of-school youth and integrate young people into a system they will use as adults. In places where school attendance rates are low, governments need to find alternative routes for communicating health information to young people. In India, many girls leave school to marry and there is no institution through which to reach them until they come for prenatal care at the time of their first pregnancy. In contrast, local health clinics in Iran make it their business to identify the young people in their immediate communities and to make sure they receive health education. Parents who elect to teach their own children are given training in how and what to teach.

Health services for youth should not only address the medical aspects of reproductive health, but also relationships and values, Peer educators may complement clinical efforts by providing young people with someone to talk to, and act as a link to sources of information and services.

Youth-friendly services are needed to reach young people with information and treatment. In clinics, as in schools, special training is needed of adult health care providers, who often impose their values on young clients, or are insufficiently sensitive or supportive to make the most of a young person's brief contact with the health system. An effort to sensitize health workers to young people's needs not only for information and services, but also for privacy and understanding is necessary.

Recruiting NGOs to support and expand on reproductive health initiatives is utmost important.

Gender inequities that expose young people to sexual and reproductive risk must be eliminated. Girls experience sexual coercion, risky pregnancy, botched abortion and STIs in large part because of gender inequities that condition their sexual encounters. Boys, who are frequently urged into experimentation by others' expectations about what it means to be a man, have difficult acting on the basis of their own feeling and often and up taking more sexual risks. Reproductive health programs need to question these unstated, yet basic notions that detract so significantly from the health of young people.

Specific goals, including financial objectives, should be set in the pursuit of youth reproductive health. Aiming high is always important, particularly when the objective is to benefit one-half of the world's people. Young people are dependent on the accountability of adult policymakers, program directors, clinicians, teachers and parents. Now is the time to act to safeguard the future of young people everywhere.

References

1. Agence France Press, "More than 10 million 15–24 years old living with HIV / AIDS; UNICEF, "Geneva", June 12, 2001.
2. Ahuja A, and Tiwari S: Awareness of Pubertal Changes Among Adolescent Girls, *The Journal of Family Welfare*, 1995, 41 (1); 46-50.
3. Alan Guttmacher Institute, Indo a New World; Young Women's Sexual and Reproductive Lives, New York, AGI, 1998.
4. Arora R, Rajaram P, Gowri, *et al* 1992: Population Based Menstrual Disorders in Pondicherry—A preliminary study, *Journal of Obstetrics and Gynaecology*, 42; 492-497.
5. Ashford, Lori S. 1001: New Population Policies: Advancing Women's Health and Rights, Population Bulletin, 56 (91):1-44.
6. Bali P, Gulati N and Murali I, 1972: A Perception Study Among Rural School Children Regarding Conception and Family Planning, *Indian Paediatrics*, 12 (7) : 575-579.
7. Bansal RK, 1992: Sexual Behaviour and Substance Use Patterns Amongst Adolescent Truck Cleaners and Risk of HIV / AIDS, *Indian Journal of Maternal and Child Health*, 3 (4): 108-10.
8. Bhatt RV, 1978: An Indian Study of the Psychosocial Behaviour of Pregnant Teenager Women, *Journal of Reproductive Medicine*, 21 (4): 275-78.
9. Chhabra, S, 1992. A Step Towards Helping Mothers with Unwanted Pregnancies. *Indian Journal of Maternal and Child Health*, 32 (2) 41-42.
10. Chhabra S, Gupte N, Mehta A and Shende A, 1988: Medical Termination of Pregnancy and Concurrent Contraceptive Adoptation in Rural Indian, Studies in Family Planning, 19 (40): 244-47.
11. Chowdhury NN and Mukherjee K, 1979: Sociological Implications in Pregnancy in Unmarried Teenagers, *Journal of Obstetrics and Gynaecology of India*, 29(2): 308-12.
12. Das DK and Mishra OP: Outcomes of Teenager, Pregnancy *Indian Journal of Preventive and Social Medicine*, 1993, 24 (23): 111-114.
13. Developing Countries, United Nations, New York, USA.
14. Francis PJ, Gill JS and Choudhary S: Knowledge, Briefs and Attitudes Regarding AIDS, STDs and Human Sexuality Among Senior Secondary Students in Delhi, *Indian Journal of Community Medicine*, 1994; 19(1): 17-20.
15. Gandhi AB, Kakodkar PC and Raval MY: The Role of Audio-visual Programmes in Creating Awareness About Reproductive Health in Adolescent Girls; *Journal of Obstetrics and Gynaecology of India*, 1993; 43:257-261.

16. Gopalan C, 1990: Women and Nutrition in Developing Countries—Practical Considerations In : H M Wallace, and K Giri (eds.) Health Care Women and Children in Developing Countries, 252-63. Oakland, California, Third Party Publishing.

17. Grover VL: Final Report on a Study of Reproductive Health Awareness and Sexual Behaviour Among Adolescents in Delhi; Report Submitted to ICMR, New Delhi, 1998.

18. Grover VL, 1995: Changes in Sexual Behaviour in Response to Increased Risk Awareness Project No. 91311 BSDA,. Final Report Submitted to Task Force for Social Science Research on Reproductive Health, World Health Organization, Geneva, Switzerland.

19. INCLEN Research; Adolescent Health <http: / / www.inclen.org / research / ah.html>.

20. International Conference on Population and Development (ICPD) in Cairo in 1994.

21. International Institute for Population Sciences (1995) National Family Health Survey (MCH and Family Planning), India 1992-93, Mumbai, International Institute for Population Sciences, Mumbai, India.

22. Jejeebhoy SJ (1996): Adolescent Sexual and Reproductive Behaviour—A Review of the Evidence from India, ICRW Working Paper No. 3, International Centre for Research on Women, Washington, DC, USA.

23. Jejeebhoy S, 1998: Adolescent Sexual and Reproductive Behaviour—A Review of the Evidence from India, Social Sciences and Medicine, 10: 1275-1290.

24. Jejeebhoy SJ, and Rama Rao SS, 1995: Unsafe Motherhood—A Review of Reproductive Health In: M. Das Gupta, L Chen, and TN Krishna (eds.) Women's Health in India, Risks and Vulnerability, 122-52. Oxford University Press.

25. Kanani S and Consul P, 1990: Nutrition Health Profile and Intervention Strategies for Underpriviledged Adolescent Girls in India: A Selected Review, *Indian Journal of Maternal and Child Health*, 13 (1): 1-3.

26. Kanbargi R and Kanbargi S, 1996: Sexually Transmitted Diseases in Bangalore City—Some Findings from an Exploratory Study, *Journal of Family Welfare*, 42 (1): 30-37.

27. Klanger B, Tyden T and Ruusuvaara I, 1993: Sexual Behaviour among Adolescents in Uppsala, Swedan, *Journal of Adolescent Medicine*, 41: 468-474.

28. Klein JR and Lith IF, 1981: Epidemiology of Adolescent Dysmenorrhoea, *Pediatrics*, 1981; 68 (5): 661-64.

29. Malhotra R, Kaur P and Nath M: Assessment of Knowledge and Attitudes of High School Students Regarding Family Planning: A Need of the Day, *The Journal of Family Welfare*, 1984; 31 (2): 57-60.

30. Masuna Mamdani, 1999: Adolescent Reproductive Health—Experience of Community Based Programmes, Published in Implementing a Reproductive Health Agenda in India: The Beginning Edited by Saroj Pauchory, ISB No. 87834-098x, Population Council, New Delhi, India.

31. Morell Virginia: Attacking the Causes of Silent Infertility, *Science, 269*, 11 August, 1995.

32. Morris DL, Berenson AB, Lawson J and Wiemann CM: Comparison of Adolescent Pregnancy Outcomes by Prenatal Care Source, *The Journal of Reproductive Medicine*, 1993; 38 (5): 375-379.

33. Nair P and Grover V, 1999: A Study of Reproductive Health and Sexuality Amongst Female Adolescent Population in a Rural Area of Delhi. (Unpublished).
34. Nand AR: Addressing the Reproductive Health Needs of Adolescents in India; Directions for Programmes, 1999. Secretary, Family Welfare, Ministry of Health & FW, Govt. of India, Nirmal Bhavan, New Delhi.
35. National AIDS Control Programme, India: Country Scenario, an update National AIDS Control Organization, Ministry of Health and Family Welfare, Government of India, Delhi, Dec, 1996.
36. National Family Health Survey, 1992-1993, India International Population Reports, Meeting the Needs of Young Adults, Family Planning Programs, Serial J: 1996, No. 41:1-30.
37. Okako Tervil: At Least 700 Kenyan Girls Each Day, Nairobi, Kenya, Pan African News Agency, July 26, 2000.
38. Pandhi RK, Khanna N, and Sekhari R., 1995: Sexually Transmitted Diseases in Children, *Indian Pediatrics*, 32 (1) : 27-30.
39. Pathak KB, and Ram F, 1993: Adolescents Motherhood—Problems and Consequences, The Journal of Family Welfare, 39 (1): 17-23, NHFS11, 1998-99.
40. Punia RK and Kaur P: Knowledge and Opinion of Unmarried College Girls About Family Planning, Indian Journal of Public Health, 1986; 30 (2): 107-111.
41. Purandare VN, and Krishna UR, 1974: Pregnancy and Abortion in Adolescence, Paper Presented at a World Health Organization Meeting on Pregnancy and Abortion in Adolescence, Geneva, June 24-28, WHO, Geneva.
42. Ramachandran P, 1989: Nutrition in Pregnancy, In C Gopalan, and S Kaur (eds.) Women and Nutrition in India, New Delhi, Nutrition Foundation of India.
43. Reddy Rani P, Rani U, Raghavan SS, *et al.*: 1992: Adolescent Pregnancy, Journal of Obstetric and Gynaecology of India, 1992, 42:764-767.
44. Sarin U, 1988: Teenage Pregnancy, Indian Journal of Preventive & Social Medicine, 19 (1): 30-32.
45. Sharma A, and Sharma V: Sexual Knowledge and Practices of College Girls in Rural Gujarat, India, Indian Journal of Family Welfare, 1996; 42(3): 19-25.
46. Sharma V and Sharma A.1992: Health Profile of Pregnant Adolescent Among Selected Tribal Population in Rajasthan, India, Journal of Adolescents Health, 13(8): 696-99.
47. Singh MM, Gupta SS, and Reeta Devi: Knowledge and Attitudes of High School Girls Regarding Population and Family Planning Issues. Indian Medical Gazette, 1998; 117-120.
48. Solapurkar ML, and Sangam RN, 1985: Has the MTP Act in India Proved Beneficial? Journal of Family Welfare, 31(3): 46-52.
49. Sundari Ravindran TK, 1996: From Rhetoric to Action, Seminar 447: 43-49.
50. Temin, MJ, Friday EO, Omorodian FO *et al* 1999: Perception of Sexual Behaviour and Knowledge about Sexually Transmitted Diseases Among Adolescents in Benin City, Nigeria, International Family Planning Perspectives, 25(4), 186-190.

51. The Center for Health and Health Care in Schools, "School-Based Health Centers; Results from a 50-State Survey, School Year 1999-2000, htm, last accessed 5/2/01. Government of India, Ministry of Human Resource Development, Department of Education (1999). Selected Educational Statistics, New Delhi, Government of India.
52. UNDP/UNFPA/WHO/World Bank, Improving Sexual and Reproductive Health Through Research; An Investment for the Future: Special Programme of Research, Dept. of Reproductive Health and Research, WHO, Geneva.
53. UNFPA website, Responds to adolescents, <http://www.unfpa.org/adolescents>2004, Briefing pack on population issues, UNFPA.
54. United Nations Children Funds, 1990, Children and Women in India. A Situation Analysis UNICEF, New Delhi, India.
55. United Nations Population Fund (1996) the State of the World's Population, New York, UNFPA.
56. United Nations Population Fund (1998), India Country Paper, Paper presented at the South Asia Conference on the Adolescent, New Delhi.
57. United Nations, 1989, Adolescent Reproductive Behaviour, Vol. 11, Evidence from.
58. Verma M, Chhatwal J and Mathew E: Safe Motherhood when to begin. *Indian Paediatrics*, 1994, 31:901-905.
59. World Health Organization, Regional Reproductive Health Strategy for South East Asia, Regional Office for South East Asia, New Delhi.
60. World Health Organization, Reproductive Health in the South East Asia Region, 50 years Commemmorative Series 5; New Delhi, 1998.
61. World Health Organization, Adolescence, The Critical Phase, Challenges and Potentials, Regional Office for South East Asia, New Delhi, 1997.
62. World Health Organization, Operational Research on Reproductive Health Scientific Working Group, Report of the first meeting, (2-4 Sept, 1996), Regional Office for South East Asia, New Delhi, 1996.
63. Youth Coalition for ICPD (International Conference on Population and Development) http://www.youthcoalition.org

CHAPTER

5 Sexual Behaviour of Adolescents

Vijay Grover

INTRODUCTION

The sexual behaviour of adolescents determine their vulnerability to sexually transmitted diseases (STDs) including acquired immuno deficiency syndrome (AIDS). The topic of sexuality is in focus today. It is because of the alarming increase in the incidence of AIDS and STDs. Youth in urban juvenile justice systems may form a "core group" of STD transmitters, core group in industrialized countries are characterized by young age, low socio-economic status. Poor access to medical care, illicit drug use and high prevalence and incidence of STDs. It is self evident, therefore, that young people are not homogenous in context for sexuality. Sexual behaviours, indeed the meaning of sexuality itself varies across groups and, also over times, both in society and in individual relation.

The scientific study of human sexual behaviour is relatively recent, with a few efforts in developing countries at the beginning of the century. Better known are US studies that took place much later than Germany and England. Statistical works of Kinsey and laboratory research by Masters and Johnson in the 1950s and 1960s.[1] During the past two decades in the Western world, there has been an explosion of research and publications on human sexuality including programs of sex education and academic courses in colleges.

Not so in Pattern 111 countries where academicians were aware of the work elsewhere but became involved only after the 1970s. The first scientific inquiries in Asia and the Pacific were carried out by Westerners, particularly by anthropologists, who proved different cultures and discovered different sexual customs.[1,2]

Anthropologists Cherry and Charles Lindholms (1980), for example, studied the Pakistan community in Pakistan within the context of an Islamic culture. More recently, foreign researchers, have conducted the studies. Outside funding from International organizations has played an important role in the emergence of these studies.[3]

The behaviours that have been reported may appear permissive, but they do not imply liberal values and attitudes. Adolescents, constitute a large proportion of the world population. They are our future generation. Only in recent years, adolescence has been identified as a separate age group. The term adolescence is derived from the Latin word "Adolescere", which literally means "to grow to maturity". This is a transition between pubescence and terminates with adulthood. Pubescence refers to biological changes of adolescence that precedes sexual maturity. Puberty is defined as a period of transformation from a stage of reproductive immaturity to a stage of full reproductive competence and when the individual changes from a sexual to a sexual being. Adolescence is a distinct phase of development. Its characteristics depend on the ways in which biological, psychological and social factors combine to fashion the maturation... patterns involved. The developmental process are characterized by periods of rapid change, interspersed which is often uneven biologically influenced, early maturation, may lead people to have social expectations of the adolescents that they are not yet ready to fulfill.[4]

The average adolescent is faced with the resolution of a number of development tasks. Including the following grossly divided three stages of development.

1. **Early adolescence** (10 to 14 years): Characterised by rejection of family desire for autonomy and preoccupation with body image.
2. **Middle adolescence** (15 to 17 years): The emphasis shifts to tasks. This is the time of very strong peer allegiance, the adolescents at this phase are risk takers and consider themselves invincible. Lack of knowledge about sex and its various aspects makes them most vulnerable to the hazards of unwanted pregnancy, unsafe abortion and risk of contracting sexually transmitted infections including STD and HIV infections, and
3. **Late adolescence** (18 to 19 years). It is that period where their rethinking becomes more abstract and separate from realism.

This general sequence is, however, affected by socio-economic and cultural conditions which may delay development through lack of opportunity.[4] A global overview of reproductive health outlines major challenges for action.

Sexuality is fundamental activity of human life, an important feature of health, happiness, individual development and indeed for the preservation of the human races. Human sexuality depends, not only on biological and physiological but psychological and social factors. It is a dynamic concept which is changing very fast in several ways in different parts of the world. Surely it is linked with the culture of the land, probably also with the degree of affluence and the freedom permitted by the society we live in. Human sexuality is an integral part of human personality.

According to the World Health Organization (WHO) "sexual health is the integration of the somatic, emotional, intellectual and social aspects of sexual being in ways, that are positively enriching and that enhances personality, communication and love." It influences the thoughts, feelings, interactions and actions and contributes to the energy that motivates people to find love, contact, warmth and intimacy and thereby achieve and maintain mental and physical health. The foundations of a healthy and fulfilling sexuality are established during childhood and adolescent period. The ability of growing people and adults, both males and females, to maintain general health is directly affected by sexuality and relationship between sexes. This can be strengthened by making such information and education about sexuality available to young people and the health of community should provide such information and services that would promote and maintain healthy sexuality throughout life.[5]

Problems of Growing Up and Adolescents

Adolescence is a period of masked rapid physical, emotional, psychological and cognitive changes which influence the social environment and this in turn are influenced by it. The process of growing up resulting from psychological changes make it necessary for them to build self image, to redesign behavioural patterns with parents, peer group and the members of opposite sex. It demands to examine prevailing values and norms and to establish individual identities, because of sexual development under the influence of hormones and associated changes, they often get bewildered by strong urges. These problems get further aggravated by the fact that the period of abstinence is increased as the age of onset of puberty has been advanced as a result of better nutrition and urbanization. On the other hand the legal age of the marriage is increased, thus the gap is widened. Social environment provides constant sexual stimulation but the rigidity of social moves create conflicts leading to anxiety, sexual frustration, deviant sexual behaviour, promiscuity, unwanted pregnancy, teenage motherhood and alarming increase in sex crimes and STDs. The situation gets further complicated by the sex related myths and misconceptions that are prevalent among the teenagers. For understanding human sexual behaviour, it is necessary to understand the psycho-sexual development of human being from infancy to childhood, through adolescence to childhood. The normal physical growth and maturation of adolescents may be adversely affected by inadequate diet, untimely or inappropriate physical stress on the growing body or pregnancy before a young girl is fully mature. Due to new liberal policies of the Government of India for foreign television media, unchecked broadcasting of violence, sex, and advertisement on smoking and alcohol product has been a great concern today.[6-10]

The problem behaviour includes alcohol and drug abuse, cigarette smoking and sexual precocity. Adolescence is one of the most fascinating period of life during which risk taking may serve to fulfill developmental needs related to autonomy, mastery and individualization. Organized constellation of risk behaviour have major implications for designing intervention to reduce risk behaviour. They call into serious questions for intervention and change efforts for promoting healthy overall lifestyles rather than continue to focus upon behaviour like smoking, drinking or substance abuse. Risk taking must be considered as one of the characteristics of adolescent period. There is growing evidence to suggest that problem behaviour cluster together.[11,12,13]

In developed countries individual risk behaviour has been studied extensively and it is observed too that there is an increasing trend of smoking[12,13] and alcohol[14] and sexual intercourse leading to adolescent pregnancy and sexually transmitted diseases[15,16] and violence.[17] Similar trends are documented in developing countries also.[16,18] The role of socio-cultural forces in adolescent development and risk taking behaviour has been mentioned.[16,17,6,7,19,20] A multifold increase in the audio-visual media is in the process of transforming over socio-cultural environment. So mass media plays a significant role in development of risk behaviour in adolescents. There is a very fast growing mass communication technology. It has been observed that children and adolescents spend many hours with electric and audio-visual sets and get influenced.[8] Due to new liberal policies Government of India for foreign television, media, increased broadcasting of violence, sex and advertisement on smoking and other products has been a great concern.[6-10]

The prevalence rates of high risk behaviour consuming alcohol, pre-marital sexual intercourse and using Bhang (cannabis) among male adolescents in South Delhi village were reported to be 32.2%, 25%, 12.5% and 11.5% respectively.[20]

The sexual behaviour of population is not uniform, sexuality as well as sexual practices vary according to age, marital condition, sexual performance, physical or mental disabilities or general health status. Furthermore, as the normative values imposed by a social group define the boundaries of practices and that is deemed accepted.

STD/AIDS continues to be an urgent and growing challenge to the health and well beings of individuals, families and nations. No country can claim to have stopped the epidemic or prevented the introduction of STD/AIDS into new communities. The major mode of transmission of HIV infection and AIDS worldwide is sexual transmission. The dimension of sexual behaviour that increases the risk of intercourse, large numbers of lifetime and current sex partners, high risk characteristics of sex partners.

The formation of families has had a tremendous impacts on the human sexual behaviour. The social nature of human beings led them to form societies. The complexity of human interaction in these societies increased and this had to be structured into certain patterns to avoid these patterns of behaviour. The family is ideally suited for this kind of training.

Sexual behaviour is a complex phenomenon. It includes the ideological aspects of individuals, groups, communities and cultures. There are biological aspects of, and there are psychological aspects too. All these lead to the formation of coginitive aspects of sexual behaviour as well as the framework of the behaviour itself. These aspects of behaviour itself. These aspects will be taken up in a little more detail. Many biologists and sociologists would claim that human behaviour is solely formed by the interaction of genes with the environment. Hence, human sexuality is an integral part of being human. There are many arguments sexuality is an inherent part of being human. There are many arguments against this kind of deterministics framework. Such an approach can not account for differences in sexuality in **Darwinian populations**.

It must be remembered that culture is a form of extra genetic transfer of information from generation to generation. Through the cultural background of experiences and behaviour, the young could be trained to behave in socially compatible ways. In order to force people to stick to cultural norms of behaviour, social sanctions against 'deviant' forms of behaviours were imposed.

Further it is useful to note that Freud looked at the sexual behaviour of a person beginning from a very early stage in the formation of a fetus. This is probably true. However, to go on and claim that is the sole 'traumatic' agency for future conflicts would be to ignore the ability of human beings to learn and to adapt to changing circumstances. However, this was too limited an idea to account for behavioural changes in later life. Erik Erikson 'seven stages' was also unable to patch up the faults in the original theory.

According to the World Health Organization, sexually transmitted diseases (STDs) are defined as a group of communicable diseases, transferred predominantly by sexual contact.[21] Earlier, STDs were untreatable since there were few drugs, if at all, that could cure such diseases. Further, the prevalence of sexual contact that is a hallmark of the disease also made people chary of voicing their complaints and symptoms. Hence, morbidity and mortality increased from many of these diseases. Over the years, with the advent of antibiotics, many of these are being treated.

Since 1980s AIDS has been the most serious threat ever known to man. In its relentness march, AIDS has already affected millions across the globe. AIDS prevention and control needs to be strengthened urgently. Here the role of health and reproductive health education can not be emphasized strongly enough and should be accorded top priority among families.[22]

This makes very clear that human sexual behaviour and its relationship to AIDS and STDs has to be studied in the present social context.

At present, especially in the urban area, large number of people group together leading to an immense complexity of social relations. The rural families break up into nuclear families or smaller units.[23] The complexities of social relations make the individual decide between a variety of choices. It is a fast changing world and the family is no longer able to enculurate their young into responsible adults. The family is at strain trying to adapt to newer situations.

These reasons lead to the peer group often becoming a bigger force in the enculturation of individuals, especially with respect to sexual behaviour. This independence itself create a feeling of 'macho-ness' of having to demonstrate visibly their prawness in sexual matters. This leads to a laxity in sexual behaviour with associated high risk of being infected with STDs and AIDS.[24-26]

During adolescence, there is a sudden onrush of hormones from various endocrine glands. Secondary sexual characteristics start to develop and the body structure also changes. Time is required to adjust physically and mentally to these changes. Meanwhile, adolescents are physically often gawky and clumsy as they have not yet adjusted to the physical changes in their body. Emotionally, they have not yet achieved much control over their hormones. Hence, they are ripe for high risk sexual behaviour. Attention getting and sensation seeking behaviour is a hallmark. Led by the passion of their hormones, the use of condoms is low among this high risk population.[47-63]

In this present situation, the mass media uses sex to the hit either in the name of entertainment or advertisement. This creates some kind of conflicts, where elders teach them one thing, the legitimized mass media plays upon these hormonal and biological urges and propounds a conflicting view.[64] This also leads to an increase in violence related to sexual encounters.[65-70]

The other concurrent features which tend to clouds the judgements with regards to the use of drugs and alcohol.[71-74,75,76] With this kind of global pattern, it would be important to note here that due to poverty, lack of knowledge and counseling and the great number of people in urban areas, the spread of AIDS in the developing countries would be expected to be quick and disastrous.[77-83]

Adolescent Sexuality

In the Indian context, Dube outlines the process through which Hindu girl's gender is constructed through rites and rituals, socialization and so on. Sex is mainly socially constructed.[84] Adolescent is the period when awareness and feeling towards members of the opposite sex are heightened and play an important role in social and sexual conduct. In Indian traditional family norms still hold that any talk about sexuality is a taboo, and only a few accurate sources of information on sexuality exist. In urban areas, the comparatively liberal views of individuals as a result of exposure to the mass media and the prevailing co-educational system have resulted in considerable intermingling between the sexes.[85]

Francis et al., (1993) pointed out in their South Delhi study of students that the source of knowledge about sex was mostly obtained from books, friends and media, parents (14%) and from friends (2%). The students have no reliable means of obtaining correct information about these subjects.[87]

The results of Delhi ICMR Study (1998) observed that only 14% of urban male adolescents admitted having had experiences of sexual intercourse and 12% of slum male adolescents, where as in only 1.8% of female adolescents it was reported.[88] Madras Study (1993) reported that 32% of all males and 35% of all females had their first sexual experiences during adolescence. But whereas the first pre-marital sex experience occurred for only 6% of female sample and for about 49% of all males.[89] Knowledge of adolescents about sexual relation, sexual intercourse and their attitudes towards sex and sexual behaviour are still inadequate.

Baseline behavioural surveillance surveys were conducted among general populations aged 15-49 years, by National AIDS Control Organisation (NACO) in female sex workers, men having sex with men and injecting drug users in a sample representative of the entire country, during 2001-2002. 26,716 respondents aged 15-24 in the general population, 2,081 female sex workers, 561 men having sex with men and 287 injecting drug users were aged less than 24 years were included in this nation wide surveillance program. More than half the respondents (54.8%; 95% CI: 48.9-60.7) were aware that consistent condom use and having sexual relationships only with uninfected faithful partners protected against HIV transmission. Rural females in Assam, Bihar, Jharkhand, Gujarat, Nagaland, Orissa, UP had lower levels of awareness.

More than 35% males aged more than 19 years from Andhra Pradesh reported indulgence in casual partners. In Chattisgarh, Arunachal Pradesh and Mizoram more than 40% rural males aged more than 19 years also reported indulgence in casual sex.[90]

52% of respondents reported using condoms in last casual sex, while 34% reported that they used a condom with all casual partr.ers in a one year recall period. Consistent use of condom was much lower and ranged between 24% and 45% across different sub population.[90]

In view of the drawbacks highlighted above and because of the fact that adolescents and young adults are prone to take 'risks', it is important to undertake a more survey of adolescents in the country on a similar pattern in a comprehensive manner. Such a survey will bring out the risk behaviour more accurately.

Pre-marital Sexual Behaviour

Studies on adolescent sexual behaviour in different parts of the world show that young people's pre-marital sexual encounters are generally unplanned, infrequent and sporadic. A much higher percentage of men report having pre-marital sex than women. While pre-marital sexual behaviour among adolescents and youth remains poorly explored in India, the available evidence suggests that between 20 and 30 percent of all males and upto 10 percent of all females are sexually active during adolescents before marriage (Pelto, 1999; Jejeebhoy 91, 92). Sexual awareness seems to be largely superficial. Social attitudes clearly favour cultural norms of pre-marital chastity particularly for women. Double standards exit whereby unmarried adolescent boys for more likely than adolescent girls to be sexually active, their movements are less likely to be supervised (NACO, 2001, 90). Boys generally engage in more risky sexual behaviours than girls, and many cultures are more tolerant of male adolescent sexual activity or may even encourage it. Also adolescent boys tend to use alcohol and drugs more often than girls, which can lead to sexual risk taking.

The role of manhood promoted in many societies may discourage young men from showing affection or other emotions while encouraging them to seek, success and power. Such pressures may promote boys to act aggressively, leading to injuries, accidents and homicides (O'Neil, 1995, 93).

Sarin (1986) in his study on unmarried pregnant girls between the age 15 to 20 years (almost 90%) mentioned that they were forced to have sex in more than 62.5% of the cases. He also indicated that none of them were aware of contraceptive.[94] Another study in South Delhi School Children also reported that about 60% of male students were involved in sexual activities with commercial sex workers or older women in their neighbourhood. Girls were also observed to be sexually active, although fewer than boys.[87]

Studies of attitudes towards pre-marital sex suggest once again that while the large majority of adolescents hold conservative attitudes to pre-marital sex, there are clear indication of changes.[89-96] The most common age at first sexual intercourse was 16 to 20 years for both boys and girls. One fourth of the boys started earlier i.e. in the age of 11 to 15 years, whereas, only 6.3% of the girls has first sexual intercourse in the age of 11 to 15 years.[87]

Marriage

In developing countries a much higher proportion of adolescents marry at early age. An increasing proportion of such marriages are entered into as a result of pregnancy indicating pre-marital sexual activity. The legal age of marriage in India is 18 years. Yet adolescent marriages are prevalent due to old custom, tradition and lack of awareness of the legal aspects of marriage. In India early marriage has long been a custom and remains common in rural areas. Regardless of whether pregnancy takes place inside or outside marriage, there are serious biomedical hazards, especially below 17 years and where living conditions are poor and access to health services inadequate. The risk to pregnant girls in early adolescence are especially high.

According to most studies, media and peer group has an important role in dissemination of sex related information (Moses 1983, Francis 1994, Thakore, 1998).[95,87,96] Mother is also an important source for sex related information in Delhi Study.[88] But other research data available reveal the limited role of parents in the enhancement of sexual knowledge for children. Only 18% and 13.4% of adolescents in Moses (1983) and Francis (1994) study consulted their parent about sex.[95,87] These surveys were conducted on boys and girls and the results obtained were their combined opinions. Nair & Grover observed that girls have very little access to sex related information and hence derive much of it from friends, parents, media and relations. There were 28% girls who admitted talking to friends about sex.[99]

Masturbation and Nocturnal Emission

Masturbation is sexual gratification by the stimulation of one's own genitals. Mutual masturbation involves stimulating another person's genitals. It is a safer sex, any sexual activity between two uninfected people is safe. Any activity which does not involve the entry of infected material into the body is safe e.g., use of sterile equipment, masturbation.

In ICMR study it was reported that nearly 52% of urban school male students agreed that they practiced masturbation, and only 30% of slum students did so. The experience was pleasure for 24.6% of urban and 6.6% slum students. For 10.4% urban and 13.3% slum students, masturbation was a regretful or sinful activity. They were quite disturbed about it.[88] Their knowledge was not based on facts.

In contrast to Delhi study, Mumbai study (2001) in male adolescent school students they observed that only 7.5% shared ingnorance, 18% were regularly masturbating where

91 (81.98%) said that they never practiced it till date. 90% of the total respondents opined that masturbation was not a healthy practice. The reasons furnished for the same were varied, but majority (70%) of them said that it causes weakness in the body, makes one's body weak because of which one may not be able to perform the sexual act successfully in future.[100] A study in adolescent males in rural Maharashtra also reported nearly one third i.e., 84 (33.6%) of the males (150 married and 100 unmarried) accepted indulging in masturbation and had several notion about the same.[96] Some of the boys often have misconception related to potency, masturbation and other sexually related issues, nor do they have reliable sources of information to depend on.[101]

A little more than one third urban and slum male students have no knowledge about nocturnal emission. About 49% of urban male students and 38% of slum students admitted that they were aware of night emission in Delhi study. The outcome of their knowledge of nocturnal emission also reflected their poor knowledge and need for sex education. The proper information flow and education will help younger generation to use this practice for their better development and direct their energy from other anti social activities etc.[88]

There is a paucity of data related to sex behaviour of adolescent girls in India but many studies have been conducted to highlight this aspect among teenager in developed countries (Klanger 1993, Thomas 1998).[97-98]

Knowledge of Contraception

In 1998-1998, National Survey on Fertility and Family Planning Practices in India also suggested that 59% of adolescents were aware of condoms.[103] In contrast to National Survey, Delhi study included only adolescent students groups. Delhi study reported that majority of the study group did not have clear knowledge of contraceptives. Condoms were the most commonly known contraceptives? (5%). Equal proportion (65%), (66%) urban and slum students were well aware of condoms. Wide variations in the knowledge of urban girls for condom 48.8% and slum girls 28% was noticed. Only 5.3 adolescents knew about oral pills.[88]

Awareness about vasectomy (42%) as a terminal method was significantly higher than tubectomy (25% to 32%) in urban students. In practice no contraceptives were used by sexually active adolescents who participated in Delhi Study. Findings of their study are consistent with the study conducted in South Delhi with the only difference that in ICMR study a small group was sexually active, whereas South Delhi Study a large number of students aged 16 to 18 reported to be sexually active. But in the later study, the knowledge about contraceptives was present in higher proportion of students.[87]

The level of awareness of oral pills was known to only 3% in Delhi rural female adolescent while knowledge of condoms and intra utrine contraceptive device (IUCD) was known to 53.7% and 20.7% respectively (Nair & Grover 1999).[99]

HIV/AIDS

The problems of HIV/AIDS has assumed a pandemic proportion, it has affected most of the countries of the world including India in a sense the AIDS pandemic has ushered a new era in the way sexual relations are prescribed and acted upon. The number of diagnosed AIDS cases among adolescents and young people severely.

Underestimates the threat posed by HIV infection given the long incubation period of the disease. At least half, and probably the majority of infected people will develop AIDS within 10-15 years of becoming infected during their teens. Worldwide between 20% to 25% of HIV infection are estimated 5 million people are infected with HIV. WHO estimates that by turn of the century majority of these infected with HIV will be in the age group of 15 to 34 years. Adolescents are both important and a potential resource for prevention of HIV infection. AIDS is a threat to them personally and to the community at large. The school children and youth who are yet to develop or are in the process of inculcating behavioural pattern with regard to sexuality can be easy and accessible target groups for education on health and safe behavioural practices. The concept of reproductive health has thus been widened since the rapid spread of AIDS pandemic.[103]

Majority of KAPB studies have been conducted in India on adolelscents. Majority of male (94%) and female (90.2%) adolescents knew about AIDS in Delhi study. The urban adolescents knew all the correct modes of transmission falling in the range of 79% to 90.6%, only slum girls were lagging behind in this aspect.

The proportion of adolescent students who had received sex education or counseling was small in both areas alike (23.5% urban and 21.6 slum). More than 75% of adolescents felt the need of sex education and counseling at school level also the need was felt more by boys as compared to girls. The priority subjects chosen were safe sex, contraceptive and decision making on sex related issues. Majority of the adolescents nearly 70% felt that needs for availability of a counseling facility at school. Again, the proposition of boys was significantly higher than that of girls.[88]

Attitudes towards STDs

Much can be done to promote and well being of adolescents of both sexes and to protect them to a greater degree. A second major potential consequence of unprotected sexual activity in adolescence is the acquisition of an STD, often with devastating effects on future fertility. The incidence of STD among adolescents has increased markedly.[21] STDs are the most common group of communicable diseases reported in majority of countries. They continue to occur at unacceptably high levels among young people. Changes in sexual behaviour as a consequence or urbanization, mass communication and ease of travel are factors that have contributed to this public health problem. Young people between the ages of 10-24 years constitute both an important target group and a potential force for the prevention of STD. STDs are a challenge to reproductive health where access to adequate diagnostic and treatment facilities is limited. Three major obstacles to the control of these diseases among adolescents are the ignorance of the young people of the symptoms of STDs, particularly in women, and the reluctance of young people to ask for help because they expect to be met with anger and hostility.[5]

In a study on South Delhi, 83% reported having had knowledge of STDs, but only 35% knew that there was treatment for STD,[87] while in a WHO study conducted in STD clinic of GTB Hospital, Delhi reported 36% of STD patients did not have the knowledge of STDs and only 56% knew about the curability of most of STDs.[102] Because of stigma attached to these diseases, and because adolescents are most likely to be frightened and inexperienced in seeking treatment for them, a special effort must be made to ensure a confidential approach.

Recognition of adolescent health (AD) as a separate discipline is the most imperative. A structural modification of the terms sex education or reproductive health awareness which are stigmatized, should be replaced by the term 'family life education (FLE) and place of sex education in adolescents, the term 'adolescent education (AE) should be used.

The various studies on adolescent sexual behaviour indicate the importance of the felt need.

It is important that teachers, like many other adults, find discussing sexual matters with young people difficult and embarrassing (Jejeebhoy, 1998, Grover, 1998).[92,98] However, a supportive school environment can help teachers to overcome some of their worries. The discipline for 'Adolescent Health' hereby should resolve to support and encourage the development of responsibility towards sexuality on the part of adolescents to support and encourage an awareness and acceptance by adults that sexuality is a part of adolescent development; to affirm the need for families to be involved in their children's sexuality education; to support innovative efforts to delay the age of onset of coitus in adolescents but to affirm the importance of self exploration, and intimacy; to increase awareness of problems of sexual abuse and to provide services to young people. Education about safer sex practices must be continued.

School health services need to be strengthened, apart from regular health check up. Focus should be on providing relevant information on health awareness like dietary habits, counseling on health, life styles, hobbies and recreation, relationship with family members and teachers. Adolescent health is emerging as a new and essential health area. Adolescents are the adults of tomorrow. The role of information, education and communication (IEC) is critical both in sensitizing the community on the special needs of this select group as also in the empowerment of the group with correct knowledge, attitudes and practices.

The media campaign should also focus on spreading the knowledge about STDs and HIV/AIDS, route of transmission and methods of preventions. The message should be simple, precise and clear cut. A National Health Policy for adolescents has to be developed by Policy Makers and Program Organizers.

There is further need for quantitative and qualitative community based studies for the assessment of the services required for the adolescents. Research is needed that explores the opinions of sexually active youth about the risk they face concerning unwanted pregnancy and HIV/STDs and to explore the ways in which young people cope with these risks and the constraints they face in changing behaviour (WHO, 2001).[104, 105]

REFERENCES

1. Kinsey AC, Pomeroy WB and Martin CE, 1948. Sexual Behaviour in Human Male, WB Sounders, Philadelphia, Pennsylvania and London, England.
2. Kinsey AC, Pomeroy WB, Martin CE and Gebhard PH, 1953: Sexual Behaviour in Human Female, WB Saunders, Philadelphia, Pennsylvania and London, England.
3. Lindholm, Cherry and Charles, 1980: Life Behind the Veil. Science Digest Special, 42, Summer.
4. Young People's Health – A Challenge for Society. World Technical Report Series 731, 1986, World Health Organization, Geneva.
5. Global Reproductive Health – Binneal Report, 1990-1991, World Health Organization.
6. Friedman L, Herbert and Edstorm, G Karim, 1983: Adolescent Reproductive Health—An Approach to Planning Health Service Research, World Health Organization, Geneva.
7. Gupta SC, 1995: Media, Culture and Mental Health; Indian Journal of Clinical Psychiatry, 22:1.
8. Derksen DJ, Strasberger VC, 1994: Children and the Influence of Media, Primary Care 21 (44): 747-58.
9. Aberol U, Khan N, Srivastava P, 1993: Role of Parents in Children's Television Viewing, Childhood, 1:212-219.
10. Malik A, 1995: Is Television Guilty? The Hindustan Times, July 23, Sunday Magazine.
11. Looney JG, Oldhan DG, 1989: Normal Development in Kaplan H, Sadock BJ, (eds) Comprehensive Text Book of Psychiatry, Vol. 11, Baltimore, USA: Williams and Wilkins.
12. United States Surgeon General, 1989, Reducing the Health Consequences of Smoking, 25 Years of Progress: A Report Surgeon General, Washington DC, USA.
13. Hann N, Asghan A, Owen W, Asal N, 1995: Smoking Health Hazards in High School. Jokla State Med. Assoc. 88 (6): 247-51.
14. Giesbrecht N, Fisher H, 1985: Alcohol Related Causualities Proceedings of an International Symposium, Toronto, Canada, ARF Bull.
15. Kay LE, 1995: Adolescent Sexual Intercourse Strategies for Promoting Abstinence in Teens. Postgraduate Medicine, 97 (6): 121-7.
16. The Health of Young People. A Challenge and a Promise, WHO (1993), Geneva.
17. The Health of Young People – "A Challenge and a Promise" WHO (1994), Geneva.
18. Dickstra RFW, 1989: Suicide Behaviour in Adolescents and Young Adults: In International Picture, Crisis, 10 (1): 16-35.

19. Jeanneret O, Sand EA, 1993: International Violence Among Adolescents and Young Adults: An Epidemiological Perspective, World Health Statistics Quarterly, 46, 34-51.

20. Irwin CE, Millstein SG, 1986: Biopsychosocial Correlates of Risk Taking Behaviour During Adolescents, Journal of Adolescents Health Care, 7: 828-968.

21. Spirak H, Prothrow S, Hansman AJ, 1988: Dying is no Accident Adolescent, Violence and Intention Injury, *Pediatric Clin North Am*, 35:1339-47.

22. Expert Committee on Veneral Diseases and Tryeponematosis. Technical Report Series No. 736, World Health Organization, 1986.

23. Wing, Clive and Chowdhary S, 1994: A Family Guide to HIV and AIDS in India, Population Prakashan, Bombay.

24. Roland A, 1991: Sexuality, the Indian Extended Family, and Hindu Culture, *J Am Acad Psychonal, Winter*, Vol. 19, No. 4: 595-605.

25. World Health Organization, 1987 Concept of Sexual Health, Regional Office, EVR/ICP/ MCH-821, Copenhagan.

26. Oswald H, and Pforr, 1992: Sexuality and AIDS: Attitudes and Behaviour of Adolescents in East and West Berlin, *J Adolesc*, Dec, 15 (4), 2373-97.

27. Werdetin L J, Malby M and Olsen, 1992: An Update on Knowledge and Sexual Behaviour Among Students in Greenland, *Scand J Soc, Med*, Sept. 62 (7), 271-9.

28. Santelli JS and Beilenson P, 1992: Demographics of Adolescents Sexual Behaviour, Contraception, Pregnancy and STDs, *J Sch Health*, September, 62 (7), 271-9.

29. Newcomer S and Baldnein W, 1992: Demographics of Adolescents Sexual Behaviour, Contraception, Pregnancy and STDs, *J Sch Health*, September, 62 (7): 5-70.

30. Fitzpatrick C, Mckenna P and Hone R, 1992: Teenage Girls Attending a Dublin Sexually Transmitted Disease Clinic, A Socio-sexual and Diagnostic Profile, *J Med Sci*, 161 (97): 460-2.

31. Leland NL and Barth RP, 1992: Gender Differences in Knowledge Intentions and Behaviour Concerning Pregnancy and Sexually Transmitted Disease Prevention Among Adolescents. *J Adolesc Health*, Nov 13(7): 589-99.

32. White SD, and Deblassic RR, 1992: Adolescence Sexual Behaviour, *Adolescence J Spring*, 27 (105): 183-91.

33. Morris LCW, Aral SO, 1993: Measuring Adolescent Sexual Behaviour and Related Health Outcomes, Public Health Rep, 108 Suppl, 1:31-6.

34. De Souza RP, De Almeida AB, Wagner MB, Zimerman II, De Almeida SB, 1993: A Study of the Sexual Behaviour of Teenagers in South Brazil, *J Adolesc Health*, Jun, 14(4): 336-9.

35. Dickson N, Paul NC, and Herbison P, 1993: Adolescents Sexual Behaviour and Implications for an Epidemic of HIV/AIDS Among the Young, *Genitorium Med*, Apr, 69 (2): 133-40.

36. Turner RA, Irwin CE, Ji Ischman JM and Milstein SG, 1993: Autonomy, Relatedness and the Initiation of Health Risk Behaviour in Early Adolescence, *Health Psychol*, May, 12 (3):200-8.

37. Stanton B X Li, Black M, Ricardo I, Galbraith J, Kaljie L, Feigeman S, 1994: Sexual Practices and Intentions Among Preadolescent and Early Adolescent Low Income Urban Africans, *Paediatrics*, June, 93 (6 Pt. 1): 966-73.

38. Nagy S, Adcock AG and Nagy MC, 1994: A Comparison of Risky Health Behaviours of Sexual Active, Sexual Abuses and Abstaining Adolescents, *Paediatrics*, Apr, 93(4): 570-5.
39. Greenblatt M: Homeless Adolescents Hosp, *Community Psychiatry*, Dec, 44(12): 121177-80.
40. Waiter HJ, Vanghan RO, Ragin DF, Gohali AT, Kasen S, Fullilove RE, 1993: Prevalence and Correlates of AIDS – Risk Behaviour Among Urban minority High School Students, *Prev Med*, Nov, 22 (6): 813-24.
41. Hanna KM, 1994: Adolescents and the Risk of AIDS in Kansas, Jan. 69 (1): 6-7.
42. Chand S and Francis J, 1994: Study of Delhi Children, NGO-AIDS Cell, AIIMS, New Delhi as in Kalpana Jain Survey. Delhi Kinds Sexually Active, The Independent March 1.
43. Arnette JL, Balle-Jenson, 1993: Culture Bases of Risk Behaviour—Danish Adolescents, *Child Dev*, Dec, 64(6): 1842-55.
44. Braveman PK, Strasbinger VC, 1993: Adolescent Sexual Activity, *Clin Paediatr Phila*, Nov, 32 (11): 658-68.
45. Creatsas GK, 1993: Sexuality—Sexual Activity and Contraception During Adolescents in Cure, *Opin Obstet Gynaecol*, Dec, 5 (6): 774-83.
46. Klanger B, Tyden T and Ruusuvaara, 1993: Sexual Behaviour Among Adolescents in Uppsala. Sweden, *J Adolesc Health*, Sept. 14(6): 468-74.
47. Tyden T, Narden L, Ruusuvaara L, 1991: Swedish Adolescents Knowledge of Sexually Transmitted Diseases and Their Attitudes, Midwifery, Mar, 7 (1): 25-30.
48. Lema VM, 1990: Sexual Behaviour, Contraceptive Practice and Knowledge of Reproductive Biology Among Adolescents Secondary School Girls in Naindi, Kenya in East Africa, *Med. J*, Feb, 67(2) 86-94.
49. Fliser AJ, *et al.*: 1993: Risk Taking Behaviour of Cape Peninsula High School Students Part VIII: Sexual Behaviour, S Afri, *Med J*, July, 83(7): 495-497.
50. Whatley J, *et al.*: 1989: Problems of Adolescents Sexuality, *J Soc Med*, Dec, 82 (12): 732-734.
51. Ross Michael W, 1992: Attitudes Towards Condoms and Condom Use: A Review, International Journal of STD and AIDS, Jan - Feb, Vol. 3: 10-16.
52. Giesecke, Johan, *et al.*: 1992: Sexual Behaviour Related to the Spread of Sexually Transmitted Diseases: A Population Based Survey International J STD and AIDS. Vol. 3; 255-260.
53. Di Clemente, Ralph J, *et al.*: 1993: Comparison of AIDS Knowledge and HIV Related Sexual Risk Behaviour Among Adolescent Health, Vol. 14: 231-236.
54. Bertrand, Jane T, 1991: AIDS Related Knowledge, Sexual Behaviour and Condom Use Among Men and Women in Kinshasa Zaire American, *J Public Health*, Vol. 81, No. 1, Jan, 53-58.
55. Forman, David and Clain, Chivers, 1989: Sexual Behaviour of Young and Middle Aged Men in England and Wales, British Medical Journal, Vol. 298, 29th April, 1137-1142.
56. Wielandt H and Hansen UM, 1989. Sexual Behaviour, Contraception and Unintended Pregnancy among Young Females, ACTA Obstet Gynaecol, Scand, Vol. 68: 255-259.
57. Morris L, 1992. Sexual Experience and Use of Contraception Among Young Adults in Latinamerica. MMWR Surveill. Summer, 28 Aug, Vol. 41(4): 27-40.
58. Barker GK, and Rich S, 1992: Influence on Adolescent Sexuality in Nigeria and Kenya-Findings from Recent Focus Group Discussions, *Stud Fam Plann*, May-June, Vol. 23 (3): 199-210.

59. Pendegast RA, Durant RH, Gaillard GI, 1992: Attitudes and Behavioural Correlates of Condom Use in Urban Adolescent Males, *J Adolesc Health*, Mar, 13(2): 133-139.

60. Di Ciemente RJ, Durbin M, Siegel *et al.*: 1992: Determinants of Condom Use among Junior High School Students in a Minority, Inner City School District, *Paediatrics*, Feb., 89 (2): 347-359.

61. Lagana L and Hayes DM, 1993: Contraceptive Health Programmes for Adolescents—A Critical Review, Adolescence, Summer 28 (110): 347-359.

62. Adinma JI and Okeske AO, 1993: The Pill—Perception and Usage Among Algerian Students, Adv. Contracept, Dec, 9 (40): 341-349.

63. Davis AJ, 1994: The Role of Hormonal Contraception in Adolescents, *Am J Obstet Gynaecol May*, 170 (Pt 2): 1581-1585.

64. Dunne MP *et al.*: 1994: Age Related Increase in Sexual Behaviour and Decrease in Regular Condom Use Among Adolescents in Australia, Int. J. STD and AIDS, Jan-Feb, 5(1): 41-47.

65. Harnett, PH and Misch P, 1993: Developmental Issues in the Assessment and Treatment of Adolescent Petrators of Sexually Abused, *J Adolesc*, Dec, 16 (4): 397-405.

66. Mclean AL, Flamingam BJ, 1993: Transition Marking Behaviour of Adolescent Males at First Intercourse, Adolescence, Fall, 28 (111): 579-595.

67. Wielandt HL, Wermuth MR, Pedersen, 1988: Contraceptive Use in a Sample of Young Danish Females, ACTA Obstet Gynaecol Scand 67(4): 319-321.

68. Strasburger VC, 1992: Children, Adolescents and Television, *Paediatr Rev*, April 139 (4): 144-151.

69. Stonim, Nevo V, 1992-93: AIDS Related Knowledge, Attitudes and Behaviour Among Juvenile Delinquents in Israel Public Health Rev, 20 (3-4): 241-250.

70. Garg BB, *et al.*: 1988: Sexually Transmitted Diseases in Children, *Indian J Sex Trasm Dis*, Vol. 7: 11-13.

71. Epps KJ, Haworth R, Swaffer T, 1993: Attitudes Towards Women and Rape Among Male Adolescents Convicted of Sexual Versus Non-sexual Crimes, *J Psychol*, Sept, 127 (5): 501-506.

72. Klierman LV, 1993: Adolescent Pregnancy and Parenting Controversies of the Past and Lessons for the Future, *J Adolescent Health*, Nov, 14 (7) 553-561.

73. Trad PV, 1993: Adolescent Pregnancy—An Intervention Challenge in Child Psychiatry, *Hum Dev*, Winter, 24 (2):99-113.

74. Holden GW, Nelson PW, Velasquez J, Hitchie KL, 1993: Cognitive Psychological and Reported Sexual Behaviour Differences Between Pregnant and Non-pregnant Adolescents, Adolescence, Fall, 28 (111): 557-572.

75. Robbins, Cynthia, 1989: Sex Differences in Psychosocial Consequences of Alcohol and Drug Related Behaviour, Journal of Health and Social Behaviour, Vol. 30, March, 117-130.

76. Rosenthal D, Moore S and Buzuwell S, 1994. Homeless Youth—Sexual and Drug Related Behaviour, Sexual Beliefs and HIV / AIDS Risk, AIDS Care, 6 (I): 83-94.

77. Shafer MA, Hilton JF, Ekstrand M, Kaogh J, Gee L, Di Giorgio, 1993: Relationship Between Drug Use and Sexual Behaviour and the Occurrence of Sexuality Transmitted Diseases Among High Risk Male Youth, *Sex Transm Dis*, Nov-Dec., 20(6): 307-313.

78. Levy SR, Lampman C, Handler A, Flay BR, Weeks K, 1993: Young Adolescent Attitudes Towards Sex and Substance Abuse, Implications for AIDS Prevention, *AIDS Educ Prev*, Winter, 5 (40): 340-351.

79. Fergusson DM, Lynskay MT and Horwood UJ, 1994: Alcohol Consumption and Associated Problems in a Birth Cohort of 15 Years Olds, *N Z Med J*, May 11, 107 (977); 167-170.

80. Robertson JA and Plant MA, 1988: Alcohol, Sex and Risks of HIV Infection, Drug Alocohol Depend, Oct, 22 (1-2): 75-78.

81. Anderson and Roy M, 1992: Some Aspects of Sexual Behaviour and the Potential Demographic Impact of AIDS in Developing Countries, Social Science and Medicine, Vol. 34, No. 3 : 271-280.

82. AIDS in India: Newsletter of the NACO (National AIDS Controlling Organization), June, 1993: 1-16.

83. Branham, Robert, *et al.*: 1990: Epidemiology of Sexually Transmitted Diseases: Current and Future Dimensions of the Problems in the Third World, in A Germain *et al.* (eds.) Reproductive Tract Infections N, Y: Plenin Pub: 35-38.

84. Schryver A and Meheus A, 1990: Epidemiology of Sexually Transmitted Diseases—The Global Picture, Bulletin of the World Health Organization, Vol. 68, No. 5: 639-654.

85. Pill Roisin, Peters TJ and Robling MR, 1993: How Important is Health Behaviour to the Health of Mothers of Lowèr Socio-Economic Status? *Journal Pub Health Med*, Vol. 15, No. 1, 77-82.

86. Anderson Roy, 1993: AIDS Trends, Predictions, Controversy, Nature, Vol. 303, 3rd June; 393-394.

87. Garnett GP and Anderson RM, 1993: Factors Controlling the Spread of HIV in Heterosexual Communities in Developing Countries: Patterns of Mixing Between Different Age and Sexual Activity Classes, Philos Trans. H. Socio. Lond. Biol., Oct, 29, 342 (1300); 137-159.

88. Dube Leela, 1988: On the Construction of Gender: Hindu Girls in Patrilineal India,. Economic and Political Weekly, April, 30 WS 11-19.

89. Braverman PK, Strasburger VC, 1994: Sexually Transmitted Diseases, *Clin Paediatr Phila*, Jan, 33 (1): 26-37.

90. Francis PT, *et al.* 1993: Knowledge, Belief and Attitudes Regarding AIDS, STD and Human Sexuality Among Senior Secondary Students in Delhi, Indian Journal of Community Medicine 1999, (96): 17-20.

91. Grover VA: Study on Reproductive Health Awareness and Sex Behaviour Among Adolescents of Delhi. Final Report Submitted to Task Force, Division of Reproductive Health and Nutrition, Indian Council of Medical Research, New Delhi, Report No. 5/10/68/94-RHN, July, 1998.

92. Jejeebhoy SJ, 1998: Adolescents Sexual and Reproductive Behaviour; A Review of Evidence from Indian Social Sciences and Medicine, 46 (10); 1275-1290.

93. O'Neil J, Good G, Holmes S: Fifteen Years of Theory and Research on Men's Gender Role Conflict; New Paradigms of Empirical Research. In Levant R, Pollack W, eds. A New Psychology of Men. (New York; Basic Books, 1995) 164-206.

94. Sarin U, 1988: Teen Age Pregnancy, Ind, J, Preventive & Social Med. 19(I): 30-32.

95. Moses S and Praveena C: Sex Education—Its Need and Attitude of Adolescents; *The J Family Welfare*, 1983; 30(2): 34-49.

96. Thakor HG, and Kumar P: Need Assessment for Sex Education Amongst the School Girls. *Indian J Community Medicine*, 23(2): 62-67.

97. Kalanger B, Tyden T and Rusuvara I: Sexual Behaviour Among Adolescents in Uppsala, Sweden. Journal of Adolescent Medicine, 1993, 41: 468-474.

98. Thomas HB, Censo AD and Griffith L: Adolescent Sexual Behaviour—Results from an Ontario Sample, Part-1: Adolescent Sexual Activity; *Canadian J Public Health*. 1998, 98(2): 90-94.

99. Parvathy N and Grover V, 1999: A Study of Reproductive Health Amongst Female Adolescent Population in a Rural Area of Delhi (unpublished).

100. Sharmila, S Patil, Chaturvedi, R and Malkar MB, 2001: Sexuality and Sexual Behaviour in Male Adolescent School Students, Mumbai; Http//www.bhi.org./journal/2000 4404 Oct/ review 664-htm.

101. Grover V: Changes in Sexual Behaviour in Response to Increased Risk of Awareness. Final Reports Submitted to Task Force for Social Science Research on Reproductive Health, World Health Organization, Geneva, Switzerland, Project No. 91311 BSDA, 1995.

102. Mawar N, Tripathy SP, John JK, *et al.*: Youth Sexuality Study on Behaviours Change Intentions for AIDS/HIV in College Youth, Pune, India x 11 International AIDS Conference, Geneva, 1998, Abstract No. 14333.

103. India 1998-1999. National Family Planning Health Survey (NFHS-2), International Institute for Population Science, Mumbai, India.

104. World Health Organization, Adolescence the Critical Phase, Challenges and Potentials, Regional Office for South-East Asia, New Delhi, 1997.

105. Ann Denise Brown, Jejeebhoy SJ, Iqbal Shah *et al.*: 2001: Sexual Relations Among Young People in Developing Countries; Evidence from WHO Case Studies, Department of Reproductive Health and Research, WHO, Geneva.

CHAPTER

6

HIV in Unwanted Teenage Pregnancy

Aneesha M Grover and *Mini Sood*

INTRODUCTION

The current sexual behavior among the youth is associated with significant risk to their health and well-being. The threats to their well being include the HIV and AIDS pandemic, high rates of sexually transmitted infections (STI's), and unintended pregnancies that may result in maternal morbidity and/or mortality. HIV/AIDS respects no borders, no economic class, no gender and no age. Current statistics on HIV/AIDS indicate that one-half of all new HIV infections worldwide occur among young people between ages 15 to 24. The socioeconomic and political consequences of the HIV epidemic place these youth at further risk.

Young teenage girls are at risk of experiencing negative consequences because of their physical immaturity, vulnerability to older men, and limited education, skills, finances, and other resources. Also, death from pregnancy-related health complications is two times more common among teenagers than women in twenties.

Apart from educating them about sexual abuse and the role of male partners, it is essential to impart the necessary skills and information in order to enable them to make healthy and responsible decisions about their sexual behavior. In order to protect them from sexually transmitted diseases, including HIV infection, and to delay too-early childbearing, access to confidential, low-cost, and youth-friendly contraceptive services is required.

SEXUAL BEHAVIORS AMONG TEENS

Adolescence is the time of emerging feelings, curiosity, discovery, exploration and experimentation regarding relationships. Sexual behavior is an important part of this process and is intrinsically linked with unsafe behavior and practices. Unprotected sexual intercourse and multiple sex partners place young people at risk for HIV infection, other sexually transmitted diseases (STDs), and pregnancy. It is thus important to understand the various aspects of sexual behavior among the youth in order to prevent the above consequences.

Changing trend in the sexual behavior of young teenagers

A changing trend in the sexual behavior of young teenagers has been noted. These include increased sexual activity at a younger age and increased pregnancy and abortion rates among younger teens.

Moore et al noted an increasing rate of teenagers initiating sexual activity at a young age. Sexual intercourse among teenage males increased from 20% (in 1970) to 27% (in 1985) and in females it increased from 4% to 10%.[1] Another study reported that as many as 23% of all 14-year-olds and 30% of all 15-year-olds had undergone sexual intercourse.[2]

The pregnancy rate among females at < 14 years increased from 13.5 per 1,000 females in 1973 to 17.1 in 1992.[3] The abortion rate among females at < 14 years increased from 5.6 per 1,000 females in 1973 to 8.4 in 1980, and 7.9 in 1990.[1] Although these figures are from the U.S, similar trends have been reported from other parts of the world, including the developing countries.

Consequences of early initiation of sexual activity among teenagers

Consequences of early initiation of sexual activity in teenagers are manifold. First intercourse at a young age is associated with subsequently having more frequent intercourse and multiple sexual partners, both of which increase the risk of contracting sexually transmitted diseases (STD's) including HIV.[1, 4]

It is also associated with an increased risk of drug abuse (again associated with HIV transmission).[1]

Early initiation of sexual intercourse among teenagers is frequently linked to previous sexual victimization. Many of the young teens are sexually assaulted and coerced and many teen mothers are victims of sexual violence. An observational study reported that 74% of women who had sexual intercourse before age 14 and 60% of those who had sex before age 15 had involuntary sex at some point in their lives.[2] Similarly, Boyer et al reported that 66% pregnant and parenting teens had experienced non-voluntary sexual activity and 44% had been raped.[5] One of the most significant consequences of early initiation of sexual activity is teenage pregnancy and is discussed below.

Pregnancy in Teenagers

Teenage pregnancy and early motherhood are associated with poor educational achievement, poor physical and mental health, social isolation, poverty and related factors. There is a growing recognition that socio-economic disadvantage is both a cause and a consequence of teenage parenthood.

Risk factors for teen pregnancy

The reasons why teen pregnancy exists are varied and overlapping. There are at least 100 risk factors leading to teen intercourse.[6] These factors can be categorized as:

- Community disadvantage;
- Lack of family support and supervision;
- Economic disadvantage;
- Family, peer, and partner attitudes and behavior; and
- Characteristics of teens themselves, including detachment from school, emotional distress and sexual beliefs, attitudes and behaviors.

Girls and young women from the lower socioeconomic strata are at ten times increased risk of becoming teenage mothers. Young people with below average achievement levels, those who failed to complete their schooling and those belonging to families that have experienced financial difficulties have also been found to be at significantly higher risk of becoming teenage parents.[7] Other vulnerable groups include homeless young people, children of teenage mothers, members of some ethnic minority groups and young people involved in crime.[8,9,10] Pressure from partners and friends is an important risk factor. Eight per cent of sexually experienced young women cited pressure from their partner as a factor in having sex for the first time; 7% cited pressure from their friends.[11]

Younger teens are often uninformed about contraception. A substantial portion of sexual activity among this age group is unplanned or coerced, making contraceptive use unlikely.[12] Also, they have fewer antibodies to STD's, making them more susceptible to STD's and cervical infections compared to older women.[2] Out of the 12 million cases reported, 3 million teens are affected by sexually transmitted diseases annually. These include infections with chlamydia (which can cause sterility), syphilis (which can cause blindness, maternal death, and death of the infant) and HIV.[13]

Epidemiology of teenage pregnancy

The rates of teen pregnancy vary among the different societies. Among the developed countries, the U.S. leads with rates nearly double of U.K, four times those of France and Germany, and more than ten times that of Japan.[14] However, the developing countries (including India) as a whole have higher rates of teen pregnancy than the developed countries. (Table 1).

In the developed countries teenage birth rates have declined steadily since 1991 as a result of steady targeting of teenagers by various programs.[15] Between 1991 and 2002, the rate fell by 30% (from 61.8 per 1,000 women to 43).[16] However, the rates still remain high. In 2002, 4 teenage girls in 100 had a baby. Also, about 17% of teen mothers go on to have a second baby within three years after the birth of their first baby.[15]

In the U.S, 860,000 teenagers become pregnant each year with one in three teenagers becoming pregnant before age 20, and about 425,000 giving birth.[16] Eleven per cent of all U.S. births were among teenagers (ages 15 to 19) and 67% of these among girls aged 18 and 19.[16]

Consequences of teenage pregnancy

Teenage pregnancy has important implications for the mother's and the child's health, socioeconomic consequences as well as the broader effect on the society.

Adverse effects of teen pregnancy on the mother

There are serious health risks for adolescents who have babies. Teens often have poor eating habits, neglect to take their nutritional supplements, and may smoke, drink alcohol and take drugs. They are less likely to be of adequate pre-pregnancy weight and/or to gain an adequate amount of weight during pregnancy. All these factors increase their risk of pregnancy complications and giving birth to babies with health problems like low-birthweight, prematurity and stillbirth.

Common medical problems among adolescent mothers include pregnancy-induced hypertension, anemia, premature labor, and cephalopelvic disproportion.[16] Teen mothers are twice as likely to deliver prematurely than women aged 30 to 34 (21 vs. 9 %).[16] They are also least likely of all maternal age groups to get early and regular prenatal care. In 2002, 6.6 % of mothers aged 15 to 19 years received late or no prenatal care (compared to 3.6 % for all ages).[16] Mortality due to pregnancy complications is also more than twice as likely than among mothers aged 20 to 24.[17]

Teens do not have good parenting skills, or the social support systems to help them deal with the stress of raising an infant making the life difficult for her and her child.

Later in life, adolescent mothers tend to be at greater risk for obesity and hypertension than women who were not teenagers when they had their first child.[18] Teen pregnancy is closely linked to poverty and single parenthood as the future prospects for teenagers declines significantly after having a baby. They are less likely to complete school and more likely to be single parents without proper job skills. The growth in single-parent families thus remains the single most important reason for increased poverty among these children.[19] Therefore, reducing teen pregnancy and child-bearing is an obvious place to anchor serious efforts to reduce poverty in future generations.

Unintended pregnancies and abortion

In the United States, 74 to 95% teenage pregnancies are unintended and almost 20% end in abortion.[20, 21, 22, 23] World over, 30 million legal and 20 million illegal abortions are conducted each year.[24] Complications of unsafe abortion are the leading cause of death among teenage women with 64% of maternal deaths between 1995 and 2000 accounted by illegal abortions.[25] The methods used commonly during unsafe abortion and which account for death associated with the procedure are the use of sharp objects like knife and coat hanger which perforate the uterus and insertion of contaminated materials and/or unclean instruments into the cervix.[26]

The probability of complications and death due to abortion increases with the length of gestation. Fatality rate at 8 weeks or less of gestation is 0.4 per 100,000 abortions and it increases to 7 per 100,000 at 16 to 20 weeks.[26] The main morbidity seen in women who survive an unsafe abortion is infertility.[27]

Easy access to safe abortion is thus essential to prevent injury and death associated with unsafe abortion procedures.[20, 24]

Adverse effects of teen pregnancy on the child

Children born to teen mothers suffer from higher rates of low birth weight (21% higher than the proportion for mothers aged 20-24) and are three times more likely to die in the first 28 days of life than babies born to older mothers.[28, 29,30] Other related health problems seen in these children include blindness, deafness, chronic respiratory problems, mental retardation, mental illness, cerebral palsy, dyslexia and hyperactivity.[31] Also, they experience poorer health outcomes, receive less medical care and treatment and when they do visit medical providers, most of the expenses incurred are paid by others in society.

They often receive inadequate parenting as both parents are still growing and developing themselves and are too young to master the demanding job of being a parent. Thus they often fall victim to abuse and neglect. A study showed the incidence of child abuse to be two times more common in families with teenage mothers.[31] They suffer from poor school performance with 50% more chances to repeat a grade and are less likely to complete school.[32] They also have higher rates of adolescent childbearing themselves.[31]

Adverse effects of teen pregnancy on the society

Teen mothers are more likely to drop out of school than girls who delay childbearing. A 1997 study showed that only 41% of teenagers who have children before age 18 complete school compared to 61% of teens from similar social and economic backgrounds who did not give birth until ages 20 or 21.[33] With her education cut short, a teenage mother lacks job skills, making it hard for her to find and keep a job. In addition they tend to have larger family size with more number of children. Thus, teen mothers are more likely to live in poverty than women who delay childbearing and over 75 % become financially dependent on her family or on public assistance within 5 years of the birth of their first child.[33] Young children born to unmarried teenage school dropout mothers are 10 times as likely as other children to be living in poverty.[34]

Teen pregnancy is thus an economic burden to the health care system, social support networks and the government funding agencies.

Thus, educational, social, medical, and economic difficulties are a consequence of teenage childbearing.[35]

Effect of HIV infection on pregnancy

Though HIV infection has little effect on pregnancy outcome or complications in the developed world, adverse pregnancy outcomes (both early and late) have been reported in the developing countries.[36-40] Complications of early pregnancy are related to the effects of concurrent sexually transmitted infections and include a higher rate of spontaneous abortion (1.4 -3 times) and ectopic pregnancy.[41] In late pregnancy there is a higher risk of preterm labour (double the rates seen in uninfected women), pre-term rupture of membranes, abruptio placentae, low birth weight (especially in women with symptomatic HIV infection) and stillbirths.[43,44,45] In the postpartum period, infectious complications are more common (Caesarean section is particularly associated with higher infectious morbidity, especially in women with low CD4+ counts).[46,47]

Apart from the HIV-related opportunistic infections (commonly tuberculosis and herpes zoster), bacterial pneumonia, urinary tract infections and other infections are more common during pregnancy.[48]

Thus, presence of HIV infection further increases the risks for the teenage mother as well as adds to the costs of their medical care.

Prevention of Teenage Pregnancy

As highlighted above, adolescent pregnancy is not simply a problem of teens having unprotected sexual intercourse at an early age but is related to much broader social, economic, cultural, and psychological factors, including poverty, school failure, and sexual abuse. Strategies to deal with this problem thus require multidisciplinary combined effort including the involvement of the community at large.

A substantial improvement in adolescent sexual health has occurred in the European countries.[49] Their experience in handling this problem provides guidelines to the rest of the world on how to tackle the situation. One of the primary requirements is to overcome obstacles and achieve social and cultural consensus, respecting sexuality as a normal and healthy part of being human and of being a teen. A summary of their approach to solve the problem is discussed below.

They viewed their youth as assets and not as problems. They supported education and economic self-sufficiency among them, expecting them to act responsibly. Sexuality education was integrated in school curriculum at all grade levels and convenient access to free or low-cost contraception along with sexual health information and services to the youth was provided. This caused the young people to believe it is "stupid and irresponsible" to have sex without protection and use the maxim, "safer sex or no sex". Active role of families in providing open, honest and consistent discussions with teens about sexuality was encouraged. The adults accepted sexual relationships as normal and natural for older adolescents, which is a positive component of emotionally healthy maturation.

The policy makers in the government recognized that interference of political and religious bodies in the formulation of public health policy should be avoided and these decisions should be based on findings of authentic research. The role of media as a partner in the massive, consistent, long-term public education campaigns to propagate information was recognized as the major impetus to solve the issues is the presence of a national desire to do so. Differences in culture and values of their immigrant populations from their own was also recognized and addressed separately.

Programs for prevention of teen pregnancy

Adolescents are at high risk for unintended pregnancy, with its associated maternal morbidity and mortality, and infection with HIV and other STI's, implementation of effective programs is essential. Programs are formulated and implemented to reduce the behavioral risks and improve their sexual health outcomes. Since the risk factors for pregnancy are diverse, so are the programs that have been developed to combat the problem. The risk factors for teen pregnancy can be considered to be either sex related or nonsexual. Therefore, there are three types of programs that can be implemented: those that focus on sexual risk factors, those that focus on non-sexual risk factors and those that do both.

Programs that focus on ***sexual risk behaviors*** *include*:

1. Abstinence only programs
2. Sex education programs
3. Clinic or school-based programs to provide reproductive health care or to improve access to contraception

Programs that focus on ***non-sexual risk factors*** *include:*

1. Youth development programs
2. Vocational and educational programs

Programs that focus on both ***sexual and non-sexual risk factors*** include both sexuality and youth development components.

The programs need to stress on positive behavior changes among youth (like delay in the initiation of sexual intercourse, increase in abstinence/reduction in the frequency of sexual intercourse, reduction in the number of sex partners/increase in monogamy, increase in the use or consistency of use of effective methods of contraception, increase in the use or consistency of use of condoms/reduction in the incidence of unprotected sex). All the programs should include a comprehensive sex education program providing information about abstinence, the use of contraception including condoms, contraceptive supplies, and/or referral to sexual health services. An extensive involvement of mass media strategies to reinforce the sexual health messages and encourage youth to make healthy decisions about sex is used.

The programs treat the youth holistically, acknowledging their sexual development as normal and offer them community-wide support for making healthy decisions about sex. Such programs have shown effectiveness in reducing the rates of pregnancy and STI's including HIV in the youth.

Programs based on holistic approach are effective

A World Health Organization review of 35 studies found that the programs most effective in changing young peoples behavior are those that address abstinence, contraception and STD prevention.[50] The CDC confirms that "the dual approach of delaying first intercourse among all adolescents and increasing condom use among those who are sexually active has succeeded in reducing overall risk through improvements in both behaviors."[51] Research has shown that balanced programs that discuss both abstinence and contraception, including condoms — do not increase sexual intercourse among teens.[52]

In a United Nations review of 68 studies on the effects of sexual health education on young peoples sexual behavior, "little evidence was found to support the contention that sexual health and HIV education promote promiscuity."[53] It is observed that education about both abstinence and contraception is effective in delaying the onset of first sexual intercourse and in ensuring that young people protect themselves when they become sexually active.[54-60]

Abstinence and contraceptive use

The typical age of sexual initiation among teenagers in the developed countries is around 17-18 years.[61,62] The declining teen pregnancy rates in the U.S are attributed to their better use of contraception (75%) and increased abstinence (25%).[63] Easy access to contraceptives reduces adolescents' sexual risk behaviors thereby decreasing their risk of infection with HIV or STDs and unintended pregnancy. Also, publicly subsidized contraceptive services have been shown to substantially reduce the number of unintended pregnancies and abortions among teens.

The Centers for Disease Control and Prevention (CDC) attributed the decline in teen birth and pregnancy rates to a declining level of high risk sexual behavior and increased use of contraceptives, especially barrier contraceptives among sexually active youth.[65,66]

Among the sexually active teens, there is increasing awareness and usage of any one contraceptive method at first voluntary sexual intercourse, the rates of usage increasing from 65% in 1988 to 76% in 1995 and two-thirds of males and one-third of females used a barrier contraceptive.[67, 68]

Use of barriers at first intercourse is an important measure of the teens' ability to behave responsibly and plan as they initiate sexual activity.[67] The availability of highly effective, long acting contraceptives has further improved the outlook by preventing unwanted pregnancies.[67]

Emergency contraception: A safe & effective contraceptive option for teens

Although effective use of contraceptives significantly reduces the chances of unintended pregnancies among teens, a vast number of the teenage pregnancies do occur and up to 85% of them are unintended.[69] Emergency contraception (EC) is an important contraceptive option that may prevent 50% of unintended pregnancies and 70% of abortions.[70,71]

It is thus imperative that health care professionals provide adequate information, counseling and access to emergency contraception among the teens. Adolescent women may be provided with an advance EC prescription for future use without requiring to undergo pregnancy test, pelvic exam, Pap smear, or STI/HIV test.

Further, education regarding sexual health has not increased the incidence of early initiation of sexual activity and their knowledge and access to contraception hasn't increased the sexual activity among the youth.[58-60, 72-76]

Research does not support abstinence-only education

In 1996 a program was introduced as an alternative to contraceptives which advocated abstinence as the only means to avert STD's, HIV, and teenage pregnancy by promoting "abstinence-only-until marriage."[77]

Virginity pledges, in early and middle adolescence, delayed the transition to first sex by as much as 18 months. Pledging only worked where some, but not more than about one third, of students pledged. However, when they broke the pledge, these teens were one-third less likely to use contraception at first sex than were their non-pledging peers.[78] It turned out that with respect to pregnancy, pledgers were thus at the same risk as non-pledgers. There is no longterm benefit to pledging in terms of pregnancy reduction, unless pledgers use contraception at first intercourse."

Abstinence-only programs often use fear, guilt and shame as techniques to scare adolescents into 'rejecting sex and contraception. Abstinence-only programs fail to provide honest, accurate information about contraception, if contraception is discussed at all.[79]

There is often a confusion in defining abstinence. Among the youth aged 12 to 17 who had abstinence education, young people's definitions of abstinence included many sexual behaviors while consistently avoiding only (vaginal) intercourse. Similarly, among college students, 37% described oral sex and 24% described anal sex as abstinent behaviors.[80]

Abstinence only programs also fail to address many of the antecedents of early first sexual intercourse.[81] There is no published scientific research demonstrating that abstinence-only programs have actually delayed the onset of intercourse or reduced any other measure of sexual activity among teens.[82]

The National Institute of Health Consensus Panel on AIDS stated that abstinence-only approaches to sexuality education "places policy in direct conflict with science and ignores the overwhelming evidence that other programs are effective."[83]

Successful programs are those that impart accurate, balanced, and realistic sexuality education, promote youth development and provide access to confidential and low-cost contraceptive services.

Essentials for a Program

Key to a successful teen pregnancy prevention program includes involvement of the youth actively in the designing and implementation of the programs. The programs should have clearly defined and realistic goals and objectives (like delayed initiation of sexual intercourse, increased and more effective contraceptive use, reduced rates of pregnancy and childbearing among participants, and/or increased rates of school completion). Community collaboration needs to be encouraged (by involvement of parents, neighborhood organizations, schools, health providers, youth agencies, media, business sector, religious organizations, and policy makers). The programs should be culturally appropriate and sensitive to the racial and ethnic backgrounds of the participants and should create activities that are both age and developmentally appropriate.[84]

Sexuality Education

It is essential to have ongoing sexuality education to prepare the youth for a healthy adult relationship by increasing their knowledge and helping them to explore attitudes, feelings, and values about human development, relationships, dating, gender roles, sexual orientation, sexual behavior, and healthy sexual decision-making. A balanced, realistic sexuality education which includes information on both abstinence and contraception can delay a teens' onset of sexual activity, increase the use of contraception by sexually active teens, and reduce the number of their sexual partners.[85]

Coordinated messages to target both young women and men should be given with an emphasis on joint responsibility, sexual communication, assertiveness, and refusal skills.[86, 87] Information on both abstinence and contraception and access to contraceptive services should be provided.[88] The role of males in family planning settings should be addressed as they are influential in contraceptive use and its acceptance among young women.[85,89,90,91]

High risk teenagers need to be specifically targeted and motivated. Psychosocial counseling, including treatment for sexual abuse, drug and alcohol use, and/or family distress should be addressed.[1,85,92,93]

For achieving these desired results, it needs to be given by sensitive, well-trained, and non-judgmental staff in the setting of schools where the students are taught about protecting themselves against unplanned pregnancy and infection with sexually transmitted diseases (STDs).[94]

The support provided to the youth through these programs should be long-term and consistent. Assurance of confidentiality, easy accessibility with flexible hours and affordability of services is essential. Directive contraceptive education and counseling should be imparted. The health care provider should offer to delay the pelvic examination at the first visit to allay their apprehension.

Youth Development

Youth development programs need to be comprehensive, multifaceted and assist the youth to define goals, complete school, develop life skills, be spiritually grounded and plan their futures. They meet these needs by building on their capacities, assisting them to cultivate their own talents and increasing their feelings of self-worth, and easing their transition to adulthood.[95]

Appropriate mentoring programs, provision of educational opportunities (including tutoring and access to higher education), generation of recreational activities (sports, drama, and social clubs), impartment of vocational and job skills, job placement and community service opportunities help in achieving the desired results.[96,97,98]

SUMMARY

Adolescent sexual health issues, like teen pregnancy and STDs/STIs including HIV, must be addressed with complex prevention efforts, including comprehensive sexuality education that is developmentally appropriate. Programs must take place before young people begin experimenting with sexual behaviors if they are to result in a delay of sexual intercourse. Comprehensive sexuality education is effective in providing adolescents with the tools— the knowledge, the skills, the attitudes and values— to make responsible choices about their sexual health while abstinence-only education to effectively delay the onset of sexual intercourse is ineffective.

Reducing the nation's rate of teen pregnancy is one of the most strategic and direct means available to improve overall child well-being and to reduce persistent child poverty. Teen pregnancy has serious consequences for the teen mother, the child, and to society in general.

Table 1. ***Fertility of Young Women Ages 15 to 19, 1995 & 2020***

Country	*Number of Women (in thousands)*		*Annual Births (per 1,000 women)*		*Births (in thousands)*	
	1995	2020	1995	2020	1995	2020
World	253,809	315,393	60	48	15,313	15,029
Asia, Near East & North Africa	108,346	144,388	66	45	7,180	6,550
India	43,939	54,701	71	41	3,102	2,237
Europe	27,824	25,506	34	3	952	798
United States	8,790	10,325	58	62	511	641

Source: U.S. Bureau of the Census, report ipc/95-1 *Trends in adolescent fertility and contraceptive use in the developing world* by Thomas M. Mc Devitt with Arjun Adlakha, Timothy B. Fowler & Vera Harris-Bourne. U.S. government printing office, Washington, DC, 1996.

REFERENCES

1. Moore KA, Miller BC, Glei D, *et al.*: Adolescent Sex, Contraception and Childbearing: A Review of Recent Research. Washington, DC: Child Trends, 1995.
2. Alan Guttmacher Institute: Sex and America's Teenagers. New York, NY: Alan Guttmacher Institute, 1994.
3. Henshaw SK, U S, Teenage Pregnancy Statistics. New York, NY: Alan Guttmacher Institute, 1996.
4. Darroch JE *et al.*: Adolescent Sexual and Reproductive Health: A Developed Country Comparison. New York, NY: The Alan Guttmacher Institute, forthcoming in Family Planning Perspectives.
5. Boyer D, Fine D: Sexual Abuse as a Factor in Adolescent Pregnancy and Child Maltreatment, *Fam Plann Perspect* 1992; 24 : 4-11.
6. Kirby D, (1999): Looking for Reasons Why: The Antecedents of Adolescent Sexual Risk Taking, Pregnancy, and Childbearing, Washington, DC: National Campaign to Prevent Teen Pregnancy.
7. Kiernan K, (1995): Transition to parenthood: Young Mothers, Young Fathers – Associated Factors and Later Life Experiences, LSE Discussion Paper WSP/113.
8. Botting B, Rosato M and Wood R (1998): Teenage Mothers and the Health of Their Children. Population Trends – Office for National Statistics 93 : 19-28.
9. Berthoud R (2001): Teenage Births to Ethnic Minority Women, Population Trends Summer, 104 : 12-17.
10. Joseph Rowntree Foundation (1995), Social Background and Post-birth Experiences of Young Parents, London: JRF.
11. Kaiser Family Foundation & YM Magazine, National Survey of Teens: Teens Talk about Dating, Intimacy, and Their Sexual Experiences, Menlo Park, CA: The Foundation, 1998.
12. Committee on Unintended Pregnancy, Institute of Medicine; Brown SS, Eisenberg L, Eds. The Best Intentions. Washington, DC, National Academy Press, 1995.
13. Centers for Disease Control and Prevention, Healthy Youth, Health Topics, Sexual Behaviors, Updated 4/26/04, Accessed 5/10/04.
14. Singh S & Darroch J E, (2000): Adolescent Pregnancy and Childbearing: Levels and Trends in Developed Countries, Family Planning Perspectives, 32(1): 14-23.
15. National Center for Health Statistics, Births to Teenagers in the United States, 1940-2000. National Vital Statistics Reports, 9/25/01.

16. National Center for Health Statistics, Births: Final Data for 2002, National Vital Statistics Reports, 12/17/03.
17. The National Campaign to Prevent Teen Pregnancy, Teen Pregnancy—So What? Updated 2/04, Accessed 5/11/04.
18. Brown S, & Eisenberg l (Eds.) (1995): The Best Intentions: Unintended Pregnancy and the well-being of Children and Families, Committee on Unintended Pregnancy, Washington.
19. Sawhill, IV (1998): Teen Pregnancy Prevention: Welfare Reform's Missing Component, Bookings Policy Brief, 38, 1-8.
20. Elam-Evans LD *et al.*: Abortion Surveillance, United States 1999, Morbidity & Mortality Weekly Report, Surveillance Summaries 2002; 51(SS-9):1-28.
21. Centers for Disease Control & Prevention, State-specific Pregnancy and Birth Rates Among Teenagers, United States 1991-92.
22. Morbidity & Mortality Weekly Report 1995; 44 : 677-84.
23. Abma JC *et al.*: Fertility, Family Planning, and Women's Health: New Data from the 1995 National Survey of Family Growth. [Vital & Health Statistics; Series 23, No. 19] Hyattsville, MD: National Center for Health Statistics, 1997.
24. World Health Organization, Unsafe Abortion, Global and Regional Estimates Incidence and Mortality Due to Unsafe Abortion, Geneva: The Organization, 1998.
25. Daulaire N *et al.*: Promises to Keep: The Toll of Unintended Pregnancy on Women's Lives in the Developing World, Washington, DC: Global Health Council, 2002.
26. Alan Guttmacher Institute, Sharing Responsibility: Women, Society & Abortion Worldwide. New York: The Institute, 1999.
27. Shane B: Family Planning Saves Lives, 3rd ed. Washington, DC: Population Reference Bureau, 1997.
28. Martin JA, Hamilton BE, Ventura SJ, Menacker F, Park MM, & Sutton PD (2002), Births: Final Data for 2001, National Vital Statistics Reports, 51 (2).
29. National Center for Health Statistics. Births: Final Data for 2002. National Vital Statistics Reports, 12/17/03.
30. Committee on Unintended Pregnancy, Institute of Medicine; Brown SS, Eisenberg L, Eds. *The Best Intentions*, Washington, DC: National Academy Press, 1995.
31. Maynard, RA (ed.), (1996): Kids having Kids: A Robin Hood Foundation Special Report on the Costs of Adolescent Childbearing, New York: The Robin Hood Foundation.
32. The National Campaign to Prevent Teen Pregnancy (1997). Whatever Happened to Childhood? The Problem of Teen Pregnancy in the United States, Washington, The Costs of Adolescent Childbearing, New York: The Robin Hood Foundation.
33. The National Campaign to Prevent Teen Pregnancy, Not Just Another Single Issue: Teen Pregnancy's Link to Other Critical Social Issues, Washington, D C, 2002.
34. The Annie E, Casey Foundation, 2003 Kids Count Data Book Online, Baltimore, MD, 6/11/03.
35. Kirby D: No Easy Answers: Research Findings on Programs to Reduce Teen Pregnancy, Washington, DC: National Campaign to Prevent Teen Pregnancy, 1997.

36. Bakas C, Zarou DM, de Caprariis PJ: First-trimester Spontaneous Abortions and the Incidence of Human Immunodeficiency Virus Seropositivity, *J Reprod Med*, 1996, 41(1):15-18.

37. Johnstone FD: HIV and Pregnancy. *Br J Obstet Gynaecol*, 1996, 103:1184-1190.

38. Brocklehurst P, French R: The Association between Maternal HIV Infection and Perinatal Outcome: A Systematic Review of the Literature and Meta-analysis, *British Journal of Obstetrics and Gynaecology*, 1998, 105: 839-848.

39. Langston C *et al.*: Excess Intrauterine Fetal Demise Associated with Maternal Human Immunodeficiency Virus Infection, *J Infect Dis*, 1995, 172 : 1451-1460.

40. D' Ubaldo C *et al.*: Association between HIV-1 Infection and Miscarriage: A Retrospective Study, AIDS, 1998, 12(9):1087-93.

41. Shearer WT *et al.*: Early Spontaneous Abortion and Fetal Thymic Abnormalities in Maternal-to-fetal HIV Infection, *Acta Pediatr*, 1997, Suppl 421 : 60-64.

42. Couturier E, Brossard Y, Larsen C, Larsen M, Du Mazaubrun C, Paris-Llado J, Gillot R, Henrion R, Breart G, Brunet JB: HIV Infection at Outcome of Pregnancy in the Paris Area, France, Lancet. 1992 Sep 19; 340(8821) : 707-9.

43. Taha TET *et al.*: The Effect of Human Immunodeficiency Virus Infection on Birthweight, and Infant and Child Survival in Urban Malawi, *Int J epidemiol*, 1995, 24:1022-1028.

44. Bergstrom S *et al.*: HIV Infection and Maternal Outcome of Pregnancy in Mozambican Women: A Case Control Study. *Genitourin Med*, 1995, 71 : 323-324.

45. Temmerman M *et al.*: Infection with HIV as a Risk Factor for Adverse Pregnancy Outcome. AIDS, 1990, 4 : 139-144.

46. Bulterys M *et al.*: Fatal Complications after Caesarian Section in HIV-Infected Women. AIDS, 1996, 10(8) : 923-924.

47. Semprini AE *et al.*: The Incidence of Complications after Caesarean Section in 156 HIV-Positive Women. AIDS, 1995, 9 : 913-917.

48. Minkoff HL *et al.*: Serious Infections During Pregnancy Among Women with Advanced Human Immunodeficiency Virus Infection, *Am J Obstet Gynecol*, 1990, 162:30-34.

49. Berne L and Huberman B, European Approaches to Adolescent Sexual Behaviour & Responsibility, Washington, DC: Advocates for Youth, 1999.

50. Grunseit A and S Kippax: Effects of Sex Education on Young Peoples Sexual Behaviour. Geneva: World Health Organization, 1993.

51. Centers for Disease Control and Prevention, Morbidity and Mortality Weekly Report, 47 (36): 749-52, September 18, 1998.

52. Kirby D, School-Based Programs to Reduce Sexual Risk-Taking Behaviors: Sexuality and HIV/AIDS Education, Health Clinics, and Condom Availability Programs, Santa Cruz, CA : 1994.

53. Joint United Nations Programme on HIV/AIDS, Impact of HIV and Sexual Health Education on the Sexual Behavior of Young People: A Review Update, 1997.

54. Baldo M *et al.*: Does Sex Education Lead to Earlier or Increased Sexual Activity in Youth? Presented at the IXth International Conference on AIDS, Berlin, 6-10 June 1993. Geneva, Switzerland: World Health Organization, 1993.

55. UNAIDS, Impact of HIV and Sexual Health Education on the Sexual Behaviour of Young People: A Review Update. [UNAIDS Best Practice Collection, Key Material] Geneva, Switzerland: UNAIDS, 1997.
56. UNAIDS, Young People and HIV/AIDS: Opportunity in Crisis. Geneva, Switzerland: UNAIDS, 2002.
57. Institute of Medicine, Committee on HIV Prevention Strategies in the United States: No Time to Lose: Getting More from HIV Prevention, Washington, DC, National Academy Press, 2001.
58. Kirby D: Emerging Answers: Research Findings on Programs to Reduce Teen Pregnancy. Washington, DC: National Campaign to Prevent Teen Pregnancy, 2001.
59. Newton N, Applying Best Practices to Youth Reproductive Health. [Lessons Learned from SEATS' Experience] Arlington, VA: John Snow, SEATS Project, 2000.
60. FOCUS on Young Adults. Advancing Young Adult Reproductive Health: Actions for the Next Decade: End of Program Report, Washington, DC 2001.
61. Darroch JE *et al.*: Differences in Teenage Pregnancy Rates Among Five Developed Countries: The Roles of Sexual Activity and Contraceptive Use, *Fam Plann, Perspect* 2001; 33:244-50.
62. Rademakers J: Sex Education Research in the Netherlands. Paper presented to the European Study Tour, Utrecht, Netherlands: NISSO, 2001.
63. Darroch JE, Singh S, Why Is Teenage Pregnancy Declining? The Roles of Abstinence, Sexual Activity, and Contraceptive Use, [Occasional Report, No. 1] New York: Alan Guttmacher Institute, 1999.
64. Forrest JD, Samara R: Impact of Publicly Funded Contraceptive Services on Unintended Pregnancies and Implications for Medicaid Expenditures. Family Planning Perspectives 1996; 28:188-195.
65. Centers for Disease Control and Prevention, State-specific Birth Rates for Teenagers, United States 1990-1996. Morbidity & Mortality, Weekly Report 1997; 46 : 837-842.
66. Saul R: Teen Pregnancy: Progress Meets Politics, Guttmacher Report on Public Policy, 1999; 2 (3).
67. Abma JC, Sonenstein FL: Teenage Sexual Behavior and Contraceptive Use: An Update. Paper Presented to the American Enterprise Institute for Public Policy Research. Washington, DC: The Institute, 1998.
68. Kaufmann RB, Spitz AM, Strauss LT, Morris L, Santelli JS *et al.*: The Decline in U S teen Pregnancy Rates, 1990-1995, *Pediatrics* 1998; 102: 1141-1147.
69. Society for Adolescent Medicine, Provision of Emergency Contraception to Adolescents: Position Paper of the Society for Adolescent Medicine. *Journal of Adolescent Health* 2004; 35 : 66-70.
70. Society for Adolescent Medicine, Provision of Emergency Contraception to Adolescents: Position Paper of the Society for Adolescent Medicine, *Journal of Adolescent Health* 2004; 35: 66-70.
71. Trussell J *et al.*: Emergency Contraceptive Pills: A Simple Proposal to Reduce Unintended pregnancies, Family Planning Perspectives 1992; 24:269-73.

72. Marsiglio W, Mott FL: The Impact of Sex Education on Sexual Activity, Contraceptive Use and Premarital Pregnancy Among American Teenagers. *Fam Plann Perspect* 1986; 18:151-162.

73. Baldo M *et al.*: Does Sex Education Lead to Earlier or Increased Sexual Activity in Youth? Presented at the IXth International Conference on AIDS, Berlin, 6-10 June 1993, Geneva, Switzerland: World Health Organization, 1993.

74. UNAIDS, Impact of HIV and Sexual Health Education on the Sexual Behaviour of Young People: A Review Update, [UNAIDS Best Practice Collection, Key Material] Geneva, Switzerland: UNAIDS, 1997.

75. UNAIDS. Young People and HIV/AIDS: Opportunity in Crisis. Geneva, Switzerland: UNAIDS, 2002.

76. Institute of Medicine, Committee on HIV Prevention Strategies in the United States. No Time to Lose: Getting More from HIV Prevention, Washington DC, National Academy Press, 2001.

77. The Personal Responsibility and Work Opportunity Reconciliation Act of 1996. (P.L. 104-193, August 22, 1996.)

78. Bearman PS, Brückner H: Promising the Future: Virginity Pledges as They Affect Transition to First Intercourse, New York: Columbia University, 2000.

79. Planned Parenthood Federation of America, Inc. Fact sheet: Helping Young People to Delay Sexual Intercourse, 1997.

80. Remez L: Oral Sex among Adolescents: Is It Sex or Is It abstinence? *Fam Plann Perspect*, 2000; 32 : 298-304. [Letter], New York: Columbia University, 2002.

81. Haffner D, Whats Wrong with Abstinence – Only Sexuality Education Programs? SIECUS Report, 25 (4), April/May 1997.

82. Kirby D, No Easy Answers: Research Findings on Programs to Reduce Teen Pregnancy. Washington DC, National Campaign to Prevent Teen Pregnancy, 1997.

83. National Institutes of Health, Consensus Development Conference Statement, February 11-13, 1997.

84. Girls Incorporated, *Truth, Trust and Technology: New Research on Preventing Adolescent Pregnancy*. Indianapolis IN: Girls Inc. 1991.

85. Grunseit A, Kippax S, Aggleton P, Baldo M, Slutkin O: Sexuality Education and Young People's Sexual Behaviour: A Review of Studies. *Journal of Adolescent Research* 1997; 12 : 421-453.

86. Howard M, McCabe JB: Helping Teenagers Postpone Sexual Involvement. *Fam Plann Perspect* 1990; 22: 21-26.

87. Kirby D, Barth RP, Leland N, Fetro JV: Reducing the Risk: Impact of a New Curriculum on Sexual Risk-taking. *Fam Plann Perspect*, 1991; 23: 253-263.

88. Frost JJ, Forrest JD: Understanding the Impact of Effective Teenage Pregnancy Prevention Programs. *Fam Plann Perspect*, 1995; 27: 188-195.

89. Brindis C, *Adolescent Pregnancy Prevention: A Guidebook for Communities*. Palo Alto Calif: Health Promotion Resource Center, Stanford Center for Research in Disease Prevention, 1991.

90. Nathanson C, Becker MH: The Influence of Client-Provider Relationships on Teenage Women's Subsequent Use of Contraception, *Amer J Pub Health* 1985; 75 : 33-38.

91. Armstrong KA, Stover MA: Smart Start: An option for adolescents to Delay the Pelvic Examination and Blood Work in Family Planning Clinics. *J Adolesc Health* 1994; 15 : 389-395.

92. Berenson AB, San Miguel VV, Wilkinson GS: Violence and Its Relationship to Substance Use in Adolescent Pregnancy, *J Adolesc Health* 1992; 13: 470-74.

93. Boyer D, Fine D: Sexual Abuse as a Factor in Adolescent Pregnancy and Child Maltreatment. *Fam Plann Perspect*, 1992; 24: 4-11.

94. Advocates for Youth and Sexuality Information & Education Council of the United States. [Poll on America's Attitudes toward Sexuality Education.] Conducted by Hickman-Brown Research for Advocates and the Council between February 23 and March 3, 1999, Washington, DC: Hickman-Brown, 1999.

95. Pagliaro S, Klindera K, Youth Development: Strengthening Prevention Strategies. [Issues at a Glance] Washington, DC: Advocates for Youth, 1999.

96. Philliber S, Allen JP: Life Options and Community Service: Teen Outreach Program. In Miller BC, Card JJ, Paikoff RL, Peterson JL, *Preventing Adolescent Pregnancy: Model Programs and Evaluations.* Newbury Park, CA: Sage Publications, 1992.

97. Tiemey JP, Grossman JB, Resch NL: *Making a Difference: An Impact Study of Big Brother/Big Sisters.* Philadelphia PA: Public/Private Ventures, 1995.

98. Carrera MA, Dempsey P, Philliber W, Philliber S: Evaluating a Comprehensive Pregnancy Prevention Program, *Fam Life Ed* 1992; 11(1) : 4-9.

CHAPTER

7 Adolescence, Substance Abuse and STIs

Pragti Chhabra

INTRODUCTION

Adolescence is a period of dynamic transition in which many interrelated changes of body, mind and social relationships take place. The adolescent's body develops in size, strength, stamina and reproductive capacity and becomes more sexually defined; psychologically, adolescents begin to become more capable of abstract thinking, foresight, empathy and internal control. The non-medical use of chemical substances in order to achieve alterations in psychological functioning is termed as substance abuse. It could be licit substances e.g. tobacco and alcohol or illicit substances e.g. heroin, cocaine. The common substances of abuse are as given in the Table.[1, 2]

Class	*Examples*
CNS depressants	Alcohol, hypnotics, anti anxiety drugs
CNS stimulants	Amphetamines, cocaine
Opiates	Opium, Heroin, Morphine, Buprenorphine
Cannabinols	Ganja, Bhang, Charas
Hallucinogens	LSD, Mescaline, Psilocybin
Solvents	Petrol, paint thinner, glues
Other drugs	Antihistaminics, cough syrups
Nicotine	Tobacco and tobacco products

Substance use is increasing around the world. Tobacco, inhalants, cannabis products, alcohol and stimulants are most commonly abused drugs by adolescents in the West. In a study among pupils of the United Kingdom almost all had drunk alcohol, 36% had smoked cigarettes in the past 30 days, 42.3% had at some time used illicit drugs, mainly cannabis. Cigarette smoking was more common among girls than boys. The Youth Risk Behaviour Surveillance Study (YRBS) of the Centre for Disease Control and Prevention provide the most consistent and recent data on substance abuse by youth in the United States. The most widely used drugs among American youth from all ethnic and socio-cultural backgrounds are alcohol, tobacco and marijuana. The age group with the highest rates of illicit drug use is the 18-25 years old age group. Cocaine use peaked in 1979 while use of heroin, methamphetamine and club drugs increased in the 1990s. Poly drug use and abuse also increased in the 1990s. The extent and pattern of substance abuse among children and adolescents in India is different from the West.[1, 3] There has been a rapid change in the production, consumption and administration pattern of drug use in the developing world, especially in South and South-east Asia. Tobacco, alcohol, cannabis and raw opium have been the traditional substances of abuse in India. These are being replaced by synthetic and semi-synthetic drugs of abuse. The biggest threat besides heroin use is the use of pharmaceutical substances viz. Buprenorphine, Diazepam, anti-Histaminics and cough syrups containing codeine. Countries in the Indian subcontinent as well as different metropolitan cities of India are experiencing an increase in injection drug use. Different substances such as heroin, Buprenorphine and Dextropropoxyphene have been reported to be used by injection drug users.

Adolescence is a time of exposure and vulnerability to substance use. Experimenting drugs is a frequent phenomenon. For some adolescents, the improper use of substances will only be part of his or her development, ceasing as the adolescence matures. Others however will develop problematic usage, which may interrupt the normal process of adolescence and bring about severe consequences to the lives of these individuals.

Consumption of licit and illicit substances has increased all over the world and the age of initiation of abuse is progressively falling. Studies in student youth in India show that alcohol is the most abused followed by tobacco and tranquilizers. A multi-centered study in 1985 showed that the prevalence of alcohol abuse was 10-15%, tobacco was 8-15% and tranquilizers 1-.5%. No opiates were reported in the 1980's[4]. Most studies in the 1990's show escalation of intravenous drug use and the use of propoxyphene, diazepam, promethazin and pheniramine. Drug use is mostly seen in men. Majority are introduced between 15 to 21 years of age. No social class or ethnic group is immune. Khushwala et al. reported in a study among adolescents the overall prevalence of abuse of psychoactive substances to be 25% in slum area and 18% in college students. Abuse of tobacco was most prevalent while cannabis was used by 0.6% of the subjects[5]. In a medical college of Delhi, about one third reported alcohol use, one fourth smoked while very few reported drug use. Boys, hostellers and those educated in public schools were more likely to use these substances[6]. In a population-based study the prevalence of tobacco, alcohol, cannabis and opioid use among males was 27.6, 1.6, 0.3 and 0.4 per cent, respectively. The rates were highest in resettlement clusters followed by urban villages, unauthorized and regularized clusters. Studies in the north-eastern states and Bihar have shown an alarmingly high frequency of tobacco use .The current tobacco use, both smoking and smokeless in any form in these states ranged from 50.4% to 74.4% while in girls it ranged from 32% to 56.4%. The frequency of smoking among boys ranged from 28.6% to 40.8% and that of girls from 8.9% to 28.2%. The school students knew very little about the ill effects of tobacco use and the schools did not include much in its curriculum to educate students on ill effects of tobacco use.[7,8]

Street children and those who live and work under inhuman conditions are at high risk of substance abuse.[7] A study among adolescents in an urban slum of Lucknow, one third of the boys were smokers and the mean age of initiation was12.3 years, 13 per cent of the boys consumed alcohol while two reported intake of opiod and marijuana each.[8] A recent study in an observation home in Delhi showed that more than half of the boys aged 6-16 years had indulged in substance abuse. The agents consumed were nicotine (44.5%), inhalants (24.3%), alcohol (21.8%) and cannabis (26.4%)[9]. In a study among drug users in Kolkata the mean age of initiating drug use was 18 years, range being 8-40 years. Hashish was the 'gateway substance' with which majority of drug users initiated the habit. Injecting drug users belonged to a higher age group, were married and had a higher educational level. In a study among women drug users in Manipur, the age range of 17-30 years was reported for initiation of drug use. Most reported use of alcohol prior to using other drugs.

Risk Factors

Most drug users are initiated into drug use in the second decade of life. The reasons cited are curiosity, pleasure seeking and personal or family problems. The presence of a parent or other relative with substance abuse in the family is the most influential factor for substance abuse. Lack of achievement and poor self esteem are important correlates for substance abuse. Children living in disturbed family relations like parental separation, divorce are more prone to experiment substance use. Other risk factors are peer drug use, social isolation and unconventional behaviour patterns. In an observation home in Delhi, substance use was significantly associated with domestic violence, maltreatment of the child, nuclear families, running away from home and working status of the child.[9] Studies from other countries have also shown that family characteristics like parent's divorce, relation with parents, drug user in household etc. to be important factors associated with drug use among adolescents.[12,13] Drug use is more in the older adolescents. Personality patterns exhibited by children with substance dependence include behavioral deviance, delinquency, violence, vandalism and hostility.

Material affection and family support, non-substance abusing family members and peers, healthy behaviour patterns like involvement in work, studies, sports, religion etc. and personal characteristics of self acceptance, self esteem and low aggression act as protective factors against substance abuse.

Substance Abuse and Sexual Behaviour

Studies have shown that adolescents who engage in one problem behaviour are more likely to engage in other. Adolescents who use drugs are more likely to be sexually active and thus at a greater risk of contacting STD and HIV. Illicit drug use and alcohol consumption are risk factors for unsafe behaviour among heterosexuals and homosexuals. Studies have shown that a substantial number of drug users practice high risk sexual behaviour and should be targeted for intervention These substances include alcohol, amphetamines, amyl nitrites, cocaine and 'club drugs' such as ecstasy (3,4-metylene dioxymethamphetamine (MDMA)) and gamma hydroxybutyrate (GHB). Non-injection substance use is highly prevalent among men having sex with men. A probability sample of urban US MSM found that many participants reported using alcohol (85%) and non-injection drugs (51%) in the prior 6 months. Use of alcohol to intoxication and increased frequency of heroin and cocaine in both men and women was associated with unsafe sexual behaviour. The high-risk behaviour includes men having sex with men, multiple sexual partners, not using condoms, exchange of money or drugs for sex, partner exchanging money or drugs for sex. Almost half reported use of either alcohol or illicit drugs or both every time before having sex with casual partners.[14, 15] The casual relation between substance abuse and sexual risk remains unclear. Association between substance abuse and risk may be due to effects of age and relationship status on both substance abuse and risk. Personality disposition may also motivate people toward both substance use and risky behaviour. Substance abuse may per se enhance risk, independent of a person's stable characteristics or interact with personal characteristics such that risk is increased. In a study among a cohort of men who have sex with men, use of poppers, amphetamines, or sniffed cocaine as well as heavy alcohol use in the prior 6 months were independently associated with unprotected anal intercourse. In the conditional analysis, after controlling for partner level characteristics, consumption of six or more alcoholic drinks use of poppers, amphetamines, or sniffed cocaine just before or during sex was independently associated with unprotected anal intercourse.

Knowledge of behavioural risks for AIDS does not prompt all at risk to change their behaviour. Educators need to move beyond imparting knowledge about modes of HIV transmission to change adolescent behaviour. Persons who believe they are personally susceptible to HIV exposure, the consequences of exposure are severe, protective measures such as condom use are effective in preventing transmission, and perceive few barriers to the adoption of condom use may be more likely to adopt such behaviour to avoid HIV transmission. In a study among Massachusetts 16-19 year olds, respondents who believed condoms are effective in preventing HIV transmission and worried they can get AIDS were 3.1 and1.8 times, respectively, more likely to use condoms all the time.[16]

There are not many Indian studies relating to substance abuse and sexual behaviour in adolescence. A study among college students in Chandigarh showed that 15% of the students were sexually active. Eighty-four were heterosexual, 7.3% homosexual and 8.7% bisexual. Thirty seven per cent of heterosexuals and 3% of homosexuals had more than one partner. Condom use was 24% in heterosexuals, 11% in bisexuals and 7% in homosexuals. Hepatitis B infection was also studied as it indicates the risk of spread of Human immunodeficiency virus. There was a striking male preponderance among drug users and the sexually active.[17] This has been observed in other studies that males are prone to high- risk behaviour even in adolescence. Fifteen per cent consumed alcohol, but only 1.6% were addicted to other drugs. In urban slums of Lucknow, about 7.7 per cent of the boys had indulged in pre-marital sex. Cigarette smokers, alcohol drinkers or both had a crude OR of 5.1, 2.7 and 4.9 respectively for having sex.[8] In a study amongst adolescent truck cleaners about one-fourth of the cleaners had a history of sexual activity, commonly with prostitutes. Majority of these had engaged in unprotected sexual intercourse. Substance abuse was fairly common in these adolescents.[19] HIV was first described among injecting drug users in Manipur in 1989.[20] The sharing of injecting equipment during drug use has been one of the reasons for the rapid spread of HIV in injecting drug users as well as in other population groups in some geographical regions. More than 50 per cent of both injecting and non-injecting drug users reported having sex with sex workers amongst the urban poor of Kolkata. Condom use was insignificant while 74% of the IDUs reported sex with female sex workers and 15% of the male IDUs also reported having sex with men. The number of partners varied from 1-3 in number. Majority (71%) reported sharing injection equipment within the last six months although they perceived it to be dangerous.[10, 21] In Manipur, eighty per cent of the women drug users had sex with non-regular partners, two thirds of the injectors and non-injectors reported 'sex work' in exchange for money or drugs. Condom use with non-regular partners was inconsistent. Most of the women screened for STIs were asymptomatic while on examination 81% had abnormal vaginal discharge.[11] The HIV seropositivity rate was significantly higher in injecting drug users as compared to non-injecting drug users although HBsAg positivity was not significantly different.

At a deaddiction center at Delhi most of the subjects were intravenous drug users who injected morphine, pethidine, opium etc. more than one third of the subjects indulged in extramarital sex. Of these about one fourth had sex with sex workers, 70% reported having sex when intoxicated. Majority preferred heterosexual partners while a few homosexual partners. Re-use of syringes was common.[22] In another study in Delhi drug users were more likely to have multiple risk partners, visit commercial sex workers and have anal intercourse. The average number of sexual partners was also higher among the drug-users as compared to non-drug users. Sexually transmitted disease prevalence was also higher among the drug users.[23]

Adolescents, Substance Use and Condom Use

Increasing condom use among adolescents is an essential component of a public health strategy aimed at decreasing rates of sexually transmitted infections and the spread of human immunodeficiency virus infection. The condom use among adolescents in the western countries is increasing, but in groups who may be at highest risk for HIV and STDs it is quiet low.[24] Among residents of a Texas crisis shelter for runaway and homeless youths about one-third had never or rarely used condoms, and 42.4% did so 'sometimes'.[25] In a study, less than 25% of young men who reported intravenous drug use or sex with an intravenous drug user or had sex with a prostitute, reported condom use during the most recent episode of heterosexual intercourse.[26]

Adolescents who drank five or more drinks daily or who smoked marijuana five or more times in the past month were less likely to have used condoms in the Massachusetts study.[16] Adolescents with greater number of lifetime partners are also at greater risk for

STDs. Studies have shown that condom use is inversely related to number of lifetime partners.[24] Sixteen per cent of adolescents who used condom when not drinking reported using them less often after consuming alcohol and 25 per cent after drug use.[16] Similar findings have been reported among adult homosexuals, heavy drinkers were less likely to have used condoms themselves or to have partners who use them during anal intercourse than did moderate drinkers.

Prevention of Substance Abuse

Smoking and Alcohol Use

Cigarette smoking is linked to more than a million premature deaths each year worldwide. The relationship between smoking and increased risks to health has served as the basis to control the 'world smoking epidemic' particularly among young people.

Legislation: different regulatory measures in legislation are:

- Control of advertising and sale promotion
- Health warnings and statement of tar and nicotine contents of cigarettes
- Control of harmful substances in tobacco
- Restrictions on sales
- Restrictions on smoking and alcohol use in public places
- Restrictions on smoking and alcohol use in workplace
- Preventing young people from smoking and alcohol use
- Mandatory health education on smoking and alcohol use
- Fiscal and economic measures prohibits the sale or other provision of alcoholic beverages to persons below a certain age.

The fact that certain modes of behaviour are endemic to adolescence like experimentation, rebellion and other sociological and psychological reasons that induce the young to smoke make them impervious to laws.

Health Education: broad based anti-smoking and alcohol education campaigns for young people that include dangers of smoking and alcohol use have far reaching effects in prevention of smoking and alcohol use in the young.

Drug Use

Prohibition: provision of laws applicable to possession, selling, supplying and distribution are most relevant to adolescents.

Educational measures: promotion of awareness of the consequences of drug use and abuse are one of the mainstays of the preventive approach. It is based on the premise that education on drug use will deter drug use. It is aimed at sensitizing the public, and in particular to the most vulnerable to the adverse consequences of drug abuse.

Drug use prevention programmes are more cost effective than other interventions if properly carried out. Drug use prevention programme is targeted at both users and non-users and aimed at creating an environment where non-users are induced not to start drug use, while users are inspired to discontinue or reduce drug use. A prevention activity could be done practically in every place one can think of such as home, neighbourhood, school, workplace, religious place etc. Many people should participate for it to be effective. Prevention should not rely on shock tactics which was popular all over the world some times ago. Young people with attitudes and beliefs favourable to drug use are more likely to use them than are young people with unfavourable or neutral attitudes. Strengthening negative attitudes towards drug use or shifting attitudes from neutral to negative is easier than reversing positive attitudes. The main target is getting younger and younger for drug use prevention programmes. The simple purpose of primary prevention is to communicate message to prevent non- user from starting drug use. The message should influence not only knowledge and attitude but also behaviour.

School based programme: children and young people are vulnerable to drug use. But youth is also a period during which knowledge, beliefs, attitudes, values and skills are acquired. Development of effective education programme that will help individual practice of risk reduction behaviour is a primary avenue for prevention of drug use and other health related problems among school youth.

Community based programmes: have an effect on delaying onset and decreasing prevalence rates. Most of the community-based programmes emphasize less on medical approach and more on psychological methods of treatment. These should include health education and counseling, health promotion, demand reduction, harm minimization, life skills training, behaviour self regulation and rehabilitation.[27]

Treatment and Rehabilitation: motivation for treatment is a key factor in success of the treatment. Confidentiality should be maintained and voluntary access should be encouraged. Long-term treatment is not only a medical problem but also needs cooperation of psychologists and sociologists.

Steps in medical care include:

Identification of drug addicts and their motivation for detoxification

Detoxification (requires hospitalization)

Post detoxification counseling and follow-up based on clinic and home visits

Rehabilitation:

In India, the Narcotic Drugs and Psychotropic Substances (NDPS) Act, 1985 provides the framework for drug abuse control.

- the act deals with supply reduction activities
- provision for health care of drug dependent individuals.

It authorizes the Central Government to take necessary measures for identification, treatment, aftercare, rehabilitation and prevention education. As a follow up of the Act, the Narcotics Control Bureau (NCB) was created in 1986 to coordinate all activities for administration and enforcement of the Act.

REFERENCES

1. UNDCP World Drug Report, New York; Oxford University Press Inc. 1997.
2. Tripathi BM, Lal R: Substance Abuse in Children and Adolescents. *Ind J Pediatr* 1999; 66 : 569-75.
3. Mc Miller P, Plant M: Drinking, Smoking and Illicit Drug Use Among 15 and 16 Year Olds in the United Kingdom, *B M J* 1996; 313 : 394-7.
4. Mohan D, Sundaram K, Ray *et al.*: Multi-centered Study of Drug Abuse Among University Students, Report Submitted to Ministry of Welfare, Govt. of India, 1987.
5. Kushwaha KP, Singh YD, Rathi AK *et al.*: Prevalence and Abuse of Psychoactive Substances in Children and Adolescents, *Ind J Pediatr* 1992; 59 : 261.
6. Grover V, Aggarwal OP, Kumar P: Prevalence and Pattern of Tobacco, Alcohol and Drug Abuse Among Students of University College of Medical Sciences, Delhi.
7. The Global Youth Tobacco Survey Collaborative Group. Tobacco Use Among Youth: A Cross-country Comparison. Tobacco Control 2002; 11 : 252-270.
8. Sinha DN, Gupta PC, Pednekar MS: Tobacco Use Among Students in the Eight North-Eastern States of India. *Ind J Cancer* 2003; 40 : 43-59.
9. Mohan D, Chopra A, Sethi H: A Rapid Assessment Study on Prevalence of Substance Abuse Disorders in Metropolis Delhi. *Ind J Med Res* 2001; 114 : 107-14.
10. Awasthi S, Pande VK, Sexual Behaviour Patterns and Knowledge of Sexually Transmitted Diseases in Adolescent Boys in Urban Slums of Lucknow, North India. *Indian Pediatr* 1998; 35 : 1105-09.
11. Pagare D, Meena GS, Singh MM, Saha R: Risk Factors of Substance Abuse Among Street Children from Delhi, *Ind Pediatr* 2004; 41 : 221-26.
12. Panda S, Saha U, Pahari S *et al.*: Drug Use Among the Urban Poor in Kolkata: Behaviour and Environment Correlates of Low HIV Infection, *Natl Med J India* 2002; 15 : 128-34.
13. Bijaya AL, Sadhana Devi N, Foley E: Interface Between Drug Use and Sex Work in Manipur. *Natl Med J India* 2001; 14 : 209-211.
14. Patton LH: Adolescent Substance Abuse: Risk Factors and Protective Factors, *Ped Clin N Amer* 1995; 42: 283.
15. Tavres BF, Beria JU, Silva de Lima M: Factors Associated with Drug Use Among Adolescent Students in Southern Brazil, Rev Sade Publica 2004; 38 : 1-9.

16. Seidman SN, Sterk-Elifson C, Aral SO: High-risk Sexual Behaviour Among Drug Using Men. Sexually Transmitted Diseases1994; 21: 173-180.
17. Colfax G, Vittinghoff E, Husnik M J *et al*.: Substance Use and Sexual Risk: A Partcipant and Episode Level Analysis Among a Cohort of Men who have Sex with Men, *Am J Epidemiol* 2004; 159 : 1002-1012.
18. Hingson RW, Strunn L, Berlin BM, Heeren T: Beliefs About AIDS, Use of Alcohol and Drugs and Unprotected Sex Among Massachusetts Adolescents. *Am J Pub Hlth* 1990; 80 : 295-299.
19. Kaur U, Sahni SP, Bambery P *et al*.: Sexual Behaviour, Drug Use and Hepatitis B Infection in Chandigarh Students, *National Med J India* 1996; 9: 156-159.
20. Islam SK, Hossain KJ, Kamal M, Ahsan M: Prevalence of HIV Infection in Drug Addicts of Bangladesh: Drug Habit, Sexual Practice and Lifestyle, *Int J STD AIDS* 2003; 14 : 76-4.
21. Bansal RK: Sexual Behaviour and Substance Use Patterns Amongst Adolescent Truck Cleaners and Risk of HIV/AIDS, *Indian J Matern Child Health* 1992; 108-10.
22. Sarkar S, Das N, Panda S *et al*.: Rapid Spread of HIV Among Injecting Drug Users in North-Eastern States of India, *Bull Nutr* 1993; 14 : 91-105.
23. Panda S, Chatterjee A, Bhattacharjee S, Ray B, Saha MK, Bhattacharya SK: HIV, Hepatitis B and Sexual Practices in the Street-recruited Injecting Drug Users of Calcutta: Risk Perception Versus Observed Risks. *International J STD and AIDS*, 1998; 9 : 214-218.
24. Grover VL, Ghosh A, Kannan AT, Singh J: Sexual Behaviour of Intravenous Drug Users of Delhi 1997; 27: 83-88.
25. Sharma AK, Aggarwal OP, Dubey KK: Sexual Behaviour of Drug Users: Is it Different? Prev Med 2002; 34: 512-5.
26. Joffe A: Adolescents and Condom Use, A JDC 1993; 147: 746-753.
27. Sugerman ST, Hergenroeder AC, Chacko MR, Parcel GS: Acquired Immunodeficiency Syndrome and Adolescents: Knowledge, Attitudes and Behaviours of Runaway and Homeless Youths. A JDC 1991; 145: 431-436.
28. Sonenstein FL, Pleck JH, Ku LC: Sexual Activity, Condom Use and AIDS Awareness among Adolescent Males, *Fam Plann Perspect*, 1989; 21: 15-158.
29. Drug Demand Reduction Report, New Delhi; UNDCP Regional Office for South Asia. 1998.

CHAPTER

8 Microbiological Aspects of HIV

Dr. (Mrs) N.K. Bhatia

INTRODUCTION

On June 5, 1981, first cases of illness were reported from Los Angeles in five young homosexual men with Pneumocystis carinii pneumonia and other opportunistic infections. In July, 1982, AIDS was reported in hemophiliacs. In January 1983, first cases of AIDS were documented. Later in 1983, cases of AIDS were reported from Central Africa. In mid 1992, state and territorial health department reported over 2,35,000 cases of AIDS and 1,44,000 AIDS related deaths to the Centre for Disease Control. In early 1998, 306 million people worldwide are estimated to be living with AIDS.

AIDS surveillance data along with homologous surveys direct towards controlling HIV infection and provide accurate picture of HIV epidemic December 1, is celebrated as World AIDS Day (WAD) to pay tribute to those who have AIDS and to those who have died of AIDS.

In India, seroprevalence rates are as follows:

High risk group	*Size*	*Seroprevelence rate*
Female sex worker Intravenous drug users	0.5-1 million 15000-50,000	2-30% 30-50%
Intermediate risk group Male and female with multiple sex partners	1-5 million	5 per 1000
Low risk group Male, female and children	800 million	1 per 10000 to 1 per 1000

In India, seroprevalence rate has risen from 102 per thousand in 1992 to 26.2 per thousand in 2000. Maharashtra is leading the tally of positive cases. Seroprevalence is highest in North-eastern state of Manipur with 161.2 per thousand.

There is epidemic of HIV despite progress in clinical science and Highly Active Antiviral therapy (HAART). A long awaited preventive vaccine remains elusive target.

HIV progresses very rapidly in infancy, 50% of infected children die by 2 years of age and more than 90% die by 5 years of age.

In adults about 60% of infected individuals will develop AIDS in 5-10 years and vast majority of infected individuals will develop AIDS eventually.

Patterns of Epidemics

I.	America	Homosexual men I.V. drug users. Since 1980, transmission by heterosexual contact	Infection occurred in late seventies and full blown AIDS in 1980
II.	Sub-Saharan Africa Latin America (specially Caribean Land)	Homosexual promiscuity and perinatal	Spread began in 70's 25% of 20-40 years of age, 90% prostitutes
III.	East Europe Middle East, North Africa, Asia, Australia, New Zealand, India	Heterosexual I.V. drug users	Female sex workers are 2-30% infected I DU 30-50% are infected.

HIV Virus

AIDS is life threatening disease caused by HIV virus which belongs to family Reteroviridae (Re-reverse, tr – transcriptase) subfamily lentivirinae, Genus lentivirus.

Isolation of aetiological agent of AIDS was first reported in May 1983 by Luc Montagnier and colleagues from Pasteur Institute, Paris. They isolated a retrovirus from W. African patient with persistent generalised lymphadenopathy. They called it Lymphadenopathy Associated Virus (LAV).

In March 1984, Robert Gallo and colleagues from National Institute of Health, Bethesda (USA) reported isolation of retrovirus and called it HTLV-3.

In 1986, it was named as HIV. HIV is spherical enveloped virus 90-120 nm in diameter with three layers. In the centre there are two identical copies of SS RNA (92 kb each) associated with reverse transcriptase and surrounded by matrix protein followed by host cell membrane derived lipid bilayer envelope from which projects 72 glycoprotein peplomers.

Two antigenic types of HIV have been identified – HIV_1 which is original LAV/ $HTLV_3$ and HIV_2 which is less virulent strain and was isolated from West Africa in 1985 though sporadic cases have been reported from other parts of the world. HIV_2 appears to be slower than HIV_1 infection. Pandemics occur due to HIV_1. Clinically HIV_1 and HIV_2 are indistinguishable. Most HIVs are variants of HIV_1. HIV_1 has further groups and subtypes HIV_2 is divided into five sub-types (A to E).

This diversity has challenged the development of HIV vaccine.

Animal Lentiviruses

Simian AIDS Virus (SIV) is more closely related to HIV_2 than HIV_1. It causes natural infection in mangabeys, vervets and African green monkeys, SIV infection is asymptomatic in primates.

Nonprimate virus includes Feline T lymphotropic virus (FTLV) which causes AIDS like syndrome in cats.

Bovine lentivirus (BTLV) causes wasting disease with CNS defects in cattle. HIV_1 does not cause disease in animals. Experimental infection in chimpanzees resulted in antibody response but no clinical illness. Rhesus monkey is susceptible to HIV_2 infection.

HIV_1 is divided into 3 groups.

1. HIV – 1 M (Major group)
2. HIV – 1 O (Outlier)
3. HIV – 1 N (New virus)

1. HIV–1 M (Major group)

It comprises eight subtypes (clades) A to H according to molecular sequencing and also four recombinant forms (AE, AG, AG1 and AB). Recombination occurs where multiple clades of virus coexist in same region. Most clades are represented in Sub-Saharan African which indicates HIV originated in African continent.

India has predominantly HIV_1M Subtype C. Subtype C is usually acquired by heterosexual contact. Though Subtype C in South Africa led to explosive homosexual epidemics. Subtype A and B are less frequent. Western countries have HIV_1 M subtype B. Subtype B is associated with homosexuals and Intravenous drug users.

Subtype E prevalent in Thailand.

2. HIV_1 O (Outlier)

It is divided into 9 subtypes

3. HIV_1 N (New virus)

Structure and Genetics Map of HIV

HIV has outer envelope which consists of lipid bilayer with 72 spikes of gp 120 and gp 41. Glycoproteins 120 protrudes out on the surface of virus and gp41 is embedded in lipid matrix.

Interior to lipid bilayer are the matrix, internal capsular and nuclear capsid proteins. Core contains two copies of single stranded RNA and viral enzymes reverse transcriptase, integrase and protease, all essential for viral replication and maturation. Proteins p7 and p9 are bound to the RNA and are believed to be involved in gene expression.

HIV has structural and regulatory genes coding for structural and regulatory products respectively – pol, env and gag are structural genes and others are regulatory genes.

HIV Genome

HIV has three structural genes (gag, pol, env) and five other small non-structural genes – tat, rev, nef, vif, vpr, vpu and vpx.

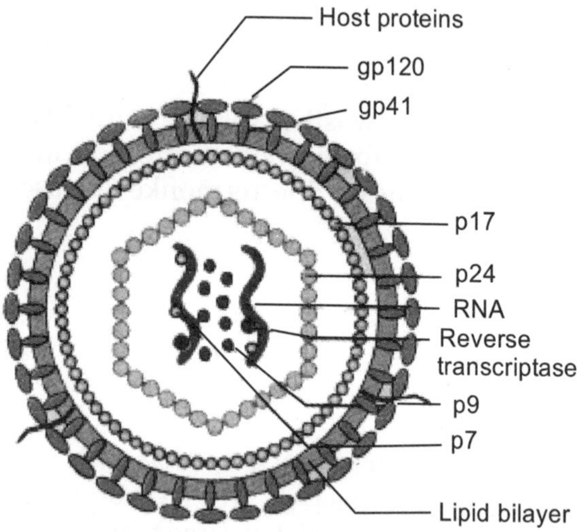

Sketch of HIV virus

Products of these genes act as antigen gag (group specific antigen) genes encodes core or capsid and matrix proteins which is expressed as precursor protein p55. The p55 precursor protein is cleaved into four proteins p17, p7, p9, p24 which constitute core and shell of virus. p24 antigen can be detected in serum during early stage of infection till the appearance of anti p24 antibody. The decline in anti p24 antibody from serum indicates progress of illness and warrants active antiviral therapy, pol gene encodes reverse transcriptase (polymerase), protease, endonuclease, integrase. It is expressed as p100 which is cleaved into 3 proteins Viz. p31, p51 and p64.

env encodes virion envelope peplomer protein and transmembrane protein. It encodes glycoprotein 160 which is cleaved into two envelope components gp120 (surface spike) and gp41 (Transmembrane pedicle protein). The divergence amongst different strains of HIV reside in env gene.

Non-structural and Regulatory Genes

1. tat (transactivation gene) – tat gene specifies a transactivating factor that in collaboration with cellular protein enhances expression of all viral genes by increasing production of active messengers.
2. rev gene (regulation of virus) – It is required for expression of gag, pol and env gene but not tat and rev. gene.
3. nef gene (negative factor) – The nef gene downregulates the transcription of HIV genome by action on its NR (negative regulatory) region. This gene may be responsible for regulation of latent state of virus.
4. Vif (Viral infectivity factor) gene – The gene product of Vif confers infectivity to the virus.
5. Vpr gene
6. Vpu (in HIV_1) and Vpx (in HIV_2)

These genes code for small viral proteins of unknown functions.

HIV_2 displays 40% nucleotide homology with HIV_1, therefore, it is only weakly reactive with HIV_1. HIV_2 differs from HIV in its envelope. The core polypeptides displays some cross reactivity. HIV_2 lacks Vpu gene. It has Vpx gene. HIV_2 is more closely related to simian. Immunodeficiency virus (SIV) with which it has 75% homology.

Major antigens of HIV_1 and HIV_2 are

1. Envelope antigens Spike	HIV_1 gp120	HIV_2 gp140
Transmembrane pedicle	gp41	gp36
2. Matrix protein antigen	p17	p16
3. Capsid protein antegen	p24	p26

Antigenic Variation

Variations of core and envelope antigens of HIV occur frequently. Variations occur due to mutation, deletion and insertion. Even in the same individual there is emergence of variant strain. There are five hypervariable regions in gp120 part of env gene. The greatest diversion amongst different HIV strains is due to env gene (pol and gag are less variable). Main hope for dealing with wide epidemics is development of effective and affordable preventive vaccine.

Resistance

HIV is delicate and thermolabile (inactivated at 50°C in 10 minutes, 56°C in 30 minutes and in one second at 100°C). It can't survive outside living host and live virus survives within blood up to 8 days. It is susceptible to common disinfectants. On the treatment with 35% isopropyl alcohol, 70% ethyl alcohol, 1% lysol, 0.5%formaldehyde, 2% gluteraldehyde, 3% hydrogen peroxide 1% household bleach or sodium hypochlorite, 2.5% Tween 20, it can be inactivated in 10 minutes at room temperature.

Because of lipid membrane, envelope is susceptible to detergents. Therefore standard washing with detergents and hot water are adequate for decontaminating clothes and household utensils. For treatment of medical equipments 2% solution of gluteraldehyde is useful. It withstands lyophilisation hence lyophilized blood product (factor VIII) is heated at 68 °C for 72 hrs and liquid plasma is heated at 60° for 10 hrs.

Mode of Transmission

There are three modes of transmission

1. Sexual
2. Parentral
3. Perinatal

80% of cases are due to sexual mode, 10% are due to parentral and 10% are due to perinatal transmission. Risk is higher in passive (receptive) partner. Sexually transmitted disease like genital ulcers in syphilis, chancroid or herpes facilitate transmission of HIV infection. Risk of transmission in patients with genital discharge caused by gonorrhoea, chlamydial infection, trichomoniasis and vaginosis is four fold. Thus early diagnosis and treatment of STD. contributes to control HIV.

Parentral transmission occurs through blood transfusion. Therefore each unit of blood should be tested for AIDS. If blood is found positive it should be incinerated. Transmission of HIV has been recorded in few recipients of blood transfusion even when blood transfused was found negative for HIV antibodies. This occurs when blood is collected in the window period, that is time between exposure to virus and development of detectable levels of antibody. This period varies between one to three months.

Therefore blood screening is not 100% safe. Infection can also be transmitted by blood products like plasma, serum and cells from HIV positive individual as well as AIDS cases. It can also be transmitted from the donors of bone marrow, semen, organs like cornea, kidney, heart etc. Therefore donors of various fluids and organs should be screened for AIDS. AIDS can be transmitted by syringes. So, HIV is more common in intravenous drug users who share needles and syringes. HIV is also transmitted by use of unsterile needles, needle stick injury and barber's razors. Perinatal (vertical) transmission may occur through placenta before birth. It may also occur from genital secretions during birth and from mother's milk after birth.

Replication of Virus

HIV attaches via gp120 envelope glycoprotein (Surface spike) to CD4 antigen complex which is primary HIV receptor on CD4 + T lymphocytes (helper/inducer) and cells of macrophage lineage. The spikes of gp120 of viral envelope bind to CD4 proteins of T helper lymphocytes. Antibodies to CD4 proteins block the virus binding sites. Attachment to CD4 is not sufficient for viral infection. Second receptor component is probably necessary for viral entry and is mediated by gp 41. All the CD4 protein expressing cells are susceptible to HIV infection like 40% blood monocytes, tissue macrophages, 5-10% B lymphocytes, dentritic cells in lymphnodes, Langerhans cells in skin, microglia in brain, certain muscle and connective tissue cells.

Nucleocapsid of virion enters host cell by pinocytosis and envelope is left behind. After binding of gp120 to CD4 protein gp41 terminus of virus is exposed. Host cell membrane fuses with viral membrane. Infected cell expresses increased level of gp120 proteins on the surface which causes fusion of CD4 proteins of uninfected neighbouring cells and formation of multinucleated syncitial cells. These syncitial cell die leading to depletion of uninfected cells. After entering the cells nucleocapsid releases its RNA into cytoplasm. The viral reverse transcriptase act an RNA dependent DNA polymerase and makes ss DNA copy of genome RNA. ss DNA is made double stranded by the same enzyme which now act as DNA dependant DNA polymerase. The ds DNA moves to the nucleus of cell and several such molecules become integrated as provirus at random sites in host cell chromosome causing latent infection. Provirus is transcribed by cellular RNA polymerase either for production of mRNA which is translated into proteins or production of genomic RNA for insertion into progeny virus. In latent infection integrated proviral DNA remains silent without transcription or expression of most viral proteins. Certain factors can convert latent stage to productive HIV infection. During viral replication naked virus buds from infected cell and acquire lipoprotein envelope from host cell membrane and glycoproteins are virus encoded. First cells to become infected may be resident tissue of macrophage or submucosal lymphocytes in genital tract or rectum. Virus then transports to draining lymph node where it replicates 2-3 weeks after infection. Patient develops viremia, fall in CD4+T-lymphocytes and glandular fever like illness. Since HIV infects cells expressing CD4 antigen, the virus is found in CD4+T lymphocytes and also in monocyte macrophage cells which act as reservoir for virus. Macrophage carry virus into CNS across blood brain carrier. Virus is also present in plasma due to lysis of activated lymphocytes. Within a month or so viremia declines to near undetectable levels and illness subsides. This is brought by CD8+cytotoxic T lymphocytes, natural killer cells and antibody dependent cell mediated cytotoxicity (ADCC) Cell mediated response to all antigens decrease due to destruction of T4 cells. This is followed by asymptomatic period of 1-15 years when small number of circulating CD4+cells are producing virus and only low titres of virus are present in blood. Many infected cells can be detected in lymph nodes. There is follicular hyperplasia in these lymph node with expansions of germinal centres by increase in B lymphocytes. B cell expansion cause hypergammaglobulinemia. Finally T lymphocytes decrease in number in paracortical area and lymphnodes become involuted. When CD4 + T cell count falls below 400/ul, a large number of virions spills over from degenerating lymph node to blood and opportunistic infection with various microorganisms may develop

CD4 + T cells fall due to:

1. Viral cytolysis of CD4 + T cells
2. Infected CD4 + T cells can fuse via gp120 with upto 100 uninfected CD4 + T cells forming a unit called syncitium. This will lead to death of entire unit.
3. Immunocytolysis of infected T cells by cytoxic T cells, NK cells, ADCC and antibodies or compliment mediated lysis.
4. HIV may infect stem cells and then there will be no replacement.
5. Autoimmune destruction of infected CD4 + T cell.

The helper cells (CD4 + T cells) provide positive signal to B cells so that they produce specific antibodies and suppressive cells (CD^{8+} T cells).

When virus enters in host cells it remains hidden in the cells for a short period of time during which no antibodies can be detected in the blood. This is known as window period which lasts for 2-3 weeks and is rarely longer than 6 months. Virus is detectable in window period in small proportions of CD4 cells by DNA hybridization. So a seronegative patient can transmit virus. In a resting cell there is little transcription of virus and cell activation results in transcription of HIV and mRNA. 2 weeks after infection before any antibodies are detectable, free P24 antigen and reverse transcriptase antigen circulate in blood. This period of antigenemia may be significant feature when infection is acquired by transfusion of blood that contain free virus and infected cells. About one month after infection, acute infection antibody titre becomes detectable and levels of antigen decrease within few days and antigen disappears from blood and remains absent throughout asymptomatic phase. This disappearance of viral antigen with antibodies formation indicates immuno suppression of viral multiplication.

Diminished positive signal to B cells leads to poor production of specific antibodies. This results in different types of bacterial infection in AIDS cases. Diminished signal to cytotoxic or suppresser T-cells results in defective killing of intracellular virus. This leads to failure to eliminate HIV and other viral associated infections.

Diminished signal to natural killer cells lead to impaired difence against tumours e.g. Kaposi's Sarcoma.

Diminished signal to macrophages results in impaired killing of organisms within macrophages. This results in infection by organisms like T gondii.

Diminished response to skin reactivity occurs because of non-availability of helper T cells at the site of injection of antigen resulting in poor release of mediators.

In most patients serum P24 antigen and viral replication remains suppressed during first few years of infection and antigen again appears in blood when damage to immune system becomes marked. Therefore p24 antigenemia corresponds to loss of anti p24 antibody with chronic HIV disease.

Opportunistic Infections in AIDS

1. ***Bacterial infection***

   Mycobacterium Avium Complex—In this, birds are the habitat. Sputum is examined for acid fast bacilli and cultured on L.J. medium. Further Aryl sulphatase test and animal inoculation tests are done.

   Mycobacterium Tuberculosis – It can be disseminated or pulmonary infection. It is diagnosed on the basis of smear for acid fast bacilli

   Salmonella – Recurrent Septicemia occurs.

2. ***Viral infections***

   — Cytomegalovirus — In this, heptatis and pneumonitis occurs. CM inclusion cells are demonstrated in urine, saliva or body fluids. Also culture of human fibroblasts is performed.

   — Herpes simplex virus – Mucocutaneous ulcerations smear are stained by aqueous solution of toluidine blue for 15 sec or by Giemsa. Multinucleated giant cells and inclusion bodies are seen.

   — Varicella zostes virus

   — Ebstein bar virus

3. ***Fungal infection - Oropharyngeal***

   — Candidiasis – Oropharyngeal candidiasis is diagnosed by gram staining and culture on Sabaraud's Dextrose Agar.

   — Cryptococcosis – Cryptococcus neofomans is present in soil and also faeces of pigeons. It causes meningitis in human beings capsulated budding cells are seen in CSF. It can be cultured on Sabaraud's Dextrose Agar.

   — Pneumocystis carinii pneumoniae – It is diagnosed by trophozoites and cysts. Cysts contain 6-8 trophozoites and are present in the lumen of alveoli. These can be demonstrated in the bronchoalveolar lavage or transbronchial biopsy by silver methamine and H & E stain.

   — Coccidioidomycosis – It is dimorphic fungi which occurs as yeast in tissues and in culture it occurs in mycelial forms. Tissue form is spherule (15-17 μ) in diameter filled with endospores.

It can be cultured on SDA.

   — Aspergillosis

   — Histoplasmosis

4. ***Parasite***

   — Toxoplasmosis.

   Toxoplasma gondii is caused by oocysts contained in cat faeces. It causes CNS involvement. It is diagnosed by demonstration of intracellular protozoa is CSF or brain by giemsa staining, culture of exudate in mice and demonstrates of antibodies.

— Cryptosporidiosis
— Isosporiasis
— Microsporidiosis
— Generalised strongyloidosis

5. ***Malignancies*** - *Kaposi's Sarcoma*
— B cell lymphoma
— Non Hodgkin lymphoma

6. ***Skin disease***

Clinical Features

Group I – Acute illness – It occurs in 50% cases. It is characterized by malaise, fever, sore throat, rash, lymphadenopathy. Peripheral smear shows lymphocytosis with fair number of abnormal monocytes. Acute HIV infection is often mistaken for mononucleosis. Infection of Central Nervous System occurs due to initial viremia or traffic of infected cells into the brain.

Group II – Asymptomatic HIV infection. It includes all infected persons who are usually well but HIV antibody positive.

Group III – Persistent generalized lymphadenopathy (PGL) – It is characterised by lymph node enlargement at two or more extragenital sites for three months or longer without any other explanation for lymphadenopathy.

Group IV – AIDS and ARC (AIDS Related Complex) - Immune system is overwhelmed by virus. Lymph nodes involute and some patients develop illness known as ARC. They suffer from fever, night sweats, diarrhoea, muscle pain, weight loss. T4 lymphocyte count decrease, viral load increases. When T4 count decreases below 200/cu mm i.e. < 50% of normal limit, opportunistic infection rises. 35% patients progress to full blown AIDS in next 5-7 years. 35% will have one or more symptoms of HIV infection but not AIDS. Rest will have antibodies but remain asymptomatic.

HIV can also infect monocytes, macrophages (thus causing infections like T.B., Toxoplasmosis etc.) microglia, neurons, capillary endothelial cells in brain leading to CNS manifestation, membranous cells and enterochromaffin cells in intestinal mucosa leading to chronic diarrhoea and malabsorption.

Since most above cells lack CD4 antigen, HIV may be able to use alternate receptors.

Collection of Blood Samples for Testing

All the universal precautions are observed. Gloves should be worn and disposable syringes and needles should be used. To avoid soiling a piece of linen with layer of absorbing cotton pad between two layers of gauze piece or simply a big absorbent cotton may be placed below the forearm before commencing venepuncture. After collecting 5ml of blood aseptically, it should be carefully transferred to sterile plastic leak proof container preferably screw capped. The container should be labelled before venepuncture. If the vial has anticoagulant then other person wearing gloves would have to help in shaking the vial for mixing blood with anticoagulant. The cap should be tightly screwed after collection.

After drawing blood, patent should be given dry sterile cotton swab to press over site of venepuncture. Elbow should be flexed to hold the swab till the blood stops. Any blood spill is wiped off with 70% ethanol. All the swabs are placed in yellow plastic bags for disposal. If outside of vial is visibly contaminated with blood, wipe with 10% freshly prepared NaOCl solution. Blood collected in EDTA screw capped vials for viral isolation and CD4/CD8 studies.

Transport of Sample

Labelled leak proof plastic container is placed in another tightly capped unbreakable container (which should also have a label) with adequate packing material to absorb accidental leakage. It is then placed in a thermocol box with ice packs and biohazard symbol. Performa with details – name, age, sex, h/o contact etc. should accompany. For virus isolation if specimen cannot be transported immediately it should be frozen in deep freezer. Blood collected in EDTA vial, should be transported within 24 hrs.

Antibody Profile

First antibody to be detected is IgM usually 1 week after infection. These antibodies are against gag, core or envelope proteins. IgM reaches peak and decline later during following weeks. One week after disappearance of IgM, IgG appears and reaches plateau within a few months. IgG antibodies to gag (P24) and env (gp 160, gp 120, gp 41) protein appear first followed by antibodies to HIV enzymes. IgG persists throughout the life of infected person. HIV antibodies may not be detected during high viremia due to being complexed to antigens HIV RNA as well as DNA are detectable in all the patients before HIV specific IgM and IgG appear P24 Antigen can also be detected in most patients before IgG and IgM. In case of vertical transmission transplacental antibodies in neonates persist for more than 15 months.

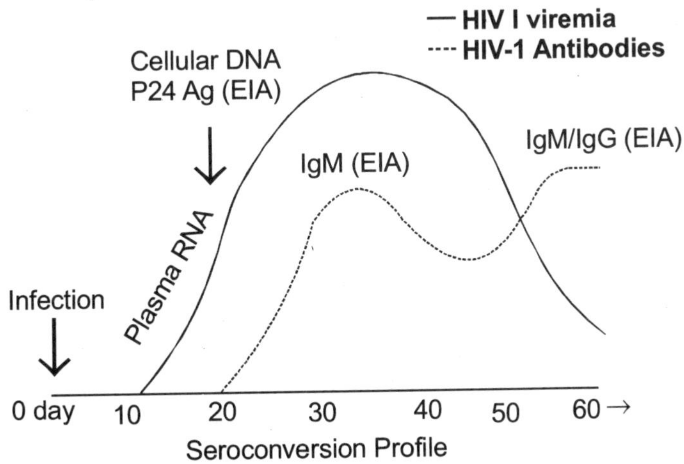

Seroconversion Profile

Lab Diagnosis

According to HIV testing policies and guidelines World Health Organisation, Regional Office for South East Asia, New Delhi and National HIV Testing Policy, HIV testing is recommended only for selected purposes.[1–12]

These includes:-

1. Screening of blood including blood products for blood safety and organs and tissues for transplantation.[7]
2. Epidemiological Surveillance particularly for HIV sentinel surveillance for epidemiological purposes using unlinked anonymous HIV testing methodology where all the personnel details of the person being tested are removed from the blood samples to hide patients identity.
3. Diagnosis of symptomatic infections among those clinically suspected to have AIDS.
4. Early diagnosis of HIV among asymptomatic patients who would like to know their HIV status. Voluntary testing in India is carried out in patients with high risk behaviour after counselling with informed consent and strict maintenance of confidentially with pretest and post test counselling.
5. To determine vertical transmission, nucleic acid amplification tests are done after counselling.
6. In health care worker for accidental exposure like needle stick injury.[12]

Forcing someone to undergo medical testing of any kind is an invasion of privacy and a violation of human rights.

HIV Testing

1. Screening tests E/R/S
   (a) ELISA
   (b) Rapid Tests
      - Dot blot assay
      - Particle agglutination test like gelatin/RBCS/latex/micro-beads
      - HIV spot test and combs test
      - Fluorometric microparticle technologies

   (c) Simple tests – These are based on ELISA principle but take only 1-2 hrs.
2. Supplementary tests
   - Western blot
   - Immunofluorescent test
3. Confirmatory tests
   - Virus Isolation
   - P24 Antigen detection
   - Detection of nucleic acid by in situ hybridization or PCR

Samples

Blood:

- ELISA
- Rapid HIV tests
- Immunofluorescence assay
- Western blot
- Immunoblot
- Recombinant immunoblot assay

Fluids

- Oral HIV antibody ELISA
- Urinary HIV antibody ELISA

Other Tests

- P24 assay
- Peripherel blood monocyte culture
- Peripherel blood monocyte HIV DNA detection
- Plasma virus load by RTPCR, DNA, NASBA

Incubation period/window period is 3-5 weeks of infection. In this period, antibodies can not be detected. IgM antibodies appear first in 3-4 weeks after infection and disappear in 8-10 weeks. IgG antibodies appear late about 5-6 weeks after infection and persists throughout. Transplacental antibodies in neonates persist for more than fifteen months and sometimes, upto eighteen months.

Screening Tests

These are done to screen antibodies against HIV. These are highly sensitive and easy to perform. These are not very specific. These are of three types.

ELISA: It is highly sensitive and specific test. It requires expensive equipments. Test procedure takes four hours.

Classification of ELISA

(a) **Based on Antigens**

First generation ELISA: During beginning of 1985 only first generation ELISA test were available where HIV lysate was used as antigen. These were highly sensitive but not very specific.

Second Generation ELISA: By 1988, more specific tests were developed based on recombinant antigens.

Third Generation ELISA: In these synthetic peptide is used an antigen.

Fourth Generation ELISA: Mixture of synthetic peptides and recombinant glycopeptides is used as antigen.

(b) Based on Principle

Indirect ELISA – It is competitive ELISA.

Antigen Sandwich ELISA – It is Antigen and Antibodies capture ELISA.

ELISA is commercially available as kits. The detection of anti-HIV antibody is mainstay of diagnosis in India. Antibodies appear in circulation between 2-6 weeks after primary infection and persist throughout life. Antigen is prepared from HIV cultivated in continuous T-Lymphocyte Cell- Lines or by Recombinant Technique (recombinant antigen usually gag and env) and synthetic peptides. Antigen is coated on microtitre wells to which serum is added. HIV antibody of serum binds to viral antigen. Unbound serum is washed away. The antihuman goat Immunoglobulin linked to soluble enzyme (alkaline phosphatase, horse radish peroxidase or B galactosidase) is added and incubated at 37° C for 1 hour. The well is washed. The suitable solution of substrate is added (The enzyme splits the substrate) and left at room temperature till the positive control develops a colour. It is read by ELISA reader. ELISA has 99.5% sensitively commercially and specificity of 95% or more. ELISA kits contain both HIV_1 and HIV_2 results of ELISA are interpreted as

- Reactive
- Non-reactive
- Partially reactive

Sensitivity means detecting those who truly have condition. Specificity excludes patients who don't have the condition. Although ELISA is extremely sensitive but it is not optimal with respect to specificity. Therefore positive ELISA or inconclusive ELISA must be confirmed with more specific tests. The most commonly employed confirmatory test is Western blot test which takes the advantage of multiple antigens of HIV.

False positive ELISA occurs in:

- Hematological malignant disorder
- Auto immune diseases – Rheumatoid arthritis, SLE etc.
- Primary biliary cirrhoses
- Passively transferred antibodies
- Renal transplantation
- Steven Johnson syndrome
- DNA viral infection
- Multiple myelomas
- Alcoholic hepatitis

- Hepatitis B vaccine
- Chronic renal failure
- Antibodies to class II leucocytes

False negative ELISA occurs in:

- Window period
- Malignant disease
- Bone marrow transplantation
- Immuno suppressive treatment
- Replacement transfusion
- B cell dysfunction
- Advanced disease
- Kits which detect P24 antigen of HIV

Rapid Tests

These includes particle agglutination (gelatin, RBCs, latex microbeads), immunofilteration (dot blot) or immunochromatography (comb assay, HIV spot test) and others.

These tests have total reaction time of less than 30 minutes. They do not require expensive equipment but are more expensive tests than ELISA.

Single use diagnostic system (SUDS) for HIV-1 (Abbot laboratories) is the only FDA approved rapid test available for use in USA.

Simple Tests

These are not as fast as rapid tests. They take 1-2 hours. They also do not require expensive equipment. These tests are also based on ELISA principle.

Supplementary Tests

These tests also detect antibodies against HIV. These are recommended for validation of positive results of screening tests. Supplementary tests are often referred to as confirmatory tests which is not a correct nomenclature as these do not confirm the results of screening tests but provide additional information only.

These include:

1. Second and third generation ELISA/Rapid/Simple
2. Western blot
3. Immuno blot
4. Immunofluorescence assay
5. Rapid immuno blot assay

ELISA/Rapid tests are used as supplementary tests to confirm the status of reactive samples in developing countries. This is because western blot and immuno blot assay are more expensive.

Electroblotting is of three types: *Southern blot* – Named after Edward Southern who invented the procedure for analysing fragments of DNA.

Northern blot – Named factiously. It is employed to analyse transfer RNA.

These two tests are employed to detect antigen by known antibody.

Western blot Assay – Western blot is highly sensitive and specific assay. This is used as supplementary test to confirm results of reactive sample in developed countries.

In this assay, HIV protein from detergent disrupted purified virions are separated according to their electrophoretic mobility and molecular weight by polyacrylamide gel electrophoresis, then blotted on to nitrocellulose membrane by standard blotting procedures. The membrane is then cut into strips having full complement of viral proteins. A serum sample found positive by screening test is incubated with the strip followed by washing. Antibody to HIV protein attach to separated viral antigen on the strip. The strip are washed and treated with enzyme conjugated antihuman immunoglobulin antibody. Enzyme substrate is subsequently added. The substrate changes colour in the presence of enzyme and permanently stains the strip. Position of band on strip indicates the antigen with which antibody has reacted.

Usually bands with multiple proteins are formed in a typical case. Antibody to core protein (P24 and P31) and envelope protein (gp41, gp120/160) are commonly detected.

Fall in titre of anti p24 antibodies indicate poor prognosis.

Criteria to Interpret Positive HIV1 Western blot

American Red Cross Society – Three or more bands from each gene-gag, pol and env.
Consortium for retrovirus –

Two or more bonds p24 or p31/34 and gp41 or gp 120 or 160.

WHO – Two env bands with or without gag or pol

Centre for Disease Control (CDC) –

Any two – p24, gp 41, gp 120/160

Recently criteria given by manufacturer of the test is followed.

Interpretation of western blot is sometimes difficult when bands are formed at one to two sites seen as p24 or gp120. This result may be obtained in early infection but may also be nonspecific. A completely reactive result is useful.

Explanation of Indeterminate Western Blot

1. Antibodies cross react with one of the proteins of HIV cross reaction occurs with P24 or/and P55.
2. Patient in process of classic antibody response.

If indeterminate western blot occurs then confirm by PCR and repeat Western blot to confirm whether indeterminate result is pattern of evolution.

Indeterminate western blot is obtained in HIV infected as well as non-infected individual. In infected case, indeterminate Western blot occurs in early seroconverter and individuals with terminal AIDS due to low levels of HIV antibodies. Developments of antibodies to all structural and regulatory proteins of HIV-1 takes between few weeks to several months after acute infection.

Sometimes indeterminate western blot results in HIV non-infected individuals who have other human retroviruses, antibodies to mitochondrial, nuclear, T cell leukocyte antigen, high concentration of bilirubin in serum, hypergammaglobulinemia due to polyclonal gammopathy and normal human ribonucleoproteins. Patients giving indeterminate results need to be retested 8-12 weeks later. Consistent indeterminate results need to be confirmed by virological test given later. Alternate supplementary/confirmatory test is Immuno - fluorescence Assay to resolve discordent results. Usually IFA and western blot are concordant. Western blot and IFA are expensive, time consuming and require expertise.

Immuno fluorescent Test – This is rarely used because it requires fluorescent microscope and technical expertise. In this HIV infected cells are acetone fixed on to the glass sides and then reacted with test serum followed by fluorescein conjugated anti human gamma globulin. A positive reaction appears as apple green fluorescence of cell membrane under fluorescent microscope.

Rapid immunoblot assay uses recombinant HIV antigen. Immunoblot uses synthetic peptide antigens. For these two tests, different antigens are spotted in different areas and strips are prepared.

For HIV2 detection P36 is used.

Other Serological Tests Are:

1. *Fujerbio Agglutination Test:* It is simple and convenient test in which antigen coated gelatin particles are agglutinated with antibodies in patients serum. It also gives false positive results.
2. *Karpas Test:* It is simple inexpensive slide immunoperoxidase test. HIV infected cells are fixed on Teflon coated slide wells to which patient's serum is added and allowed to react. Then horse radish peroxides labelled anti human immune globulin is added. Finally suitable substrate is added. Positive test develops a colour.

   Interpretation is subjective
3. Immunofluorescent test and Radio immuno precipitation assay can be done to detect anti P24 antibodies which are liable to subjective error. This test is less frequently done.

Saliva HIV Testing

Many workers have shown that saliva is an acceptable and often favourable alternative to serum for HIV antibody testing because blood of HIV infected individual is a hazardous substance. It can occasionally lead to HIV infection among health care workers.

Saliva is safer medium than blood for four reasons:

1. HIV is rarely found in saliva
2. Concentration of HIV is very low
3. There appears to be factors in saliva that inhibit infectivity
4. Saliva is specially useful in HIV testing among intravenous drug users who have collapsed blood vessel and those who refuse to give blood samples oral fluids contain IgG antibodies against HIV concentration of antibodies is greater than concomitent serum levels. Performance of the test during sero conversion is not clear. ELISA test for saliva has 98% sensitivity and 99.4% specificity. FDA USA has approved oral saliva test called orasure (Epitope, Inc).

A cotton swab is inserted in mouth for 2 minutes to collect transudate Swab to place in transport container containing antibacterial preservative.

Urine HIV Testing

IgG antibody capture particle adherence tests are used (e.g. GAC PAT, GAC ELISA, SUDS) and standard commercially available EIA tests. Various studies report that urine based antibody screening was comparable to serum tests. So urine is alternative medium in patients unwilling to provide serum.

Home HIV Testing

Home access system has been approved by FDA. It uses standard EIA and confirmatory western blot from blood collected by patient at home. From preliminary studies it is apparent that home collection of HIV antibodies screening along with pre-test and post test telephonic counselling is viable alternative to conventional virus antibody screening in clinics. After pretest counselling on phone patient collects blood at home with lancet and places on test card and mails the card to testing center where testing is done and the results are obtained by client on phone with post test counselling. The client's identification number is the number assigned to specific test kit. Post test counselling of negative test is given through prerecorded matter where as in case of positive results the client is referred to counsellors.

Confirmatory Tests

These tests confirm HIV infection in those who is either seropositive or has equivocal results from various serological tests.

Virus Isolation

Virus can be isolated from peripheral blood lymphocyte by co-cultivation with normal healthy donor's lymphocytes in the presence of mitogens and T cell growth factor (intaleukin 2). Isolation of virus takes 3-6 weeks and must be conducted under strict biocontainment. The presence of virus is detected by assays for reverse transcriptase and P24 antigen in supernatent fluid of culture. Less readily HIV can also be isolated from plasma, CSF, genital secretions and various organs like brain and bone marrow. Culture is rarely used. It is done mainly for research purposes like drug sensitivity and vaccine study.

Disadvantage

1. It is labour intensive
2. It is expensive
3. It takes weeks for result
4. It exposes workers to high concentration of HIV.

Detection of P24 Antigen

Shortly after HIV infection (i.e. 2 weeks, after infection) and before the detectable antibodies response free P24 antigen and reverse transcriptase may be detectable in sera. This early period of antigenemia is difficult to identify P24 is detected upto 3-5 months. P24 antigen in serum is detected by ELISA in 30% patients during window period, 10% asymptomatic patients and 50-60% of AIDS patients. P24 is core antigen and is detected in serum, plasma, CSF and cell culture supernate. Presence of P24 antigen in CSF means CNS involvement by HIV.

Uses –

1. Diagnosing infection during window period or late stage
2. To diagnose infection in neonates
3. Resolving discordant serological tests
4. Monitoring response to antiretroviral therapy
5. Detection of window period infections in blood donors
6. Research

Commercial EIAS are available. Sample is incubated in the presence of anti P24 antibodies. Enzyme reaction results in development of colour.

EIAS primarily detects uncomplexed P24 antigen in CSF, plasma, serum and cell culture. As the antibody response builds up, antigen becomes negative. Late in infection P24 Ag may reappear with onset of clinical features which correspond to loss of anti P-24 antibody. Patient with persistent P24 antigen in blood progress more rapidly to AIDS than those without it. Serum levels of P24 is useful guide to monitor viral suppression particularly when patient is on AZT therapy.

Disadvantages

1. HIV-2 cannot be detected
2. Limited sensitivity especially in neonates less than 1 month old.
3. Not possible if there is rise in P24 antibodies as immune complexes are formed.

P24 antigen lacks, specifically and sensitivity. Anti P24 antibodies are better marker of progression than P24 antigen.

Recently ultrasensitive low HIV1 P24 antigen detection assays are available. Presence of P24 antigen means increased level of viremia and increased risk of progression. P24 antigen is often present in infected newborn of positive mother.

Federal Drug Agency, USA has not approved use of P24 antigen for blood screening.

Detection of Viral Nucleic Acid

HIV1 DNA

It can be detected by insitu hybridization and polymerase chain reaction (PCR). PCR can detect proviral DNA during window period and can differentiate latent from active viral transcription and can quantitate the copy number of HIV DNA (e.g. viral load assay). It can differentiate between HIV$_1$ and HIV$_2$. HIV infection can be detected by detection of viral genes HIV$_1$ gag or pol gene (pro virus) by probing and amplifying PCR. Amplified product is detected by hybridization with enzyme or radio labelled specific oligonucleotide probes. This test gives advantage of detection of virus during window period before the appearance of antibodies in serum and during extended period of viral latency. It is extremely sensitive 96-99% although false positive reactions can occur. Sensitivity is low in patients with higher CD4 counts, low infected peripheral blood monocytes and those on anti-retroviral therapy.

It has important role in diagnosis of babies born to infected mother and patients with double infections. HIV1 DNA PCR is used to resolve indeterminate serological test or western blot tests in high risk patients and minimize window period in transfusion services. It reduces window period to 10-15 days in transfusion services in USA.

HIV1 RNA

It is detected in plasma (HIV$_1$ DNA detected in PBMC) HIV$_1$, RNA is used for diagnosis of primary HIV infection where there is increased viremia and serological tests are negative. Quantification of HIV$_1$ RNA is done to monitor the progress of disease and response to anti HIV treatment. Quantification is done by RT-PCR, NASBA (Nucleic Acid Sequence Band Amplification) and nucleic acid hybridization, branched DNA signal amplification, DNA hybridization and calorimetric detection and multiplex transcription mediated amplification system (Gene probe).

High viral load i.e. > 30,000 copies of HIV$_1$, RNA/ml predict rapid progression to AIDS and death. Less than 10,000 copies/ml predict slow progress. More than 10^5 HIV$_1$ RNA within six months of seroconversion are ten times more prone to AIDS within 5 years. Viral load should be undetectable within 3-6 months of treatment. If not it means change in regime is required.

Sl. No.	*Viral markers*	*Window period*	*Acute infection*	*Asymptomatic phase*	*AIDS & ARC*
1.	Virus isolation	++	+	–	+
2.	Antigen P24 RT	–	+	–	+
3.	Antibodies				
	Anti P24	–	+	+	+
	Anti gp 120, gp41				
	ELISA	–	+	+	+
4.	Western Blot	–	+	+	+
			Partial p24 and/or gp 120	Full pattern	Absence of p24 antibodies

Non-specific tests include:

1. TLC, DLC – In full blown AIDS leucopenia occurs with lymphocyte count <400/cu mm. There is pancytopenia
2. Assay of T lymphocyte subsets
   In AIDS CD4 falls below 200/cu mm. Normal CD4; CD8 T cell ratio is 2:1. It is reversed to 0.5-1:1. The count of CD4 lymphocytes rises with treatment.
3. Platelet count – There is thrombocytopenia
4. IgG and IgA levels are increased
5. Skin test for cell mediated immunity:
   CMI is diminished as is evident from tuberculin skin test
6. Elevated serum transaminases

Surrogate markers supporting diagnosis of HIV in adults:

1. Increase prolactin
2. Decrease dehydroepiandrosterone concentration
3. Antibodies to HIV1 virion infectivity factor proteins
4. Increase Serum IgE concentrate

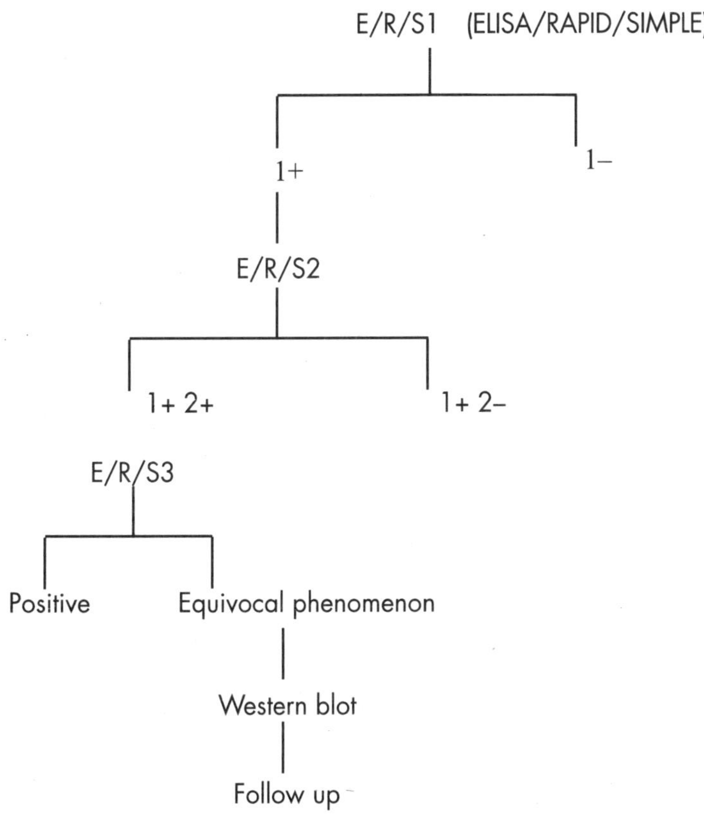

Indirect prediction of HIV:

1. ↓ CD4 cells
2. ↑ Serum neopterin
3. Indicator disease for AIDS
4. ↑ β_2 microglobulin
5. ↑ IL2 receptors

Strategies for HIV Tests

Strategy I

Serum is tested with one E/R/S test and if reactive sample is considered positive and infected, if non-reactive, it is considered negative. This test should be highly sensitive so that no false negative results occur. Thus strategy is used for transfusion safety (Blood, also organ, tissue, sperm etc). Donor is not informed, and the unit of blood tested positive is incinerated. If the donor wants to know the status, he is counselled and HIV testing is performed as per strategy III.

Strategy II

Serum reactive with one E/R/S test is retested with second E/R/S test with higher specificity based on different antigen preparation and/or different test principle. If found reactive on second E/R/S test also it is reported positive otherwise it is negative. This test should be of higher specificity.

This strategy is used for HIV surveillance and to diagnose HIV in patients with AIDS indicator disease.

Strategy III

Kit should be of highest specificity. The serum reactive with 2nd E/R/S test is retested with 3rd E/R/S. The third test is based on different antigenic preparation or test principle.

The serum reactive with all the three E/R/S tests is reported positive. The serum non- reaction with 3rd E/R/S is considered equivocal/borderline. Such individual is retested after 3 weeks. If sample provides an equivocal results, the person is considered to be HIV antibodies negative.

For asymptomatic HIV infection, it is necessary to confirm diagnosis with three tests. Symtomatic infection with opportunistic infection may be subjected to two tests. Cross reacting antibody positive with EIA as well as western blot are associated with rheumatoid arthritis, polyclonal granulopathy, SLE, syphilis, malaria etc. Results which remain indeterminate for upto 1 year should be considered negative. Sample reactive in all the three tests is reported positive for HIV antibodies.

Diagnosis of Paediatric HIV

Detection in a woman done before and during pregnancy. Early in utero transmission is rare. Transmission occurs in third trimester. In a baby maternal anti HIV antibodies persist upto 18 months of age. Cord sample should not be tested because there is risk of contamination with mother's blood. At birth virological tests have 30-35% sensitivity. Days to weeks after birth sensitivity is 50-70%. In young infants infection is detected by virological assays. Serological markers (IgM and IgA) are not reliable because of transient presence of these markers as well as unpredictable time to transmit HIV from mother to child.

Sensitivity	1-14 days age	1-4 months age
DNAPCR	41%	88.5%
P24 Antigen	39.5%	79.8%
RNA PCR	31.5%	96.5%
Viral culture	41%	90%

Birth to 18 Months Age

Viral Assays

- HIV DNA PCR
- HIV RNA PCR
- Virus culture
- P24 assay is less sensitive for HIV1 diagnosis in infants and has more false positive among those less than 1 month of age.

DNA PCR is positive in 40% infected infants at 48 hours after birth and 93% infected children by 14 days of age. HIV_1 RNA is more sensitive but sensitivity and specificity of the test to diagnose neonatal infections need to be defined.

If the virological tests are positive within 48 hours after birth, transmission is considered positive intrapartum. In the absence of breast feeding, if the virological tests are negative within 48 hours after birth but positive after 1 week of life, infection is considered in utero. HIV transmission carries additional risk during breast feeding. Breast fed infants need to be tested again after 18 months or till breast fed. Current practice is to test infants born to HIV infected mother at the age of 48 hours, 1-2 months and 3-6 months.

Two or more negative serological tests 1 month apart at 6 months of age in non breast-fed infant excludes HIV.

After 18 months of age, disease is diagnosed by similar methods as in adults i.e. HIV specific antibodies, by screening and later confirmed by E/R/S assay. Mother to child risk is 25% in absence of anti-retroviral drugs. If mother and infant are administered AZT as per PACTG 076 guidelines, mother to child risk is reduced to 4-8%. Surrogate markers – Progressive decrease of CD4 cell count in absence of any other cause.

Diagnosis of perinatally HIV infected infants less than 18 months of age

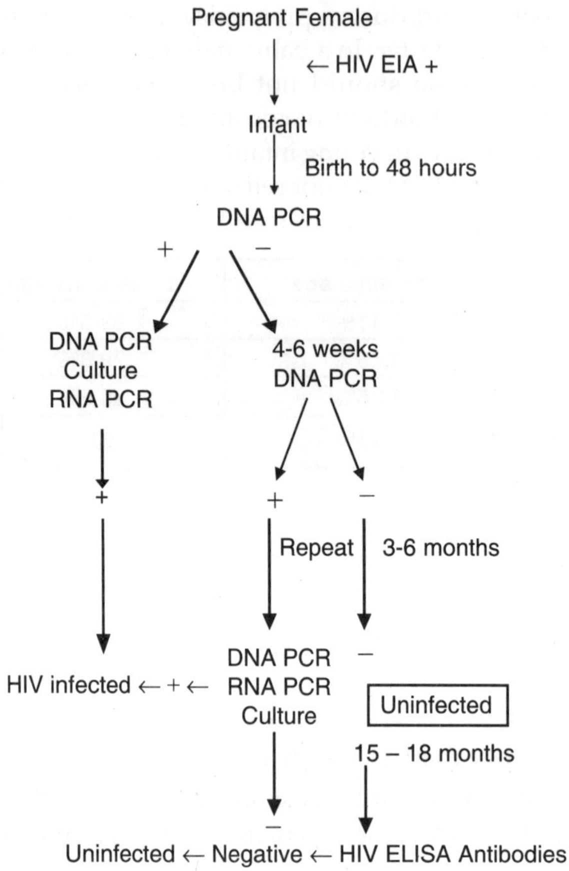

Anti-retroviral Therapy

New anti-retroviral drugs combined with updated treatment strategies have now achieved efficient inhibition of HIV replication in most of the patients. Classes of drugs include both nucleoside and nonnucleoside inhibitors of the viral enzyme reverse transcriptase and inhibitors of virus proteases. However, eradication of HIV is not achieved with existing anti HIV drugs and despite major advances there remain many challenges in clinical management of HIV infected individuals.

A major drawback of highly active antiviral therapy (HAART) is selection of resistant mutants. Monitoring of antiviral therapy is achieved by measuring viral load using nucleic acid amplification techniques.

Basic Regimen

Azidothymidine also known as Zydovudine is drug of choice. It is nucleoside which is converted by cellular thymidine kinase and other intra cellular enzymes into an active phosphorylated form which prevent viral DNA synthesis by displacing viral RNA from reverse transcriptase.

ZDV	–	300 mg BD or 200 mg TDS × 4 weeks
Disadvantage of ZDV	–	Myelosuppression
	–	patients become refractory to drugs after prolonged therapy.
Lamivudine	–	150 mg BD × 4 weeks

Expanded Regimen

Basic regimen + Indinavir 800 mg TDS × 4 weeks

Alternate drugs – dideoxynosine and dideoxycytidine are under evaluation. These have same pharmacological action as ZDV (AZT).

There is very little information on safety of ZDV during Ist trimester of pregnancy or on the safety of other anti-retroviral drugs taken during pregnancy. To know whether the exposed health care worker has acquired HIV infection following exposure, HIV testing should be done at the time of exposure and 6 weeks and 12 weeks following exposure.

Post-exposure Prophylaxis

Health care workers are normally at low risk of acquiring HIV infection during management of infected patients. Absence of vaccine or effective treatment makes health care worker apprehensive. Most exposure don't result in infection. The risk of infection varies with amount of blood/bodyfluid/other potentially infected material, the time of exposure, the number of viruses present in patient's blood and whether PEP was taken within recommended time. Risk of transmission of blood borne virus to health care worker by percutaneous exposure is 0.05 –0.4% for HIV, 9-30% for HBV and 3-10% for HCV.

Following exposure wash needle stick cut with soap and water. Don't put pricked finger in mouth. Don't squeeze to encourage bleeding. Flush exposed areas like nose, eyes, mouth or skin with plentys of water. Administration of PEP to health care worker depends on exposure code (EC).

EC is divided into 3 categories EC1, EC2, EC3 depending on the nature of exposure. If exposure to blood or body fluids or instrument contaminated with one of the substances, no PEP is required when the skin is intact. If mucous membrane and skin integrity is compromised and small volume is contacted (few drops/short duration) then it is exposure code 1. If large volume (several drops or major splash) and larger duration contact (several minutes or more) then it is exposure code 2. Also, if percutaneous exposure i.e., less severe exposure e.g., solid needle, superficial scratch, then it is exposure code 2. More severe exposure e.g. large bore needles, deep punctures, visible blood on devise or needles used in patient's artery or vein, then it is EC3.

HIV status code of exposure source is classified into following categories.

HIV SC1	–	HIV positive, low titre exposure e.g. asymptomatic or increased CD4 count.

HIV SC2 – HIV+ve – Higher titre exposure e.g. advanced AIDS, primary HIV infection, high viral load and low CD4 count.

HIV status unknown – Status of source unknown

HIV negative – No PEP required.

EC	*HIV SC*	*PEP*
1	1	May not be required
1	2	Basic
2	1	Basic
2	2	Expanded
3	1 or 2	Expanded

Both risk of infection and side effect of drugs should be carefully considered when deciding PEP exposure. Based on limited information, ziduvidine taken during 2nd and 3rd trimester of pregnancy has not caused serious side effects in mothers or infants.

Vaccine

Since there is no effective treatment against AIDS there is need of effective vaccine. The development of vaccine is difficult due to the following reasons:

1. HIV can mutate very rapidly. There is increased risk of mutation of env gp of virus.
2. There is possibility of recombination between different HIV strains.
3. There is prolonged asymptomatic period which provides sufficient time for antigenic drift to occur.
4. Paucity of suitable animal model
5. Antibodies may be insufficient CM I may be necessary.
6. Virus normally enters through mucous membrane therefore vaccine induces IgA antibodies and submucosal lymphocytes.
7. Virus enters the body not only as free virions neutralisable by antibodies but also as infected leucocytes in semen or blood in which virus or provirus is protected against antibodies as well as T cell mediated cytolysis.
8. Virus can spread from cell to cell by fusion to produce syncitia.
9. Virus establishes life long latent infection hiding from antibodies.
10. HIV infects cells of immune system notably CD4 +T lymphocytes and cells of monocyte/macrophage lineage.

An attenuated virus vaccine is unlikely because HIV is lethal virus, it establishes latent infection, it is difficult to assess attenuation and there is likelihood of subsequent mutation. Killed vaccines are not very effective inducers of cytotoxic T cell responses gp 160, 120, 41 produced by recombinant DNA technology in mammalian cells or in insect cells using Baculovirus as vector have been tested with very limited success. Gene coding for gp120 of HIV has been inserted into vaccinia virus. Inoculation of gp 120/vaccinia hybrid virus elicits both antibody mediated and cell mediated immunity against gp 120 peplomer. Research is on for synthetic/recombinant vaccine.

Procedures for HIV Testing

Unlinked Anonymous Testing

Its objective is public health survillance of HIV infection. It is a method for measuring HIV prevalence in selected populations with minimal bias. It involves use of blood already collected for other purposes. Therefore selection bias remain minimum.

Voluntary Confidential Testing

It is done for diagnostic purposes at VCTC (Voluntary Counselling and Testing Centres). It is related to counselling, informed medical consent and confidentially. Confidentially encourages more and more people practising high risk behaviour to come forward for HIV test.

Mandatory Testing

It is done without consent and result could be linked to identify a person. It is recommended for ensuring blood safety and screening of donors of semen, organs or tissues to prevent transmission of HIV in recipient of biological products.

Compulsory Testing

To determine HIV antibody status without individual's consent and with legal sanctions to enforce compliance e.g. (rape cases or court's orders.) Mandatory testing of patients admitted in hospital for surgery is no substitute for standard work precautions that need to be adopted for every patient in the hospital or health care setting. HIV testing is encouraged in health professional who perform exposure prone invasive procedures and also hemophiliacs. All antinatal cases may be given information on risk behaviour and then invited to undergo voluntary testing. ANC testing must be promoted in increased prevalence areas. HIV testing is very important in those with high risk behaviour (unsafe sex, gay, bisexual man, multisexual partners, substance abuse, professional workers etc). It is essential to motivate client to confide a friend or spouse or parent etc. However, confidentiality is very important to prevent victimization or discrimination. Some code is devised to indicate HIV positive status rather than writing on case sheet/OPD card.

Counseling

Informed consent is taken which includes pretest discussion of issues like nature and consequence of proposed test (counseling).

Pre-test Counseling

Knowledge about HIV is imparted to the client so that client can make informed decision and is emotionally and psychologically prepared to accept HIV test result. It is important because of serious social and personal consequences.

Client is given knowlege about:–

- HIV transmission
- Implication of HIV positive result
- Implication of HIV negative result (window period) and repeat testing
- Emphasis is given on anti-retroviral drugs and non availability of cure and vaccine.

Client is empowered to make informed decision about HIV testing and to accept the result.

Post-test Counseling

HIV test report is communicated to right person in right way under right circumstances. (one to one interaction). It is aimed at reiterating the updated knowledge about HIV to empower the client to make decision on management and behaviour modification.

Indian National Testing Policy

1. No individual should be made to undergo mandatory testing for HIV.
2. No mandatory HIV testing should be imposed for employment for providing health care services.
3. Any HIV test must accompany pre-test and post-test counselling.
4. Informed consent and confidentially are important issues when HIV testing is undertaken for diagnostic purposes.
5. HIV testing protocol should be commensurate with objective of testing and appropriate strategy should be followed to achieve the said objection.
6. Testing is a part of overall prevention and control programme.
7. Testing should be technically sound and appropriate.
8. Test procedure must be appropriate to field situation.
9. Test procedure should be cost effective.
10. Lab procedure must be monitored to ensure quality.
11. Quality assurance should be practised to avoid false positive and false negative results.

HIV Testing and Counseling

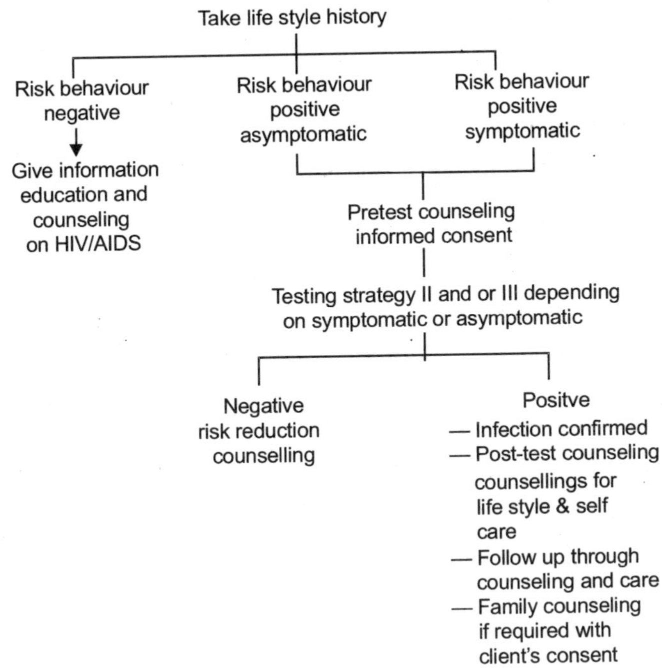

Prevention

WHO has recommended following measures:

1. *Sexual contact:* Safer sex should be practised by using condoms to prevent transmission of virus by exchange of body fluids.
2. *Sharing needles:* Contaminated needles, syringes, shaving kits and other skin piercing instruments should not be shared with others.
3. *Blood/organs:* All blood and blood products should be screened. Autogenous blood transfusion is useful before anticipated surgery. Semen donation, cornea, bone marrow, kidney and other organs should also be screened.
4. *Control of infection:* Universal precautions are to be followed which include screening of individual at risk and to identify HIV infected patients. Carriers are to regularly followed up.
5. Isolation of AIDS patients and initiation of treatment against viruses and opportunistic infection should be done.
6. Risk factor identified. Positive health behaviour needs to be actively encouraged.

7. Drug injectors who are unable to stop using drugs should be told where they can obtain sterile needles and syringes or how to disinfect equipment used for injection. Some countries or cities have needle and syringe exchange programme. Avoid injections unless necessary. Use disposable syringes and needles.

Precautions for Health Worker

There are recommendations for prevention of HIV transmission in health care settings of United States Centres for Disease Control. Observe Universal precautions in care of all the patients. Use barrier precautions to prevent skin and mucous membrane exposure when contact with blood and other body fluids. Gloves should be worn for touching blood/body fluids/articles soiled with blood/body fluids. Masks and protective eye wear should be worn during invasive procedures. Gowns and aprons should be worn. Hand washing is very important. Hands should be washed before wearing gloves and after removing gloves. All health care workers should take precautions to prevent injuries caused by needles, scalpes etc. To prevent needle stick injuries, needles should not be recapped. Health Care Workers who have opened lesions or weeping dermatitis should refrain from patient care. Waste should be disposed safely. Immunization against HBV is provided.

Do's & Don'ts

1. Give up high risk behaviour i.e., multiple sex partners.
   Don't have vaginal/anal/oral sex with prostitutes.
2. Use condoms.
3. HIV positive or sexually promiscuous or IDU should not donate blood/serum/ breast milk/other organs.
4. Don't share needles, syringes or blades.
5. Get STD treated.
6. HIV positive should not marry. If married don't indulge in sex without condom. If HIV positive female becomes pregnant, get pregnancy terminated otherwise baby will develop AIDS/become AIDS orphan. (No forcible abortion or sterilization on grounds of HIV status of women.) Prevent future pregnancies.

   Message

   Absteinence before marriage and infidelity after marriage is must.

REFERENCES

1. Lopex-Bernaldo de Quiros JC, Delgado R, Garcia F, Eiros JM, Ortiz de Lejarazu R, Microbiological diagnosis of HIV Infection. Enferm Infecc Microbiol Clin, 2007 Dec; 25 (10): 632-638.
2. Dax EM, Arnott A : Advances in Laboratory Testing for HIV Pathology, 2004 Dec; 36(6): 551-560.
3. Struelens M, Delforge ML, Denis O, Liesnard C, Rodriguez-Villalobos H: The Microbiology Department, *Rev Med Brux* 2003; 23 Suppl 2: 107-110.
4. De Simone JA, Pomerrantz RJ: New Method for the Detection of HIV, *Clin Lab Med*, 2002 Sep; 22(3): 573-92.
5. Kelley VA, Caliendo AM: Successful Testing Protocols in Virology, *Clin Chem*. 2001 Aug; 47(8): 1559-62.
6. No Author Listed. FDA Review of Viral Load Test Kits. Food and Drug Administration. *BETA*. 1996 Mar; 13.
7. Busch MP: Testing Blood Donors for HIV: Current Controversies. Immunol Invest. 1995 Jan-Feb; (1-2): 147-54.
8. Rouzious C: Virologic Diagnosis of Human Immunodeficiency, *Rev Prat*, 1991 Feb; 41(4): 324-6.
9. Lynch JR, Brown JM: The Polymerase Chain Reaction; Current and Future Clinical Applications. *J Med Genet*. 1990 Jan; 27(1)2-7.
10. Nakamura RM, Bylund DJ, Rooney KE: Current Status of Clinical Laboratory Test for the Human Immunodeficiency Virus. *J Clin Lab Anal*. 1990; 4(4): 295-306.
11. Richeldi L, Barnini S, Saltini C: Molecular Diagnosis of Tuberculosis, *Eur Respire J Supp*. 1995 Sep; 20: 689s-700s.
12. Murno CL: The Impact of Recent Advances in Microbiology and Immunology on Perinatal and Women's Helth Care, *J Obstet Gynecol Neonatal Nurs*. 1995 Jul-Aug; 24(6):525-31.

CHAPTER 9

Clinical Features of STDs and Gastrointestinal Manifestations in HIV/AIDS

Parvathy Nair

Clinical Features of STDs

Sexually Transmitted Diseases (STDs), are among the most common infectious diseases in the world today. More than 20 STIs have now been identified. Most of the Sexually transmitted diseases are asymptomatic particularly in women. But an asymptomatic person who is infected can pass the disease on to a sex partner. Complications caused by STDs tend to be more severe and more frequent for women than for men, in part because the frequency of asymptomatic infection means that many women do not seek care until serious health problems have developed. The following table classifies the sexually transmitted disease according to symptomatology.

S. No.	*Symptoms*	*Disease*
1.	Abnormal vaginal discharge/Leucorrhoea	Bacterial vaginosis, chlamydia, gonorrhoea, herpes, trichomoniasis, Candidiasis
2.	Burning Micturation/Dysuria	Chlamydia, gonorrhoea herpes, trichomoniasis
3.	Mennorhagia/Abnormal menstrual cycles	Chlamydia, gonorrhoea
4.	Post Coital Bleeding	Chlamydia, gonorrhoea
5.	Swollen and/or painful testicles	Chlamydia, gonorrhoea
6.	Pelvic pain	Chlamydia, gonorrhoea
7.	Blisters or sores on the genitals, anus	Herpes, syphilis

(Contd...)

8.	Persistent vaginal candidiasis	HIV infection/AIDS
9.	Warts or bumps on the genitals, anus	Human papillomavirus
10.	Pruritis Vulvae/Itching in Genital Area	Bacterial vaginosis, herpes, trichomoniasis, yeast infection
11.	Discharge from penis	Chlamydia, gonorrhoea, trichomoniasis

Syphilis

Many people infected with syphilis do not have any symptoms for years, yet remain at risk for late complications if they are not treated. Although transmission appears to occur from persons with sores who are in the primary or secondary stage, many of these sores are unrecognized. Thus, most transmission is from persons who are unaware of their infection.

Primary Stage

Marked by the appearance of a single or multiple sore or chancre lasts for 3 to 8 weeks. Usually accompanied by regional adenopathy. Lymph nodes are large, round, discrete, rubbery, freely movable and usually non-tender. The time between infection with syphilis and the start of the first symptoms can range from 10 to 90 days (average 21 days).

The chancre is usually firm, round, small, and painless. It appears at the spot where syphilis entered the body on the vulva, the clitoris and around the opening of the urethra, on the cervix in women and on the penis and foreskin in men. It can also appear around the anus and mouth. The chancre lasts 3 to 6 weeks, and it heals without treatment. However, if adequate treatment is not administered, the infection progresses to the secondary stage.

Secondary Stage

This stage appears 9-11 weeks after the chancre. In about 15% of cases chancres persist.

Lesion of secondary syphilis, also called Condylomatalata are moist, flat, warty-looking, bilaterally symmetric, non-indurated lesions with high concentrations of Treponema. It usually occurs on the vulva in women and around the anus in both sexes. The plantar area may show extensive involvement lesion appear as rough, red, or reddish brown spots both on the palms of the hands and the bottoms of the feet. They are relatively painless and does not cause itching.

Other lesions like split papules may appear on the corners of the mouth and nose, white mucous patches on the tongue or roof of the mouth; or bilaterally symmetric annular lesions with a clear, hyper pigmented central area of raised border.

Other symptoms of secondary syphilis may include fever, swollen lymph glands, patchy alopecia, sore throat, headaches, weight loss, muscle aches and fatigue.

The signs and symptoms of secondary syphilis will resolve with or without treatment, but without treatment, the infection will progress to the latent and late stages of disease.

Late Stage

The latent (hidden) stage of syphilis begins when secondary symptoms disappear. Without treatment, the infected person will continue to have syphilis even though there are no signs or symptoms; infection remains in the body. This would usually develop after more than 10 years. It is then that syphilis can affect the heart, and possibly the nervous system. The eyes, heart, blood vessels, liver, bones, and joints can be affected. Signs and symptoms of the late stage of syphilis include difficulty coordinating muscle movements, paralysis, numbness, gradual blindness, and dementia. This damage may be serious enough to cause death.

Congenital Syphilis

This disease process begins at 18 to 20 weeks of gestation, when the immune system is capable of responding. The disease is systemic. A stillborn fetus may result, and for those babies that have syphilis onset at delivery, the prognosis is poor.

Those who survive usually present with the disease 2 to 6 weeks after delivery. Eighty percent of these infants have the disease by 3 to 4 months of age and 20 to 60 percent have cutaneous lesions.

Lesions are similar to those seen in the adult and are often prominent in the plantar region. Bulbous and vesicular lesions may also occur. Early congenital syphilis may include bilateral symmetric mucous patches, snuffles (a profuse nasal discharge containing large amounts of Treponema); osteochondritis or periostitis in the long bones (seen in 75-100% of children and therefore a good diagnostic indicator seen on X-ray) evidenced as a moth eaten appearance at the distal ends of bones. The bone can repair completely within a year.

Late Congenital Syphilis

Patients may have any one of the following findings:

1. Hutchinson's teeth (only permanent teeth are affected) — notching of teeth, with widely spaced, peg-shaped teeth. The two front teeth can be shaped like screwdrivers.
2. Interstitial Keratitis — inflammation of the cornea; may lead to scarring.
3. Clutton's joints — arthrosis of the knee, causing bilateral degeneration.
4. Mulberry Molar-abnormality in cusp and enamel formation.
5. Rhagades – abnormal fine pattern of scarring in the lower part of the face in people who had snuffles and were not treated. The invasion of Treponema undermines the development of soft tissue.
6. Sabre shin (convex bowing of the tibia) and saddle nose from osteochondritis and perichondritis.

Gonorrhoea

Most women who have this STD have no symptoms, or very mild symptoms that are often mistaken for something else, such as a bladder infection. When a person has symptoms, they most often appear within 2 to 10 days after having sex with someone who has the STD. But, some people can take as long as a few months to show symptoms.

Symptoms in Women

Although most **women** infected will remain asymptomatic (without symptoms), women who develop symptoms will do so within 10 days of infection.

The cervix is primarily affected in woman infected with this sexually transmitted disease. Symptoms are:

1. Abnormal discharge from the vagina that is yellow-greenish colour, sometimes bloody, mostly foul smelling.
2. Irritation and/or discharge from the anus and general irritation of the outer area of the vagina.
3. Burning or pain during urination.

When the infection spreads to the fallopian tubes, some women still have no signs or symptoms. Others may experience one or more of the following symptoms, which can be an indication that the infection has progressed to PID:

1. Lower abdominal pain
2. Lower back pain
3. Pain during intercourse
4. Intermenstrual bleeding
5. Menorrhagia
6. Nausea
7. Fever

Symptoms in Men

Most men exhibit symptoms within two days to five days after exposure, with a possible range of one to 30 days. About one in five infected men may not experience symptoms of gonorrhoea. In others, the symptoms are

1. Yellowish-white discharge from the penis
2. Burning micturation
3. Increased frequency of micturation
4. Pain or swelling of the testicles
5. Inguinal lymphadenopathy
6. The head of the penis may turn red

Both men and women might have rectal or anal infection which is asymptomatic in most of the cases. If present, symptoms include anal or rectal itching, soreness, bleeding, discharge, and pain during defecation.

Gonorrhoea infections of the mouth and throat are usually without symptoms. If present, symptoms include soreness and redness in the mouth or throat.

If gonorrhoea infects the eye, men and women might experience conjunctivitis, which includes redness, itching, and discharge from the eye.

The most common symptoms in new borns include conjunctivitis and pneumonia, which usually develop 5 to 12 days after birth.

Complications

If untreated, gonorrhoea can cause complications in men, women and infants.

Complications in Men

1. Prostatitis
2. Urethral scarring, which can cause a narrowing or closing of the urethra
3. Infertility
4. Epididymitis

Complications in Women

1. Pelvic Inflammatory Disease (PID): PID can develop from several days to several months after infection with gonorrhoea. Left untreated, PID can cause infertility.
2. Chronic menstrual problems
3. Chronic pelvic pain
4. Ectopic pregnancy
5. Postpartum endometritis
6. Cystitis
7. Mucopurulent cervicitis: characterized by a yellow discharge from the cervix

Rare Complications in Both Sexes

Disseminated Gonococcal Infection (DGI) – About 1% of men or women with gonorrhoea may develop Disseminated Gonococcal Infection (DGI), which is sometimes called gonococcal arthritis. DGI occurs when gonorrhoea infection spreads to sites other than genitals, such as the blood, skin, heart, or joints. Symptoms of DGI include fever, multiple skin lesions, painful swelling of joints (arthritis), infection of the inner lining of the heart, and inflammation of the membrane covering the brain and spinal cord meningitis. DGI can be successfully treated using antibiotic regimens similar to those recommended for treating uncomplicated gonorrhoea.

Complications in New Born

Gonorrhoea can be passed from mother to newborn as the baby passes through the infected birth canal. Complications in infants include blindness, from untreated eye infections and symptoms of DGI including arthritis, meningitis and sepsis, a bacterial infection of the blood.

Chlamydia

Approximately, two-thirds of infected women and half of infected men are asymptomatic. If a person does have symptoms, they usually develop within one to three weeks after exposure to chlamydia. The period of infectivity is difficult to determine since so many people are asymptomatic.

Symptoms in Women

When the infection is limited to the cervix:

1. Vaginal discharge
2. Burning sensation during urination

If the infection spreads to the fallopian tubes, women may experience:

1. Lower abdominal and lower back pain
2. Pain during intercourse
3. Intermenstrual bleeding and post coital bleeding

Chlamydial infection of the cervix can spread to the rectum.

Symptoms in Men

Men may be asymptomatic or symptoms may be minor. When symptomatic, men may experience one or more of the following:

1. Mild irritation at the end of the penis, which disappears after two or three days.
2. Pus (thick yellow-white flud) or watery or milky discharge from the penis
3. Burning micturation
4. Pain or swelling of the testicles

Both men and women can experience proctitis, urethritis and conjunctivitis (inflamed eyelid). Most infections of the mouth and throat are asymptomatic. If present, symptoms are soreness and redness in the throat or mouth.

Complications

If untreated, chlamydia can cause complications in men, women and infants.

Complications in Women

1. Pelvic Inflammatory Disease (PID). PID is a serious infection of a woman's reproductive organs. Left untreated, PID can cause infertility.

2. Ectopic pregnancy
3. Cystitis (inflammation of the urinary bladder)
4. Mucopurulent cervicitis, characterized by a yellow discharge from the cervix

Complications in Men

1. Prostatitis (inflammation of the prostate gland)
2. Urethral scarring
3. Infertility
4. Epididymitis

Complications in Pregnant Mothers

1. Premature delivery

Complications in Infants

(Transmission from infected mother to child):

1. Conjunctivitis that can lead to blindness
2. Complications of pneumonia, which can include death

Reiter's Syndrome

Reiter's syndrome is a disorder that causes three symptoms– arthritis (joint inflammation), redness of the eyes, and urinary tract problems. Chlamydia trachomatis is one of the bacteria that can cause the disease. It usually affects men between the ages of 20 and 40. Women can develop the disorder, though less often than men and with symptoms that are milder and less noticeable.

Appendicitis can also be caused by chlamydia.

Genital Herpes

Most of those infected by genital herpes are asymptomatic or they do not recognize any symptoms they might have. Most often, the incubation period is 2 to 10 days. These first episodes of symptoms usually last 2 to 3 weeks.

Symptoms

Early symptoms are itching or burning feeling in the genital or anal area, pain in the legs, gluteal or genital area, abnormal vaginal discharge and feeling of pressure in the abdomen.

This followed within a few days by appearance of sores in areas where the virus has entered the body, such as on the mouth, penis, or vagina. Sores can erupt inside the vagina and on the cervix in women, or in the urethra of women and men. Small red bumps appear first, develop into blisters, and then become painful open sores. Over several days, the sores become crusty and then heal without leaving a scar.

Other symptoms that may go with the first episode of genital herpes are fever, headache, muscle aches, painful or difficult urination, vaginal discharge, and swollen glands in the groin area.

Recurrence – After the first outbreak, any future outbreaks are usually mild and last only about a week. Most people can except to have several (typically four to five) outbreaks or symptomatic recurrences within a year. An infected person may know that an outbreak is about to happen by a tingling feeling or itching in the genital area, or pain in the buttocks or down the leg. Sometimes, only the tingling and itching are present without appearance of sores or very small blisters appear that are barely noticeable. The frequency and severity of recurrent episodes vary greatly. While some people have only one or two outbreaks in a lifetime, others may have several outbreaks a year.

Although some people with herpes report that their outbreaks are brought on by another illness, stress, or having a menstrual period, outbreaks often are not predictable. In some cases, outbreaks may be connected to exposure to sublight.

Complications

1. Recurrent painful genital sores in many adults.
2. Herpes infection can be severe in people with suppressed immune systems.
3. Psychological distress
4. Herpes can make people more susceptible to HIV infection, and it can make HIV infected individuals more infectious.
5. Cervical cancer and genital herpes – Though is direct no link between genital herpes and cancer of the cervix it is still advisable for infected woman to have regular pap smear tests.

Complications in Infected Mothers and New Born

If a woman has her first episode of genital herpes while she is pregnant, she can pass the virus to her unborn child and may deliver a premature baby. As most infections occur during birth from lesions in birth canal, a ceaserian section is strongly advised in the affected women.

Infection in new born could be subclinical or localized to mouth, skin and eyes. But half the babies born with herpes can develop serious problems that may affect the nervous system. If the infected new born are treated immediately with acyclovir, their chances of being healthy are increased.

Genital Warts

Genital warts are often called **veneral warts** or Condylomata Acuminata and are caused by certain types of the human papillomavirus (HPV). Genital warts are growths or bumps that appear in and around the vagina or anus or on the cervix in females; or on the penis, scrotum, groin, or high in males. They can be raised or flat, rough or smooth, single or multiple, or small or large. Some cluster together to form a cauliflower-like shape. They are usually flesh-colored and painless. They are spread by direct, skin-to-skin contact during vaginal, anal, or oral sex with an infected person. In women, HPV can invade the vagina and cervix. These warts may be flat and invisible. Genital warts are particularly severe in pregnant women and in persons whose immunity has been lowered by cancer, AIDS, organ transplantation, immune suppressive medications, or certain other medications.

Complications

Because the virus can lead to changes in the cervix that may lead to cancer, it's important that this condition is diagnosed and treated. Sometimes warts can cause a woman to have abnormal pap smear. For this reason, women with warts on the cervix should have a pap smear test every six months to one year. Infants exposed to the virus in the birth canal can develop warts in the throat, which can obstruct the airway and must be removed.

Chancroid

The incubation Period is 3-5 days or less.

Symptoms in Women

The following are symptoms of chanchroid in women:

1. Soft, gray, painful vesico-pustules or sores containing pus. The sores often have ragged edges and bleed easily when touched.
2. Sores are present around or inside vagina, rectum, or other lares, may have a bad odor.
3. The sores tend to merge into large patches of damaged tissue, and are often accompanied by an infected abscess in the groin due to inguinal lymphadenitis.
4. Painful urination
5. Painful bowel movements

Symptoms in Men

1. Painful sores on foreskin, shaft or head of the penis, scrotum, rectum, or other areas, may have a bad odor.
2. Pain or swelling in groin area.

Both men and women may have no symptoms.

Complications

Increases the chance of contacting HIV/AIDS.

Trichomonas

Symptoms in Women

Women and men may have no symptoms.

The following are symptoms of trichomonas in women:

1. Discolored discharge with bad odor
2. Frequent, painful urination
3. Inflammation of the genitals (itching or burning)
4. Sometimes pain in lower abdomen

Symptoms in Men

The following are symptoms of trichomonas in men:

1. Discharge from the penis
2. Painful urination

Complications

1. Increase in risk of acquiring HIV infection, if exposed.
2. In those with Trichomoniasis and concurrent infection with HIV, increase in the chances of transmitting HIV infection to a sex partner.

Complications in Fetus/New Born

Trichomoniasis in pregnant women may cause premature rupture of the membranes and pre-term delivery.

Molluscum Contagiosum

Molluscum contagiosum is a viral skin infection from the poxvirus family that causes pearl-like bumps on the skin. The nodules are 2-5 millimeters in diameter and are painless. Molluscum contagiosum can sometimes be confused with herpes when seen on the genitals, however, the distinct difference is that molluscum lesions are painless whereas the herpes lesions can be painful. Although it is possible to have a single bump, molluscum contagiosum is typically found in multiples.

In the beginning, the dome of the bump is firm, but later it becomes softer and grayer and may drain. In most cases, this infection is found in children, seen on the face, neck, armpits, and hands. In adults, however, molluscum contagiosum can be seen on the genitals, abdomen, and inner thighs and is considered to be a sexually transmitted disease. Lesions may occur anywhere except the palms of the hands and soles of the feet.

People with normal immune systems can expect individual lesions to last anywhere from 2 to 3 months. Complete disappearance of the virus can last anywhere from 3 to 18 months. However, people who are immuno-deficient because they have an illness such as AIDS may have a rapidly worsening case of the virus.

Hepatitis

Hepatitis is inflammation of the liver. It can be caused by a variety or causes but it could be the result of a viral infection. There are many types of virus, which can cause hepatitis of which hepatitis B and C are most important. They can be transmitted by sexual route. Each of these viruses act differently.

Symptoms

About one-third of people with Hepatitis B virus are asymptomatic. Rest may suffer from symptoms like a short, mild, flu-like illness.

- Nausea and vomiting
- Diarrhoea
- Loss of appetite
- Weight loss
- Jaundice
- Pruritis

Complications in Adults

- Chronic hepatitis
- Liver cirrhosis
- Liver cancer

Possible Consequences for the Fetus and New born: Pregnant women can transmit the disease to their unborn children. Some 90% of infants infected at birth become chronic carriers and are at risk of liver disease and liver cancer. They are also capable of transmitting the virus. Infants of infected mothers can be given immunoglobulin and vaccinated at birth, potentially eliminating the risk of chronic infection.

Non-specific Urethritis

Non specific Urethritis (NSU) is an inflammation of a man's urethra. This disease does not occur in woman. This inflammation can be caused by different types of infection, the most common being chlamydia trachomatis, gonococcus; ureaplasma and mycoplasma hominis.

Signs and Symptoms

NSU may be experienced months or even in some cases years into a relationship. The symptoms of NSU may include:

1. Dysuria or burning micturation
2. White/cloudy fluid from the tip of the penis especially early in the morning
3. Feeling that you need to pass urine frequently

Human Acquired Deficiency Syndrome

World Health Organization has categorized the disease into stages based on symptomatology.

Symptoms/Clinical Features

WHO Stage-1

Early stage of infection and is characterized by:

(a) Swollen glands
(b) Fever
(c) Headache
(d) Tiredness
(e) Sore muscles
(f) Diarrhoea

WHO Stage-2

1. Repeated infections of upper airways, chest and throat
2. Mouth ulcers
3. Unintentional weight loss of < 10% body weight
4. Herpes Zooster or Shingles
5. Rashes
6. Skin diseases like sebbhoric dermatitis, prurigo
7. Fungal infection in nails
8. Cracks at corners of mouth-angular chelitis

WHO Stage-3

1. Bedridden for < 50% of days in the last one month
2. Severe bacterial infection like pneumonia or pyomyositis
3. Weight Loss of > 10% of body weight
4. Diarrhoea for more than one month
5. Fever for more than one month
6. Oral candiasis
7. Vulvovaginal candidiasis > 1 month
8. Hairy leukoplakia: White patches with what looks like hair growing out of them in the mouth
9. Tuberculosis of lungs
10. Severe infections occurring in other places in body
11. Full blown AIDS will occur within an year or two after stage 3.

WHO Stage-4

1. Bedridden for more than 50% of days last month
2. Weight loss that has progressed to severe wasting.
3. Chronic persistent diarrhoea
4. Dementia
5. The person is confused
6. Opportunistic infections occur at this stage
7. Exprapulmonary Tuberculosis
8. Cryptosporadiasis with diarrhoea > 1 month
9. Cytomegalovirus of organs other than liver, spleen or lymph nodes
10. Herpes simples, Mucocutaneous > 1 month or visceral for any duration
11. HIV dementia
12. Isosporiasis with diarrhoea > 1 month
13. Lymphoma
14. Mycobacteriosis, atypical and disseminated
15. Mycosis: disseminated Histoplasmosis or coccidiomycosis
16. Progressive multiple Leucoencephalopathy
17. Salmonella Septicemia (Non-typhoidal)
18. Toxoplasmosis of Brain
19. Wasting Syndrome due to HIV

Respiratory Conditions in HIV Infection

Lungs are the most frequently affected organs in HIV-infected patients. They suffer from many different opportunistic infections; among them, two are most frequently observed:

Pneumocystis Carinii Pneumonia (PCP) and Pulmonary Tuberculosis.

Persistence or worsening of cough and/or chest pain and/or dyspnoea make the clinician suspect of an opportunistic resp.

CHAPTER

10 HIV/AIDS and Nutrition in Adolescents

Santosh Jain Passi and *Vandana Sabharwal*

This chapter provides information on how nutrition plays an important role in the lives of HIV-positive people and helps them to lead healthier lives throughout the progression of human immunodeficiency virus (HIV)/Acquired Immunodeficiency Syndrome (AIDS) disease. Researchers suggest that the chances of infection with the HIV virus might be reduced in individuals who have good nutritional status; the onset of the disease and death might be delayed where HIV-positive individuals are well-nourished, and nutrient-rich diets might reduce the risks of HIV transmission from mother to fetus/the baby during pregnancy or after birth.

Malnutrition and HIV

Nutrition and HIV are linked. Any immune impairment as a result of HIV/AIDS can contribute to malnutrition. Malnutrition leads to immune impairment, worsens the effects of HIV, and contributes to a more rapid progression of the disease. Thus, malnutrition both contributes to and is a result of HIV disease progression.

A person who is malnourished and then acquires HIV is more likely to progress faster to AIDS because the body is already weak and cannot fight co-infections, particularly without access to ARVs and prophylactic medications. A well-nourished person has a stronger immune system for coping with HIV and fighting illness. Figure 1 illustrates the relationship between good nutrition and resistance to infection in the context of HIV/AIDS.

Timely improvement in nutritional status can help strengthen the immune system, thereby reducing the incidence of infections preventing loss of weight and lean body mass, and delaying disease progression, so that HIV has less chance to develop in a person who is well nourished.

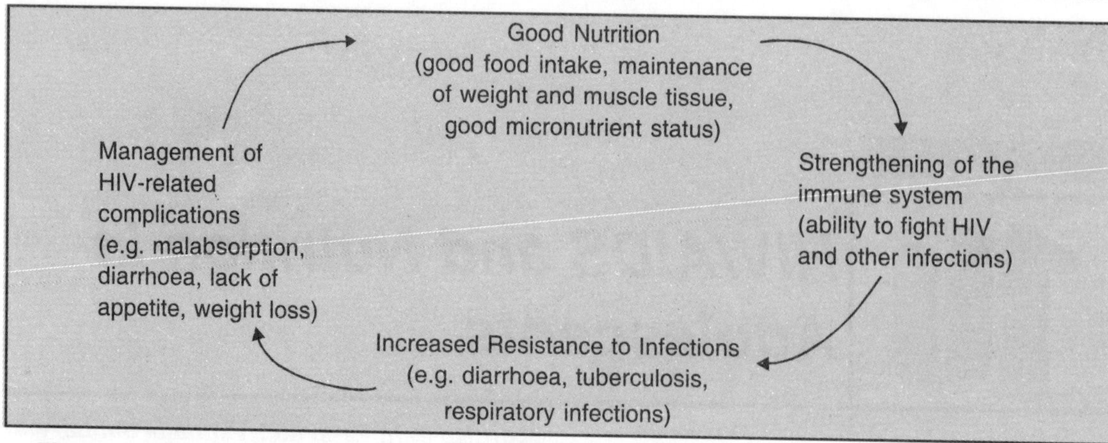

Figure 1. The Cycle of Good, Nutrition and Resistance to Infection in the Context of HIV/AIDS

Adapted from Ellen G. Piwoz and Elizabeth A. Preble, HIV/AIDS and Nutrition: A Review of the Literature; and Recommendations for Nutritional Care and Support in Sub-Saharan Africa. Washington, D.C.: Academy for Educational Development (AED), 2000.

Nutrition for HIV Positive People at Various Life Cycle Stages

Nutritional care and support helps people living with HIV to manage HIV-related complications, promotes good responses to medical treatment, and improves the person's quality of life by maintaining strength, comfort, level of functioning, and human dignity. Nutritional care and support is especially effective for those HIV-positive people who have not yet progressed to the stage requiring ARV treatment.

Nutrition and HIV/AIDS: Basic Facts

HIV infection affects nutrition through increases in resting energy expenditure, reductions in food intake, nutrient malabsorption and loss and complex metabolic alterations that culminate in weight loss and wasting common in AIDS. The effect of HIV on nutrition begins early in the course of the disease, even before an individual may be aware that he or she is infected with the virus.

Good nutrition for all individuals, but especially PLWHAs, requires the consumption of an adequate amount in the appropriate proportions of macronutrients (e.g., proteins, carbohydrates, and fats) and micronutrients (e.g. vitamins, minerals). It is important to remember that many people in resource limited settings are experiencing pre-existing malnutrition and that HIV will worsen the situation.

The nutritional needs of HIV-infected persons depend on the stage of disease progression.

Required intake levels are suggested based on the abscence or presence of symptoms such as fever, diarrhoea, weight loss, and wasting.

Energy Requirements: The HIV-infected person has additional energy needs due to:

- Energy used for HIV infection and opportunistic infections;
- Nutrient mal-absorption; and
- Altered metabolism

The various phases of the infection are marked by an increase in metabolism, increased energy needs, and nutrient depletion. These effects of infection often occur synergistically and result in weight loss and wasting. In the absence of AIDS symptoms (WHO stage 1), HIV infected persons should increase energy intake by 10 percent over the level of energy intake recommended for healthy non-HIV-infected persons of the same age, sex, and physical activity level. In the presence of symptoms (WHO stage 2 and above), HIV infected persons should increase energy intake by 20 to 30 percent over the level of energy intake recommended for healthy non-HIV infected persons of the same age, sex, and physical activity level. These recommendations are for HIV-infected persons, including those taking HIV-related medications such as ARVs.

Protein Requirements – According to WHO's Nutrient Requirements for People Living with HIV/AIDS, "Data are insufficient to support an increase in protein requirements due to HIV infection." HIV-infected persons do not require more protein than the level recommended for healthy non-HIV-infected persons of the same age, sex, and physical activity level.

At the onset of opportunistic infections, the body loses nitrogen, which suggests a need for increased protein intake if opportunistic infections remain untreated. Studies have not demonstrated, however, that improved clinical outcomes occur from increased protein intake among HIV-infected individuals. Further research is needed on the optimal protein requirements of HIV-infected persons during the course of HIV disease. HIV-infected people often have pre-existing protein-energy malnutrition. Protein-energy malnutrition.

(PEM) results from inadequate intake or poor utilization of food and energy, not a deficiency of one nutrient and not usually simply a lack of dietary protein. It may needed to address the deficiency by increasing intakes to meet the recommended levels.

Fat Requirements – According to the recent WHO guidelines, there is no evidence that fat requirements are different because of HIV infection. However, certain ARVs or certain infection symptoms such as diarrhoea may require changes in the timing or quantity of fat intake in some cases.

Micronutrient Requirements – WHO does not recommend micronutrients beyond the level of recommended micronutrients for healthy non-HIV-infected persons of the same age, sex and physical activity level. However, micronutrient deficiencies are common in areas where HIV is prevalent. Deficiencies of vitamins and minerals such as vitamins A, B-Complex, C, E, Selenium and Zinc, which are needed by the immune system to fight infection, are common in people living with HIV. Deficiencies of anti-oxidant vitamins and minerals contribute to oxidative stress, a condition that may accelerate cell death and increase the rate of HIV replication. Good nutrition is best achieved by consuming a diverse diet with foods rich in micronutrients, especially vitamins A B_6, B_{12} and selenium, iron and zinc. If the HIV-infected person presents signs of a spcific or multiple micronutrient deficiencies, the deficiency should be addressed using the standard protocols.

Nutritional Care and Support for HIV-Infected Pregnant Women and Adolescents

This section presents nutritional care practices recommended for HIV-infected pregnant women and adolescent girls, like other PLWHAs, have increased energy requirements due to infection with HIV. Attention to nutrition for HIV-infected pregnant women and adolescent girls is doubly important in order to maintain weight, prevent weight loss, and continue adequate weight gain during pregnancy. Improved nutritional status will help to maintain a strong immune system, decrease susceptibility to infections, and slow the progression to AIDS.

Energy Requirements – Energy requirements of HIV-infected pregnant adolescents and adult women vary according to the stage of the disease. ***HIV-infected asymptomatic*** pregnant adolescents and adults (WHO stage 1) should increase energy intake over the level recommended for healthy non HIV-infected pregnant adolescents and adult women by an amount equaling 10 percent of the intake level recommended for non-pregnant adolescents or women of the same age and activity level plus the additional energy (i.e., approximately 285 kcal per day) needed to support pregnancy. ***HIV-infected symptomatic*** pregnant adolescents and adults (WHO stage 2 and above) should increase energy intake over the level recommended for healthy non HIV-infected pregnant adolescents and adult women by an amount equaling 20 to 30 percent of the intake level recommended for non-pregnant adolescents or women of the same age and activity level plus the additional energy needed to support pregnancy. The amount of increased energy is the same for HIV-infected persons taking ARVs. The level of additional energy intake for the HIV infected pregnant women depends on the presence and severity of symptoms. Table 1 illustrates the changes in recommended energy intake of pregnant women based on the stage of the disease.

Protein Requirements – At this time, there is not enough evidence to suggest that HIV infected pregnant women require more protein than the level recommended for healthy non-HIV-infected pregnant woman. Meeting the protein requirements of HIV-infected pregnant women will help prevent muscle wasting and support the additional protein demands of pregnancy including the growth of the placenta and increased red blood cell mass.

Micronutrient Requirements – Micronutrients play important roles in the healthy functioning of the immune system and therefore are particularly important for PLWHAs. At the same time, in populations with high AIDS prevalence, micronutrient deficiencies are often common. Current recommendations from the expert consultation to the world.

Health Organization advises HIV-infected pregnant adolescents and adult women to consume varied diets to ensure that they meet the RDAs for micronutrients.

The results of vitamin A supplementation trials for HIV-infected women are mixed. The current WHO guidelines advise that vitamin A intake by HIV-infected pregnant and lactating women not exceed the existing RDAs. No additional vitamin A should be provided. In areas of endemic vitamin A deficiency, WHO continues to recommend administration of a single high dose (i.e., 200,000 IU) vitamin A supplement within the first six to eight weeks of delivery to the new mother. The iron/folate supplementation schedule also remains the same as for non-HIV-infected women. Although a varied, nutritionally adequate diet is the best source for micronutrient supplement is recommended. Some studies have shown improvements from specific multivitamin and mineral supplements to HIV-infected women for a range of outcomes, including increased maternal weight gain during pregnancy, increased hemoglobin concentration, HIV progression to AIDS and improved CD_4 cell counts. For children, improved birth weight, reduced postnatal transmission of HIV, and decreased mortality have been shown, particularly among nutritionally vulnerable women with advanced HIV disease. The optimal composition of multiple micronutrient supplements for HIV infected women has yet to be determined and is currently being studied.

Table 1. ***Estimated Changes in the Daily Energy Intake (kcal) of a 28 years old, moderately active HIV-infected Woman, According to the Stage in the Disease***

Stage in the disease	*Average daily energy intake for moderately active* adult women (kcal)*	*Additional energy due to HIV** kcal)*	*Additional daily energy required by the pregnancy (kcal)*	*Total (kcal)*
Asymptomatic	+ 2140	+ 214	+ 285	2639
Early symptomatic	+ 2140	+ 428	+ 285	2853
Symptomatic	+ 2140	+ 642	+ 285	3067

* Daily energy intake for a 28 years old moderately active woman Multiply Basal Metabolic Rate (BMR) by adjustment
factor for the activity level = 1305 x 1.64 = 2140 kcal

**10 percent daily energy intake increase during the asymptomatic phase = 10 percent (2140); 20 Percent daily energy intake increase at the early symptomatic phase = 20 percent (2140); and 30 percent daily energy intake increase during the symptomatic phase = 30 percent (2140).

Support for Pregnant and Lactating Women and Adolescent Girls

Additional Recommended Care Practices Food Safety and Handling – Proper food handling and safety practices for HIV-infected pregnant women are very important. Remind HIV infected women and adolescent girls that they are more susceptible to harmful bacteria and viruses in contaminated food and water as a result of their infection with HIV. Food poisoning can cause weight loss and further lower their resistance to future infections. Hygienic food handling should be accompanied by sanitary disposal of feces, good personal hygiene, including hand washing and covering of wounds, and the use of clean water for drinking and food preparation.

Psychosocial Support – HIV-infected pregnant women and adolescent girls need special care and attention. In addition to dealing with a life-threatening disease, they must also deal with the usual discomforts that can accompany pregnancy. They may also have to confront discrimination and stigmatization by their family and community. Psychosocial support from caregivers and health workers is important. Mental health interventions may be needed to address depression. Program staff should work with communities to raise awareness about the need to support HIV-infected pregnant women to improve pregnancy outcomes and the survival of the mother.

The Low Social Status of Women – Poor health and nutritional status of girls and women, especially in limited resource settings, may be due in part to gender inequality and the low status of women in certain societies. Women may need the approval of husbands or mothers-in-law to obtain nutrition and health services. Differential access to education and income generation opportunities for adolescent girls and women may be a barrier to their ability to improve dietary intake and/or treat and control infections. Community level program staff should carry out a situation analysis of women's health and nutrition and identify and address problems that affect their nutritional status, especially during pregnancy and lactation.

Food Insecurity in the Context of HIV/AIDS – In many resource limited settings that have been hit hard by the HIV/AIDS epidemic, access to sufficient food may be limited, especially for families affected directly by HIV/AIDS. Strengthen linkages and refer women to programs that provide nutritional care and support and support food security and coping strategies of HIV/AIDS-affected households and individuals.

Inequity in Intra-household Food Distribution – In many cultures, women frequently serve themselves last at meals. Husbands and male children are often the first to get food and mothers and girls eat what remains. For HIV-infected pregnant women and adolescent girls, problematic intra household food distribution patterns may compound already existing inadequate nutritional intake due to increased energy needs of HIV infection and pregnancy.

Food Taboos – Pregnant women may observe culturally dictated diretary guidelines that prohibit certain foods. These food taboos may restrict nutrient dense foods, such as eggs or a specific type of meat. Avoiding such foods deprives pregnant women of an important source of protein and micronutrients and can contribute to malnutrition. Although culturally sensitive, programs should work with communities to address taboos that may deprive women of foods they need to ensure good nutritional status and birth outcomes.

Cultural Beliefs – Fear of Having a "Big Baby". In some cultures, women restrict food intake during the final months of the pregnancy. This limits weight gain to reduce the size of the baby and, thus, decrease the risk of obstructed labour. In addition to LBW, inadequate diets can contribute to a weakened immune status of the mother with resulting increased risk of morbidity and possibly mortality of both mother and baby.

Additional Care and Support for Pregnant and Lactating Women and Adolescent Girls

High Physical Activity Workloads – Women in resource limited settings routinely have heavy workloads that do not diminish with pregnancy. To compensate for the high amounts of energy expended on household and agricultural work, in addition to the energy used by the virus and by the growing baby, HIV-infected pregnant women must increase their energy intake. Alternatively, their workloads can be reduced and periods of rest can be added to reduce their energy expenditure. However, continued physical activity at usual/moderate levels remains important for HIV-infected women to preserve lean body mass.

Nutritional Care and Support for HIV-Infected Lactating Women

Energy Requirements – The energy requirements of HIV infected lactating mothers vary according to the stage of the disease. ***HIV-infected asymptomatic*** (WHO stage 1) lactating adolescents and adults should increase energy intake over the level recommended for healthy non-HIV-infected lactating adolescents and adult women by an amount equaling 10 percent of the intake level recommended for non-lactating adolescents or women of the same age and activity level plus the additional 500 kcal to support lactation. ***HIV-infected symptomatic*** (WHO stage 2 and above) lactating adolescents and adults should increase energy intake over the level recommended for healthy non-HIV-infected lactating adolescents and adult women by an amount equaling 20 to 30 percent of the intake level recommended for non-lactating adolescents or women of the same age and activity level plus the additional 500 kcal to support lactation. The necessary energy intake increase is the same whether or not the HIV infected person takes ARVs. The level of additional energy intake for the HIV-infected pregnant woman depends on the presence and severity of symptoms. Table 2 shows the amounts of energy needed, depending on the stage of HIV/AIDS.

Protein Requirements – HIV-infected lactating women and adolescents need the same level of daily protein intake as healthy HIV-negative lactating women, which are estimated to be 1.1 g/kg body weight per day or approximately 71 g of protein per day, according the U.S. National Academies of Science in 2002.

Micronutrient Requirements – HIV-infected lactating women and adolescents need the same amounts of micronutrients as healthy HIV-negative lactating. HIV-infected lactating women should be encouraged to eat a variety of foods, including animal products, fruits, and vegetables, to help ensure adequate micronutrient intake.

Table 2. ***Recommended Energy Intake of 28 Years Old HIV-infected Moderately Active Lactating Women, According to the Stage in the Disease***

Stage in the disease	*Average daily energy intake (kcal)**	*Additional energy due to HIV** kcal)*	*Additional energy for Lactation (kcal)*	*Total (kcal)*
Asymptomatic	+ 2140	+ 214	+ 500	= 2854
Early symptomatic	+ 2140	+ 428	+ 500	= 3068
Symptomatic	+ 2140	+ 642	+ 500	= 3282

* Daily energy intake for a 28-years-old moderately active woman Multiply Basal Metabolic Rate (BMR) by adjustment factor for the activity level = 1305 x 1.64 = 2140 kcal

** 10 percent daily energy intake increase during the asymptomatic phase = 10 percent (2140); 20 Percent daily energy intake increase at the early symptomatic phase = 20 percent (2140); and 30 percent daily energy intake increase in the mid symptomatic phase = 30 percent (2140).

Nutritional Care and Support for Pregnant and Lactating Women and Adolescent Girls

Additional Recommended Care Practices

Breast Health Management – Cracked nipples, mastitis, and breast abscesses increase the risk of HIV transmission through breast milk. One should demonstrate proper latching-on techniques to prevent the development of cracked nipples and counsel on how to prevent and manage other types of breast problems such as mastitis.

Safer Infant Feeding Practices – This has been discussed latter in details.

Nutritional Care and Support for HIV-Infected Infant

Guidance is needed on feeding for infants and young children in the context of HIV/AIDS to ensure their optimal growth and development, boost immune system functioning, and reduce transmission of HIV. The recent LINKAGES/AED publication, Infant Feeding Options in the Context of HIV, published in 2004, and the most recent WHO guidelines. HIV and Infant Feeding: A Guide for Health-care Managers and Supervisors, published in 2003 are the primary sources for the recommendations. Here we discuss nutritional care for:

- Infants and young children of HIV positive women; and
- Young children with HIV disease.

Breast milk is widely recognized as the best source of nutrition for infants, and exclusive breastfeeding is recommended for the first six months of an infant's life. In addition to essential nutrients, breast milk contains antibodies and enzymes that protect against infections and strengthens the infant's immune system. However, HIV may also be transmitted to an infant during breastfeeding. On average, approximately one out of seven infants born to an HIV-infected mother will become infected through breastfeeding up to 24 months.

WHO, the United Nations Children's Fund (UNICEF) and other United Nations agencies currently recommend that HIV-positive mothers avoid breastfeeding if replacement feeding from birth is acceptable, feasible, affordable, sustainable, and safe (AFASS). If these conditions are not met, then it is recommended that HIV-positive mothers practice exclusive breastfeeding for the first months of life. If circumstances change and the AFASS criteria can be met, shortening the period of exclusive breastfeeding and transitioning as quickly as possible to another breast milk option or replacement feeding will reduce the risk of exposure to HIV.

The Caregiver's Choice of Feeding Method: HIV-positive mothers should be made aware of the risks and benefits of different infant feeding options, including the risk of transmission of HIV through breastfeeding. Mothers who can provide replacement feeding that is acceptable, feasible, affordable, sustainable, and safe are advised to do so. When these criteria cannot be met through family or community resources, particularly in resource limited settings, women are advised to exclusively breast feed. (position of the American Dietetic Association and Dietitians of Canada: Nutrition intervention in the care of persons with human immunodeficiency virus infection. Journal of the American Dietetic Association 104 (2004): (1145-1441).

AFASS: Acceptable, Feasible, Affordable, Sustainable, and Safe

These terms should be adapted in the light of local conditions and formative research. The following may serve as a starting point:

Acceptable: The mother perceives no barrier to replacement feeding. Barriers may have cultural or social reasons, or be due to fear of stigma or discrimination. According to this concept the mother is under no social or cultural pressure not to use replacement feeding; and she is supported by family and community in opting for replacement feeding, or she will be able to cope with pressure from family and friends to breastfeed, and she can deal with possible stigma attached to being seen with replacement food.

Feasible: The mother or family has adequate time, knowledge, skills, and other resources to prepare the replacement food and feed the infant up to 12 times in 24 hours. According to this concept, the mother can understand and follow the instructions for preparing infant formula and, with support from the family, can prepare enough replacement feeds correctly every day and at night, despite disruptions to preparation of family food or other work.

Affordable: The mother and family, with community or health-system support if necessary, can pay the cost of purchasing/producing, preparing, and using replacement feeding, including all ingredients, fuel, clean water, soap, and equipment, without compromising the health and nutrition of the family. This concept also includes access to medical care if necessary for diarrhoea and the cost of such care.

Sustainable: Availability of a continuous and uninterrupted supply and a dependable system of distribution for all ingredients and products needed for safe replacement feeding for as long as the infant needs it, up to one year of age or longer. According to this concept there is little risk that formula will ever be unavailable or inaccessible, and another person is available to feed the child in the mother's absence and can prepare and give replacement foods.

Safe: Replacement foods are correctly and hygienically prepared and stored and fed in nutritionally adequate quantities, with clean hands, and using clean utensils, preferably by cup. This concept means that the mother or caregiver:

- Has access to a reliable supply of safe water (e.g., from a piped or protected-well source);
- Prepares replacement feeds that are nutritionally sound and free of pathogens;

- Is able to wash hands and utensils thoroughly with soap and regularly boil the utensils to sterilize them;
- Can boil water for preparing each of the body's feeds; and
- Can store unprepared feeds in clean, covered containers and protect them from rodents, insects, and other animals.

Source: WHO, What are the options? Using formative research to adapt global recommendations on HIV and infant feeding to the local context, 2004.

When to Counsel on Infant Feeding Options

- After an HIV-positive test, but prior to delivery, to assist the mother to select the best option for her infant
- Within 10 days of delivery to assess the ability of the mother to successfully implement her infant feeding choice
- At routine postpartum visits, well-child checks, and sick-child service delivery points
- When mothers plan to change her current feeding practice

Source: WHO, HIV and Infant Feeding: A guide for healthcare managers and supervisors, 2003.

Nutritional Care Recommendations for Infants and Children of HIV-positive

As noted above, for infants of HIV-positive mothers, WHO (2003) advises that:

When replacement feeding is acceptable, feasible, affordable, sustainable and safe, avoidance of all breastfeeding by HIV-positive mothers is recommended. Otherwise, exclusive breastfeeding is recommended during the first months of life. To minimize HIV transmission risk, breastfeeding should be discontinued as soon as feasible, taking into account local conditions, the individual woman's situation and the issues of replacement feeding including infections other than HIV and malnutrition. When HIV-positive mothers choose not to breastfeed from birth or stop breastfeeding later, they should be provided with specific guidance for at least the first two years of the child's life to ensure adequate replacement feeding.

Nutritional Care Recommendations for Infants and Children

WHO Recommendations Result in the Need for the Following Actions:

- Provide HIV-positive mothers with information on different infant feeding options to enable them to make an informed choice for their infants.
- Inform HIV-positive mothers of the advantages and the risks associated with the infant feeding option they have chosen.

- Provide HIV-positive mothers with the support required to implement their choice.
- Where possible, involve the mother's partner or other members of the family in the counseling and decision-making process.

Infants at Birth through Five Months Born to HIV-positive Women: Exclusive Breastfeeding Followed by Replacement Feeding

If the mother decides to breastfeed, she should:

- Breastfeed exclusively for not longer than six months and prevent and manage breast problems and sores in the infant's mouth to prevent HIV transmission from mother to child during breastfeeding; and
- Transition to replacement feeding when it is AFASS. This means feeding infants who are not receiving breast milk with a nutritious diet that meets their nutrient requirements until they are old enough to consume a diet of family foods. From birth to six months, replacement feeding is a suitable breast milk substitute. After six months, this means giving a breast milk substitute plus appropriate complementary foods to support optimal growth and development. Exclusive breastfeeding practices for children of HIV-positive mothers are the same as for children born to HIV-negative mothers or mothers of unknown HIV status. Infants are fed only breast milk for up to six months. No other foods, teas, water juices, milks, or infant formula should be given to the infant.
- Keeping Breasts Healthy – Mastitis, nipple lesions, and breast abscesses may increase the risk of HIV transmission through breast milk. Health workers should counsel HIV-positive mothers on how to prevent, manage, and seek treatment for breast problems to reduce the risk of HIV transmission to the infant.

Prevention and Treatment of Sores in the Infant's Mouth – Sores in an infant's mouth may increase the risk of HIV transmission from breast milk. It should be shown to a HIV-positive lactating mothers how to check for sores and, if found, they should be advise them to promptly seek medical care. Where possible, refer mothers to a breastfeeding counselor or a breastfeeding support group.

Challenges Posed by Exclusive Breastfeeding in the Context of HIV– There are several challenges to ensure the successful implementation of exclusive breastfeeding by HIV-positive mothers of infants less than six months of age. These challenges include the cultural practice of early mixed feeding, lack of breastfeeding support for mothers, the common perception that malnourished mothers do not have sufficient milk to breastfeed exclusively, and limited access to food for the lactating mothers.

Compliance with Exclusive Breastfeeding – Exclusive breastfeeding for six months is rarely practiced even when programs actively promote and support it. In the context of HIV, the practice of mixed feeding may be especially harmful because of the increased risk of HIV transmission. The exact mechanisms fostering this increased risk are not known but several have been suggested: the gut may become inflamed as a reaction to new food allergens, or germs from the food and water may damage the gut, increasing susceptibility to infection by HIV carried in breast milk. Exclusive breastfeeding helps to maintain a healthy gut epithelium that acts as a protective barrier against infectious agents. Through awareness raising activities, counseling, and community mobilization, programs need to create a supportive environment in which mothers can successfully practice exclusive breastfeeding.

Feeding Expressed, Heat-treated Breast Milk

An alternative to exclusive breastfeeding is collecting expressed breast milk and heat treating it. This is accomplished by bringing it to a boil and cooling the milk immediately by standing the clean container in cold water. Untreated expressed breast milk may be stored up to eight hours at room temperature in a cool place and 72 hours in a refrigerator. Once the milk is heat treated, it must be used within an hour. The mother or caregiver feeds the heat-treated breast milk to the infant with a cup in order to avoid the risk of contamination from bottles. This method of feeding infants of HIV-infected mothers requires resources for heating and storing the milk, time to prepare the feeds, and a supportive environment to successfully feed children in this manner.

Breastfeeding by an HIV-negative Wet Nurse – This infant feeding option requires that the mother and family of the child consider wet nursing only if the wet nurse is offered HIV testing and counseling, takes the test voluntarily, and is found to be HIV negative.

She must then practice optimal exclusive breastfeeding and safer sex practices to ensure that she is not infected with HIV while breastfeeding the infant. She will need to be available to feed the infant frequently and on demand throughout the day and night and she must receive services to prevent and treat any problems such as cracked or bleeding nipples, mastitis, or abscesses that may occur.

Factors that Increase Risk of MTCT of HIV

- Mixed feeding in the first 6 months (i.e., combining breastfeeding with breast milk substitutes)
- Breastfeeding duration (i.e., long term breastfeeding increases the risk of HIV transmission)
- Improper latching and positioning during breastfeeding.
- Breast conditions (i.e., fissured and bloody nipples, mastitis, and breast abscess)
- Sores in infant's mouth
- High maternal viral load
- Maternal immune deficiency
- Maternal malnutrition
- New HIV infection

Adapted from World Health Organization (WHO). HIV and Infant Feeding: A guide for healthcare managers and supervisors, 2003.

Infants at Birth through Five Months Born to HIV-positive Women: Replacement Feeding with Appropriate Breast milk Substitutes.

HIV-positive mothers who do not breastfeed are advised to exclusively feed their infants with appropriate breast milk substitutes (i.e., replacement feeding). These can be either commercial infant formula, the most nutritionally complete substitute for breast milk, or home-modified animal milk.

Early Cessation of Breastfeeding – The risk of HIV transmission during breastfeeding continues for as long as breastfeeding is practiced. Because this risk is cumulative, early breastfeeding cessation is recommended for HIV positive mothers. A transition from exclusive breastfeeding to exclusive replacement feeding will decrease the risk of HIV transmission. The best time to stop exclusive breastfeeding varies from one situation to another and is dependent on such factors as the mother's health status, the physical environment, economic status of the household, and risk factors for disease and death due to alternative feeding practices. Health workers and mothers should discuss and decide the most appropriate time for transition to replacement feeding based on case-specific circumstances. Health workers should then provide the necessary guidance to make the transition to exclusive replacement feeding as safe as possible.

Transitioning from Breastfeeding to Replacement Feeding – Mothers usually transition gradually from exclusive breastfeeding to breastfeeding plus complementary foods after an infant is six months old. However, in cases where a mother is HIV-positive, it is recommended that the transition from breastfeeding to replacement feeding occur as quickly as possible. While some mixed feeding is usually necessary during the transition, it should be strictly avoided once the baby has switched to replacement feeding. Healthcare workers can provide guidance and support to mothers when they have decided to make the transition to replacement feeding:

- Begin by expressing breast milk to familiarize the baby with cup feeding by offering the expressed breast milk by cup between regular breastfeeds;
- When the infant has accepted cup feeding, eliminate one breastfeed at a time and replace with expressed breast milk fed by cup;
- Express and discard breast milk if breasts become engorged during the transition process. Apply cold compresses to reduce swelling;
- Once all feeds are accepted by cup, feed only breast milk substitutes;
- Health care workers can advise mothers on comforting infants with alternative methods to breastfeeding such as massaging, swaddling, carrying, rocking, singing, sleeping with and talking to the baby; and
- Counsel women on adequate protection against pregnancy in the absence of the contraceptive protection of breastfeeding. When using breast milk substitutes, mother need to be assisted in the prevention of breast engorgement, plugged milk ducts, or mastitis as lactation is suppressed in the early days following

delivery. The infant should not be allowed to suckle; breasts should be well supported but not tightly bound, and mothers can express small amounts of breast milk to relieve discomfort.

Commercial Infant Formula – Commercial infant formula is usually available as powder and needs to be reconstituted with clean water according to the instructions on the tin before being fed to the infant. Over-concentration can cause health problems such as diarrhoea, and over-dilution can lead to malnutrition due to insufficient nutrient intake.

Safe feeding of commercial infant formula includes:

- Utensils for measuring/preparing the formula;
- Clean water to prepare the formula and clean all utensils;
- Fuel in adequate amounts to boil water for reconstituting the formula and cleaning utensils;
- Resources for hand washing and food preparation hygiene;
- Ability to read or follow directions for correct reconstitution of infant formula;
- Caregiver time to prepare at least eight feedings per day if refrigeration is not available; and
- Correct use of cup for feeding prepared infant formula.

Mothers need to have access to consistent and affordable supplies of commercial formula for at least six months. WHO estimates that 20 kg of commercial infant formula are required per infant during the first six months of life for replacement feeding. Programs should assess the types and costs of replacement feeding options that are available in the area as well as the reliability of supply. Many households in resource limited settings may not be able to afford replacement foods. In such cases, programs should work to identify mmechanisms to help households access the required foods. Both commercial and home-prepared formulas require time and knowledge to prepare safe replacement feeds, and equipment and fuel to clean utensils and the preparation environment.

Home-modified Animal Milks – When commercial infant formula is not readily available, too expensive, or otherwise not acceptable, home-prepared modified animal milk can be used as a replacement feeding option. Families need to have access to at least one half liter or the equivalent of animal milk or milk product per day. Home-modified animal milk is used exclusively, and the infant does not receive breast milk. Modified animal milks can be made from fresh animal milk, evaporated milk, dried full cream milk powder, or ultra high temperature (UHT) milk. All of these milks need to be modified to become suitable for the infant by diluting with water and adding sugar so that they have protein, fat, and sugar content somewhat similar to breast milk. The quantity of water and sugar varies from one type of milk to another. Modified animal milks do not provide enough micronutrients to meet the infant/child needs, therefore micronutrients to meet the infant/child needs, therefore micronutrient supplementation is essential. Full cream dried milk powder and evaporated milk should be reconstituted using brand-specific instructions before being fed to the infant.

Table 3. *Preparation Guide for Mother/Caregiver*

Commercial infant formula	*Home-modified animal milk*
• Wash hands with soap and water.	• Wash hands with soap and water.
• Clean all utensils, containers, and cups with soap and water	• Clean all utensils, containers and cups with soap and water
• Read or have someone read instructions on the formula tin.	• Boil water vigorously for a few seconds and let it cool. Boil as much water as needed for the whole day and store in a clean, covered container.
• Boil water vigorously for a few seconds and let it cool. Boil as much water as needed for the whole day and store in a clean covered container.	• Measure the amount of water and milk needed.
• Measure the amount of milk powder needed for one feed and mix it with the correct amount of boiled water.	• Measure the exact amount of sugar and mix it with the liquid.
• Prepare fresh commercial formula before each feed if refrigeration is not available.	• Prepare formula before each feed if refrigeration is not available.
• Feed the infant by cup about 150 ml of correctly prepared formula per kg per day, divided into six to eight feeds.	• Feed the infant by cup the appropriate amount based on the infant's weight. The infant will have to learn to drink from a cup.
The infant will have to learn to drink from a cup.	• Give the infant multivitamins specially formulated for the non-breastfed child. The multivitamin can be in the form of liquid syrup (i.e., 5 ml per day) or powder. The multivitamin can be mixed with the formula or given separately.

Care Recommendations for Infants and Children

Unacceptable Options for Replacement Feeding – The following fluids are not acceptable options for use in replacement feeding of infants because of their inadequate energy and micronutrient content: sweetened condensed milk, skimmed milk, coffee creamers, soy milk, fruit, juices, sugar water, or diluted porridges.

Mothers: Complementary and Replacement Feeding Foods

Appropriate complementary feeding for children of HIV-positive mothers ages six though 23 months consists of feeding breast milk or breast milk substitutes (e.g. milk, milk products) with complementary or additional semi-solid and solid food/liquids. All infants require foods in addition to milk by six months in order to meet their nutritional requirements for energy, protein, and micronutrients. But about six months of age, infants are able to digest undiluted animal milk as well as semi-solid foods, making replacement feeding less difficult and less expensive for mothers than during their child's first six months. HIV-positive mothers have the following options for feeding their children from six months of age:

- Continued breastfeeding until transition to other options are safe and feasible (e.g., cessation of breastfeeding and transition to breast milk substitutes), plus appropriate complementary foods;
- Expressing and heat-treating breast milk plus appropriate complementary foods;
- Wet nursing by an HIV-negative woman plus appropriate complementary foods;
- Breast milk substitutes (e.g., commercial infant formula, fresh animal milk, powdered full-cream or evaporated milk, UHT milk) plus appropriate semi-solid and solid foods; and
- Appropriate semi-solid and solid foods plus clean drinking water in circumstances where milk is not available.

Current draft guidance for the ***non-breastfed child,*** recommends that children should receive four to five meals of nutritious foods each day from six months of age, with additional nutrient-rich snacks one to two times a day as desired. Meals may be a combination of milk-only feeds, other foods, or a mix of milk and food. It is optimal to include milk in the diets of children through at least the first year of life.

Nutritional Care Recommendations for Children with HIV Disease

HIV infection is often difficult to diagnose in very young children. Infants born to HIV infected mothers have HIV antibodies made by the mother's immune system that cross the placenta to the baby's bloodstream before birth and may persist for up to 18 months. Because these maternal antibodies reflect the mother's but not the infant's infection status, an HIV antibody test is not reliable for children under 15 to 18 months. More definitive tests can determine whether a younger infant is actually infected with HIV but these tests are still expensive and are not typically available in resource limited settings.

Nutritional Needs for HIV-infected Children

Increased Energy Needs

HIV-children have greater energy needs compared to healthy non-HIV-infected children. HIV infection causes increased resting energy expenditure, may reduce food intake, and causes poor nutrient absorption, loss, and metabolic alterations that result in weight loss and wasting. The energy needs of HIV infected children will vary according to the presence and severity of symptoms.

Nutritional Care Recommendations for Infants and Children

The energy requirements of HIV-infected children with no symptoms are increased by 10 percent. During the symptomatic phase without weight loss, energy requirements increase by 20 to 30 percent over the level of energy intake recommended for healthy non-HIV-infected children of the same age. When the child is both symptomatic and losing weight, energy requirements increase by 50 to 100 percent.

Protein and Micronutrient Needs – Protein and micronutrient requirements remain the same for children of the same age, sex, and physical activity, regardless of HIV status.

However, if children have pre-existing micronutrient deficiencies or inadequate protein intake, these need to be addressed and may require micronutrient supplementation and/or increased protein intake.

Pre-existing Malnutrition – Many children in resource limited settings are already underweight and malnourished. Healthcare workers will need to help families correct underlying malnutrition as well as address the additional nutritional requirements caused by infection with HIV. It is especially difficult for children to consume 50 to 100 percent more energy when they are fighting opportunistic infections and experiencing weight loss. Help caregivers to encourage children to eat additional energy-dense, micronutrient rich food when periods of illness subside. According to WHO in 2003 breastfed children who are found to be HIV-infected may benefit from continued breastfeeding as well as complementary feeding, according to the recommendations for the general population.

Management of AIDS-related Symptoms – HIV-positive children often suffer from symptoms such as thrush, fever, nausea, or vomiting, which may affect food intake and nutritional status. The dietary management of HIV/AIDS-related symptoms in children is similar to that of adults.

Other Issues to Consider

The medications HIV-positive children take to treat opportunistic infections may produce side effects such as taste changes, loss of appetite, vomiting, nausea, and diarrhoea, which can negatively affect food intake and nutrient absorption and metabolism. Therefore it is crucial to be aware of potential interactions and negative effects, and to manage such symptoms and side effects to minimize the negative impacts on the child's health and nutritional status. Medications may also affect nutrient absorption and food may affect medication efficacy.

REFERENCES

1. Abdale, F., and V. Kraak. Community-Based Nutrition Support for People Living with HIV / AIDS: A Technical Assistance Manual. New York, NY.: God's Love We Deliver, 1995.
2. AIDSLINK Eating with Hope: Taking Control of Your Life through Good Nutrition. Johannesburg, South Africa Gauteng Department of Health, Greater Johannesburg Metropolitan Council, 1997.
3. Anderson, JR. "HIV and reproduction". In A Guide to the Clinical Care of Women with HIV, edited by JR Anderson. Washington, DC.: US Department of Health and Human Services, Health Resources and Services Administration, HIV / AIDS Bureau, 2002.
4. Baker J, L Martin and E Piwoz: Time to Act: Women's Nutrition and Its Consequences for Child Survival and Reproductive Health in Africa, Washington, DC: Support and Analysis for Research in Africa Project (SARA), Academy for Educational Development (AED), 1996.
5. Bijlsma, M: Living Positively—A Nutrition Guide for People with HIV / AIDS, Mutare City, Zimbabwe: Mutare City Health Department, 1996.
6. Bonnard, P: HIV / AIDS Mitigation—Using What We Already Know (Technical Note 5). Washington, DC: Food and Nutrition Technical Assistance Project (FANTA), Academy for Educational Development (AED), 2002.
7. Castleman T, E Seumo-Fosso, and B Cogill: Food and Nutrition Implications of Anti-retroviral Therapy in Resource Limited Settings (Technical Note 7), 2nd ed. Washington, DC: Food and Nutrition Technical Assistance Project (FANTA), Academy for Educational Development (AED), 2004.
8. Clark TD, and RD Semba: Iron Supplementation During Human Immunodeficiency Virus Infection: A double edge sword? Medical Hypotheses 57 (2001): 476-479.
9. Christian P, KP West, Jr, SK Khatry, *et al.*: Vitamin A and Beta Carotene Supplementation Reduces Symptoms of Illness in Pregnant and Lactating Nepali Women, Journal of Nutrition 130 (2000): 2675-2682.
10. Dreyfuss ML, RJ Stoltzfus, JB Shresta, *et al.*: Hookworms, Malaria, and Vitamin, A Deficiency Contribute to Anemia and Iron Deficiency Among Pregnant Women in the Plains of Nepal, Journal of Nutrition 130, No. 10 (2000): 2527-2536.
11. Dreyfuss ML, and WW Fawzie: Micronutrients and Vertical Transmission of HIV-1, American Journal of Clinical Nutrition 75 (2002): 959-970.
12. Epstein L: Food for People Living with HIV / AIDS, Cape Town, South Africa—Network of Malawian People Living with HIV / AIDS and Network for Zambian People Living with HIV / AIDS, 1995.

13. Food and Agriculture Organization of the United Nations (FAO), Living Well with HIV/AIDS, Rome, Italy, FAO, 2002.
14. Fields-Gardner C, S Salomon, and M Davis: Living Well with HIV and AIDS: A Guide to Nutrition. Chicago, IL: American Dietetic Association, 2003.
15. God's Love We Deliver, Eating Tips for HIV Disease. New York, N Y: God's Love We Deliver, 1994.
16. Kennedy RD: The South African National Guidelines on Nutrition for People Living with HIV/AIDS, Pretoria, South Africa: AFRICON, South Africa Department of Health, United Nations Children's Fund (UNICEF), 2001.
17. Kennedy RD, and UE MacIntyre: Development and Testing of the South African Nutrition Guidelines for People Living with HIV/AIDS. South African Journal of Clinical Nutrition 16 (2001): 1-6.
18. Ministry of Agriculture, Animal Industry and Fisheries, Republic of Uganda and United Nations Development Programme (UNDP), Feeding Guidelines for People Living with HIV/AIDS: A Handbook for Field Extension Agents; Kampala, Uganda: UNDP, 1997.
19. Network of African People Living with HIV/AIDS. A Healthy Diet for Better Nutrition for People Living with HIV/AIDS. Nairobi, Kenya: Network of African People Living with HIV/AIDS, 1997.
20. Piwoz EG and EA Preble: HIV/AIDS and Nutrition—A Review of the Literature and Recommendations for Nutritional Care and Support in Africa; Washington, DC: Food and Nutrition Technical Assistance Project (FANTA), Academy for Educational Development Printer, 1999.
21. Wences M, M Kudrati, R Rajani and H Grosskurth: Life First—A Practical Guide for People with HIV/AIDS and Their Families. Dar es Salaam, Tanzania: American Medical Research Foundation (AMREF)/Tanzania and Kuleana, 1993.
22. World Health Organization (WHO), Energy and Protein Requirements, Report for Joint FAO/WHO/UNU Expert Consultation (Technical Report Series 724). Geneva, Switzerland: WHO, 1985.

Managing HIV Disease through Nutrition Interventions the websites

Academy of Educational Development (AED) www.aed.org

American Dietetic Association www.eatright.org/public/

Food and Agriculture Organization of the United Nations (FAO): HIV/AIDS and Food Security www.fao.org/hivaids/

Food and Nutrition Technical Assistance Project (FANTA) www.fantaproject.org

God's Love We Deliver www.godslovewedeliver.org

Joint United Nations Program on HIV/AIDS (UNAIDS) www.unaids.org

South Africa Department of Health www.doh.gov.za

United Nations Children's Fund (UNICEF): HIV/AIDS Program www.unicef.org/aids/index.html

United Nations Development Programme (UNDP) www.undp.org

World Health Organization (WHO): HIV/AIDS Program www.int/hiv/en

CHAPTER

11 Psychiatric Aspects of HIV and AIDS

M.S. Bhatia and *Ravi Gupta*

In the past few years prevalence of HIV infection as well as AIDS has increased tremendously not only in the Western world but also in India. This can be attributed to multiple factors e.g., increase in drug abuse especially intravenous drugs, breaking interpersonal bonds, morals and indulgence of younger age group in unsafe sexual practices etc.

Psychiatric sequels of HIV infection and AIDS are important parts of spectrum of illness. In a study that examined referrals from the HIV-AIDS ward, the most frequent reasons for referral were evaluation of coping problems (42%), assessment of possible depression (31%), and assessment of psychotropic medication (24.5%). The most common psychiatric diagnoses were mood disorders (36.5%), psychoactive substance use disorders (22.7%) and organic mental disorders (18.1%) (Judd et al., 1997). This data is sufficient to understand the role of psychiatrist in management of AIDS patients.

Pathophysiology of Psychiatric Disorders in HIV-AIDS

Disorder usually starts in the adolescence when indulges in unsafe sex practices or injectable drug use to curtail his stress. Many factors that appear at adolescent age may generate enough stress e.g. an individual may find that he has different sexual orientation which is not socially acceptable, he may feel that social and family support is inadequate, career ambitions and workplace expectations may induce pressure, and most importantly it is vulnerable age when psychiatric disorders like anti-social personality disorder, mood disorders, anxiety disorders emerge that add stress. In addition, this is the most vulnerable age for sexual and drug experimentation, where gateway drugs e.g., tobacco, alcohol and cannabis are consumed more often followed by hard substances viz., opioids, cocaine etc.

These factors work together in various combinations where a given factor positive feed forward another to establish a vicious cycle. Resultantly, the adolescent is exposed to unsafe sexual practices e.g., multiple sexual partners or homosexual relations; substance use e.g., injectable substance use superimposed upon psychiatric illness to enhance chances of catching HIV infection.

Psychiatric disorders that arises during HIV infection can be explained best on the "bio-psycho-social" model where all three factors act in cohesion to produce various clinical syndromes.

Biological factors play role in three different ways and one or more of them occur in combination-the affected person may be genetically predisposed to develop the illness e.g., anxiety, depression or cognitive impairment; or the inflammatory markers that are found in high levels in the body during infection may alter neuronal functioning to induce functional neurochemical abnormalities that lead to psychiatric illness; or lastly, gross neuronal damage that develops secondary to HIV infection e.g., CNS lymphoma, toxoplasmosis etc. may cause psychiatric features.

Social factors should not be underemphasized because they act as the 'second hit' to provoke full-blown symptoms in persons with various biological predispositions. Most of the infected individuals are discarded by family members, friends and social groups; denied of medical care and treatment; lose their jobs and found themselves along in distressful situation without any chance for ventilation of their feelings.

Psychological factors are consequent to biological and social problems that have been discussed. In the stressful situation, affected person usually tries to find easiest path of escape and usually indulge in the substance abuse. Drug experimentation is further precipitated by adjustment disorder, depression, cognitive impairment and psychosis. In this situation, most of the HIV infected persons indulge directly in use of hard substances, commonly injectable opioids.

Table 1. *Pathophysiological Classification of HIV Related Psychiatric Disorders*

S.No.	*Pathology and Psychiatric Disorder*
1.	Illness caused through CNS damage caused by HIV • Dementia
2.	Illness caused through infections secondary to AIDS • Generalized damage to CNS • Focal pathology of CNS
3.	Treatment emergent problems
4.	Functional psychiatric disorders • AIDS Phobia • Acute Stress Reaction • Bereavement • Depression • Anxiety • Psychosis

Vulnerable Periods for Development of Psychiatric Disorders

Certain periods in the course of HIV infection make more susceptible for psychiatric disorders (Table 2). In the present section we will discuss two such periods (at the time of HIV screening and post test) where if adequate precautions are taken, risk can be minimized. It has been found that psychological symptoms increase just before test and return to baseline (below pretest level) approximately 3 months after test. Most prevalent disorder at this point of time is adjustment disorder with anxious or depressed features.

(*a*) ***Pre-test HIV Counseling***

HIV is seen as an incurable disease and has stigma attached with it due to social discard of the infected person. Therefore, whenever any body is asked to undergo, screening test, stress develops. The said person may react with shock, anger, denial guilt and anxiety. Fears of loss of life, family, job, reputation stimulate psychological pain. Patient may become hostile towards physician. In such time pre-test counseling may help the person to overcome the situation.

Before advising screening test for HIV, physician must clarify the meaning of positive test and clarify cognitive distortions, if any. Most of the patients feel that positive test means that have developed AIDS, and it must be elucidated that, actually it shows only HIV infection and not the AIDS syndrome. At the same time it is also important to discuss the natural course of HIV infection with statistical figures. Similarly, he should be explained that negative result does not mean absence of infection and high risk behaviour of calls for another testing after some period because sero-conversion requires time.

At this time, sometimes patients develop unrealistic fears due to paucity of information, which must be cleared at that time only. Necessity of test must be discussed even if patient denies high risk behaviour.

Try to find out how he would react in case of positive result. It may provide you time to prepare the patient as well as seek a professional help. A better guide in these cases can be past reactions to stress as he is more likely to react in the same fashion. Confidentially of test is of paramount importance and it should be openly discussed with the patient who should have access to his results. Possible social and psychological implications of positive test must be discussed.

Hence, it includes a myriad of factors that assess the person's predisposition towards stress and it, if adequately done prepares a person to deal; with forthcoming events.

(*b*) ***Post-test Counseling***

This is high time for development of psychological reactivity and the test results must be carefully disclosed. If a person comes with negative result, it must be clarified that it does not provide him life-long immunity from HIV and any risk behaviour must be avoided in future. If the physician feels that repeat testing is necessary, discuss with the patient.

Situation becomes more difficult in cases of positive result. At this point of time patient requires emotional support and empathetic relationship and he should be forbidden.

Possible problems that he may face in future must be discussed and a family member must be called at this situation for providing care. Patient must be informed about measures he may take to prevent spreading infection. Few patients may become aggressive and may start cursing themselves or sometimes become revengeful to the society. These reactions should be adequately taken care of.

As the discussion explains, it is high time for possible psychological complications and tests the skills of physicians in psychological management; therefore it must be given due concern.

Table 2. ***Temporal Classification of HIV-AIDS Related Psychiatric Disorders***

S.No.	*Time of Onset of Disorder*
1.	Before catching illness • AIDS Phobia, Worried Well
2.	At the time of screening test • Acute Stress Reaction
3.	At the time of disclosure of result of test • With Negative Test • With Positive Test Acute Stress Reaction Bereavement in AIDS

Psychiatric Disorders

There are many symptoms which are quiet frequent in these patients but for which exact pathology is yet to be identified, are termed as functional disorders. Readers should not misinterpret them as disorders without any pathological basis in the brain. All the disorders described below may be functional, secondary to generalized or focal CNS damage by AIDS or may appear in response to therapy.

(*a*) ***AIDS Phobia or Worried Well***

In the recent past media has spread a huge awareness regarding HIV and AIDS. However, this has become a two edged sword. Whereon few people have started prophylaxis and changed their life style, there are a lot of people who have actually developed the fear of catching illness.

Persons exposed to a life style that make them prone for HIV infection e.g., homosexual persons, people with history of unsafe sexual practices, intravenous drug users etc. most commonly present with this syndrome. After such an exposure, they become overly conscious for physiological changes in the body, develop anxiety features amounting to a diagnosis so hypochondriasis. Sometimes the intensity may reach delusional level. Such persons repeatedly ask for screening test and best of the clinician's efforts are unable to relieve their anxiety. Negative tests are attributed to laboratory error or emergence of some new virus or their inability to form antibodies in response to infection as other people do (Maj, 1990). Confrontation and explanations of clinicians regarding their groundless conviction make them angry. Sometimes they avoid touching objects at public places, washes their hands if mistakenly touch anything or sometimes develop paranoid psychosis after an affair. Past history of psychiatric illness especially depression is common in them. Kausch (2004) described two cases that committed suicide and Chand (1998) described a case who suffered koro.

As clear from the description, treatment of these patients is challenging. Repeated reassurances are unable to improve the situation. Two treatment methods – Cognitive Behaviour Therapy (Chand, 1998) and Antidepressant Drugs, especially when phobia is the part of underlying depression are found helpful.

(b) ***Acute Stress Reaction***

It is common at the time of serological testing, more common when it turns out positive. Both these moments should be dealt carefully as explained.

Pre test counselling should include the disclosure of reason for testing, future impacts of negative as well as positive tests, explaining the differences between screening and confirmatory test, education regarding HIV infection and AIDS etc.

Post test counselling, especially it positive is a crucial moment. It brings the realization of fears which may long have been present, need to tell others, importantly their partners. Life styles that were previously concealed may be exposed to parents and colleagues for the first time.

Typical features are anxiety, depressive symptoms, guilt, panic, insomnia lasting for several weeks.

Suicidal ideation may develop. Patient may develop a preoccupation with bodily symptoms and wrongly attribute them to commencing illnesses that develop during the course of AIDS.

Under such stress patient may start abusing addictive substances. Patient may disregard medical advices for himself and those that have been provided to prevent infection of others.

These patients also perceive other changes in their life, even when they are not threatening as stressful situations and are prone to develop PTSD symptoms in response to previous life events (Koopman et al., 2002).

Situation can be handled with the help of drugs (Benzodiazapines and antidepressants) along with reassurance.

(c) ***Bereavement in AIDS***

There are multifaceted problems in the patients, their families, friends and partners. They have many reasons to develop it are: – constrains on public display of grief when homosexuality has been concealed previously, punitive responses in case of drug use etc. Patent may be unable to find out an anchor for support and emotional exhaustion is expected.

(d) ***Adjustment Disorder***

This is diagnosed according to standard DSM IV TR criteria i.e., when the expressed and perceived distress is greater than what might be expected in that situation and interferes with social, personal or occupational functioning. It is commoner in patients with past psychiatric history, lack of social acceptance. Disclosure of the test result, especially if it is positive, is the risky period. Anxiety and depression are usually found along with.

(e) ***Anxiety Disorders***

Patients with HIV report significantly more anxiety than general population (Sewell et al., 2000). Elliot (1998) described the prevalence to be 38% in AIDS patients. Most common type of anxiety disorders associated with HIV are Panic Disorders. PTSD and GAD. The underlying theme centers upon the health issues, social support, financial arrangements and risk of infecting others. Symptoms include chest pain, headache, numbness and insomnia. Obsessive rumination regarding death, past experiences and somatic symptoms are common.

While assessing these symptoms in HIV patients, attention should be paid to anti-retroviral and ancillary treatment since few drugs e.g., ddl, d4T, AZT, fluconazole, foscarnet, and isoniazid may cause anxiety symptoms (Elliot, 1998).

Treatment may range from acupuncture to benzodiazepine, depending upon the patient's preference.

(f) ***Depression***

Depression is not uncommon during AIDS, 15.5-22% patients may suffer from it (Starace et al., 2002; Komiti et al., 2003). Increasing age causes decline in the rate of depression in general population but not in these patients (Rabkin et al., 2004), and prevalence is especially high in patients not receiving HAART (Starace et al., 2002).

It is commonly associated with previous history of depressive illness, poor perceived social support and personality disorders. Being in a relationship appears to afford protection against depression while having a history of illicit drug use and current 'stress' are highly associated with depression. Interestingly, HIV-related medical variables including laboratory markers of HIV disease, duration of illness and anti-retroviral medication regimen were not related to depression (Komiti et al., 2003). Female gender, negative life events and disability have been described as risk factors in general population recently (Olley et al., 2004). Blaney et al., (2004) found that psychosocial factors significantly predicted the level of prenatal depressive symptoms in HIV infected females beyond the effects of demographic and health-related factors. Perceived stress, social isolation, and disengagement coping were associated with greater depression, positive partner support with lower depression.

It is important to treat the symptoms in the early staged as they may interfere with the treatment compliance. It is sometimes difficult to be differentiated from HIV associated

dementia, apathy secondary to AIDS. It is even more difficult to diagnose when ARC is also present. Abrams et al., (1986) and Kalichman et al., (2000) suggested that depression can be diagnosed in ill patients by paying attention to cognitive and affective symptoms and relying less on the physical complaints. Few mental changes e.g., lowered self esteem, guilt, feel defeated, suicidal ideation, crying points the presence of depression.

Routine screening to identify those currently depressed or at risk for depression should be integrated into prenatal HIV-care settings to target issues most needing intervention (Blaney et al., 2004). Treatment with SSRIs can reduce the severity of depression and improve the quality of life in HIV patients (Elliot et al., 2002).

(g) ***Sleep Disorders***

Insomnia is widespread and under diagnosed in HIV-seropositive ambulatory patients. Insomnia is especially prevalent among those with cognitive impairment and substance use. Cognitive impairment and depression are the best predictors for insomnia in these patients (Rubinstein et al., 1998)

(h) ***Suicide***

It is especially common in early and late stages of disease. Perry et al., (1990) noted that these are common at the time of serological testing but falls significantly thereafter. It tends to cluster in first 6 months after diagnosis, undermine the importance of pre and post test counseling.

Komiti et al. (2001) reviewed articles on suicide associated with HIV/AIDS and found that most studies have been done on homosexual/bisexual groups, with little data was available for heterosexual populations or women. Studies showed an increased rate of suicidal ideation, suicide attempts and completed suicide in individuals with HIV/AIDS. An increased rate of substance use and psychiatric illnesses were found in these patients. According to them, though the increased rate of suicidal behaviour in HIV-infected persons was consistent with findings in other medically ill groups with chronic, life-threatening disorders, even than, assessment of any possible direct effect of HIV/AIDS on suicidal behaviour was confounded by methodological limitations of many of the studies. They stressed the need for long term prospective studies in this field to gather more information.

(i) ***Psychosis***

There is bilateral relationship between HIV-AIDS and psychosis. Extant research had found alarming rates of the human immunodeficiency virus/acquired immune deficiency syndrome (HIV/AIDS) in persons with severe mental illnesses, with seroprevalence rates ranging from 4% to 23% (Lyon, 2001). Though patients with psychotic disorders have reduced sexual activity, they present greater frequency of sexual risk behaviours that predispose them to acquire HIV infection and other STD. The psychotic patients have significantly less knowledge about HIV/AIDS, they have a smaller proportion of stable sexual partners and greater frequency of sexual risk behaviours, such as inconsistent condom use and sexual intercourse outside wedlock (Matsuoka et al., 2003).

Psychotic features caused by HIV infection are rarely found in these patients, Many different pictures have been described, mostly not meeting any particular criteria. Many cases arise in ARC subjects. Delusions, hallucinations, bizarre thoughts, lability of mood may be present in different combinations.

(j) ***Substance Use Disorders***

It is the most important factor to be understood as it may cause or result from HIV and AIDS. As a cause, intravenous drug use is one of the important reason for transmission, it also increase the chances of unprotected sexual encounters among these people thus multiplying the risk of catching disease (Klinkenberg et al., 2004).

This is often secondary to Post traumatic Stress Disorder, since many patients with HIV AIDS are exposed to traumatic event during their life. There is reason to believe that the co-occurrence of HIV and PTSD or co-morbid PTSD and Substance Use Disorder (PTSD/SUD) may predict poorer health outcomes. There are several pathways through which PTSD or PTSD/SUD might adversely impact the health of individuals living with HIV, including participation in negative health behaviours, low levels of adherence to anti-retroviral medications, and/or a direct, deleterious effect on immune function (Brief et al., 2004).

Though the prevalence of substance use disorder declines with age in general population, such trends were not observed in HIV-AIDS population (Rabkin et al. 2004).

(k) ***Cognitive Impairment***

It is thought to represent the widespread neuronal loss caused by HIV infection in the form of encephalitis. The impairment can occur in a spectrum-from mild cognitive impairment (MCI) to frank dementia.

Initially it presents with the motor disturbance concordant with the diagnosis of sub-cortical dementia and with the advancement of disease cortical symptoms appear. Symptoms can be grouped into these categories - cognitive, motor and behaviour.

Cognitive symptoms include forgetfulness, poor concentration, and difficulty with problem solving and reading. Some people reread the paragraphs before fully understanding it. Few may complain of solved thinking. Behaviourally apathy, reduced spontancity, and social withdrawals are common, in a significant minority of patients it may present in the form of affective disorder, psychosis or seizures. Physical examination reveals tremors, impaired rapid repetitive movements, imbalance, ataxia, hypertonia, generalized hyper-reflexia, positive frontal release signs, impaired pursuit and saccadic eye movements. All possible secondary causes must be ruled out and evidence of HIV infection must be there.

Evidences of vacuolar myelopathy, neuropathy may be present; these findings are uncommon in children.

Children also develop an HIV associated neuro developmental disorder characterized by developmental delay, hypertonia, microcephaly, basal ganglia calcification. The neurological involvement most often occurs in the absence of secondary infection, and neoplasms which is not the case for adults. It usually progresses rapidly to mutism, coma and death. (ICD-10)

World Health Organization (1990) has recommended the use of operationally defined criteria for HIV dementia which are modified from ICD 10 criteria for dementia. It suggested that diagnosis is based upon-

1. Decline in memory, may not be severe enough to impair routine functions.
2. Decline in motor functions, but not entirely due to myelopathy, peripheral neuropathy or other physical illness.
3. Minimum duration of symptoms is 1 month.
4. Aphasia, apraxia and agnosia must be present.

Additionally evidence of HIV infection must be present in absence of secondary causes that can explain condition.

Prevalence

It is the commonest disorder found in HIV/AIDS. Different researchers have estimated the prevalence ranging from 8% to 60%.

Staging

AIDS-dementia complex (ADC) can be staged according to following criteria : (brew)

- *Stage 0:* Normal mental and motor function
- *Stage 0.5 (Sub-clinical):* Minimal or equivocal symptoms without impairment of work or activities of daily living. Soft neurological signs e.g., slowing of fine finger movements or primitive reflexes may be present.
- *Stage 1 (Mild):* Cognitive disturbances that compromise performance on more demanding aspects of work or activities of daily living.
- *Stage 2 (Moderate):* Cognitive deficits makes the patient unable to perform work or motor activities.
- *Stage 3 (Severe):* Patient can perform only rudimentary tasks and faces difficulty in routine work.
- *Stage 4 (End stage):* Patient is almost mute, incontinent and bed ridden.

Course

The course is typically steadily progressive though sometimes can be punctuated by abrupt progressions. Insight is relatively preserved until late in the disorder. The delayed appearance of cortical signs e.g., apraxia, agnosia favours the sub cortical nature of disease. Even in the later stages consciousness is preserved unless superimposed by delirium. Median time for death is approximately 6 months from the onset of symptoms.

Investigations

- Serum levels of vitamin B_{12} and folate must be assessed as they decrease with the illness and mimic ADC.
- EEG is often normal initially but diffuse slowing may be present later on.
- Neuro-imaging shows variable cortical atrophy and ventricular dilatation. T2 MRI shows areas of increased signal as the dementia progresses. However, main role of MRI is to demonstrate treatable conditions e.g., infections and lymphomas. Recently Paul et al. (2005) demonstrated involvement of Caudate and amygdala in patients with apathy secondary to HIV infection. Functional imaging shows areas of hypometabolism in basal ganglia and thalamus further elucidating the pathology.
- Virological markers in CSF may be correlated with the ADC. Of all markers, it is CSF viral load that best correlates with ADC severity. However, there is no critical cut-off level which is diagnostic for dementia. (Brew 1997). Approximately 50% patients have detectable p24 antigen in the CSF that is uncommon in non-demented subjects. (Brew 1994)
- In absence of other confounders CSF level of beta-2 microglobulin, neopterin and quinolinic acid correlates well with severity of ADC.

Differential Diagnosis

The diagnosis during life is essentially one of exclusion. Mild Cognitive Impairment must be differentiated from anxiety, depression, fatigue and manifestations of systemic infections.

Metabolic causes of encephalopathy and effect of psychotropic drugs must be excluded.

Psychotic features should raise the possibility of independent schizophrenia or psychosis as it is not the typical manifestation.

All possible secondary causes e.g., cytomegalovirus, toxoplasma, neurosyphilis, cryptococcal, tubercular meningitis, lymphoma and other neoplasia must be excluded by appropriate investigations.

Quality of life after HIV/AIDS

A diagnosis of human immunodeficiency virus/acquired immunodeficiency syndrome (HIV/AIDS) is a life-changing event, where persons must deal with a life-threatening, debilitating disease and its associated stigma and isolation. Studies over the past decade have shown that writing and talking about stressful and traumatic experiences, such as a life-threatening illness, causes emotions surrounding the trauma to change and to become cognitively reorganized. The result is a reduction in inhibition and change in basic cognitive and linguistic processes, which have contributed to meaningful behavioural, psychological, and physical health benefits across a variety of populations. These processes interact with each other to impair the quality of life of HIV infected persons.

Many HIV-specific instruments with established validity and reliability are available for the quantification of impairment including the Medical Outcomes Study-HIV Health Survey, HIV/AIDS Targeted Quality of Life Instrument, Functional Assessment of HIV Infection, AIDS Health Assessment Questionnaire, HIV Overview of Problems-Evaluation Systems, and Multidimensional Quality of Life Questionnaire for HIV/AIDS (Robinson, 2004).

Nixon et al. (2002) reviewed the role of exercise in HIV patients and indicated that performing constant or interval aerobic exercise, or a combination of constant aerobic exercise and progressive resistive exercise for at least 20 minutes, at least three times per week for four weeks appears to be safe and may lead to clinically significant improvements in cardiopulmonary fitness. Further more, individual studies suggest that aerobic exercise may improve psychological well-being for adults living with HIV/AIDS.

Medication Use In HIV-AIDS

It is well known that patients often after their medication regimens and that these changes may have profound consequence for their health outcomes. Russell et al. (2003) identified factors that affect medication compliance in these subjects and found that facilitators included motivation, factors of faith, routines, and other's influences. Categories of identified barriers included perceptions, psycho emotional issues, provider/clinic issues, interpersonal factors, and disease and treatment factors. This study showed medication decision making to be a complex process, influenced by often-competing life and treatment issues and affected by participant's beliefs and values.

REFERENCES

1. Abrams DI, Dilly JW, Maxey LM, Volberding PA: Routine Care and Psychosocial Support of the Patient with the Acquired Immuno Deficiency Syndrome, *Med Clin North Am*, 1986; 70: 707-720.
2. Blaney NT, Fernandez MI, Ethier KA, Wilson TE, Walter E, Koenig LJ: Psychosocial and Behavioural Correlates of Depression Among HIV-infected Pregnant Women, AIDS Patient Care STDS, 2004; 18(7); 405-15.
3. Brew BJ: AIDS Dementia Complex, Neurol Clin 1999; 17(4); 861-881.
4. Brew BJ, Paul M, Khan A *et al*.: Cerebrospinal Fluid HIV-1, p. 24, Antigen and Culture; Sensitivity and Specificity for AIDS Dementia Complex. *J Neurol Neurosurg Psychiatry* 1994; 57:784-789.
5. Brew BJ, Pemberton L, Cunningham P *et al*.: Levels of HIV-1 RNA Correlates with AIDS Dementia, *J Infect Dis* 1997; 175: 963-966.
6. Brief DJ, Bollinger AR, Vielhauer MJ, Berger-Greenstein JA, Morgan EE, Brady SM, Buondonno LM, Keane TM: Understanding the Interface of HIV, Trauma, Post-traumatic Stress Disorder, and Substance Use and Its Implications for Health Outcomes, *AIDS Care*, 2004;16 Suppl 1: S97-120.
7. Chand SP: Koro Associated with Phobia for AIDS, *Int J Psychiatry Med*, 1998; 28(3): 353-6.
8. Elliott A: Anxiety and HIV Infection, STEP Perspect 1998; 98(1): 11-4.
9. Elliott AJ, Russo J, Roy-Byrne PP: The Effect of Changes in Depression on Health Related Quality of Life (HRQoL) in HIV Infection, *Gen Hosp Psychiatry*, 2002; 24(1); 43-7.
10. Judd FK, Cockram A, Mijch A, McKenzie D: Liaison Psychiatry in an HIV/AIDS Unit, *Aust N Z J Psychiatry*, 1997; 31(3): 391-7.
11. Kalichman SC, Rompa D, Cage M: Distinguishing Between Overlapping Somatic Symptoms of Depression and HIV Disease in People Living with HIV-AIDS, *J Nerv Ment Dis* 2000; 188 (10); 662-70.
12. Kausch O: Irrational Fear of AIDS Associated with Suicidal Behaviour, *J Psychiatr Pract*, 2004; 10(4): 266-71.
13. Klinkenberg WD, Sacks S: Mental Disorders and Drug Abuse in Persons Living with HIV/AIDS, AIDS Care, 2004;16 Suppl 1:S22-42.

14. Komiti A, Judd F, Grech P, Mijch A, Hoy J, Lloyd JH, Street A: Suicidal Behaviour in People with HIV/AIDS: A Review, *Aust N Z J Psychiatry*, 2001; 35(6): 747-57.
15. Komiti A, Judd F, Grech P, Mijch A, Hoy J, Williams B, Street A, Lloyd JH: Depression in People Living with HIV/AIDS Attending Primary Care and Outpatient Clinics, *Aust N Z J Psychiatry*; 2003; 37 (1): 70-7.
16. Koopman C, Gore-Felton C, Azimi N, O'Shea K, Ashton E, Power R, De Maria S, Israclski D, Spiegel D: Acute Stress Reactions to Recent Life Events Among Women and Men Living with HIV/AIDS, *Int J Psychiatry* Med, 2002; 32(4): 361-78.
17. Lyon DE: Human Immunodeficiency Virus (HIV) Disease in Persons with Severe Mental Illnesses Issues Ment Health Nurs. 2001; 22(1): 109-19.
18. Maj M: Psychiatric Aspects of HIV-1 Infection and AIDS, *Psychol Med* 1990; 20: 547-563.
19. Matsuoka GD, Vega-Dienstmaier JM, Mazzotti G, Chavez-paz JM, Mendoza D, Miranda Verategui C, Sanchez Alfaro J: Sexual Behavior at Risk for HIV/AIDS and Sexually Transmitted Diseases in Male Patients with Psychotic Disorders. *Actas Esp Psiquiatr* 2003; 31(2): 73-8.
20. Nixon S, O'Brien K, Glazier RH, Tynan AM: Acrobic Exercise Interventions for Adults Living with HIV/AIDS, Cochrane Database Syst Rev, 2002;(2): CD001796.
21. Olley BO, Seedat S, Nei DG, Stein DJ: Predictors of Major Depression in Recently Diagnosed Patients with HIV/AIDS in South Africa, AIDS Patient Care STDS, 2004: 18(8): 481-7.
22. Paul R, Flanigan TP, Tashima K *et al.*: Apathy Correlates with Cognitive Function but not CD_4 Status in Patients with Human Immunodeficiency Virus, *J Neuropsychiatr Clin Neurosci* 2005; 17(1): 114-118.
23. Perry S, Jacobsberg L, Fishman B: Suicidal Ideation and HIV Testing, *JAMA* 1990; 263: 679-682.
24. Rabkin JG, McElhiney MC, Ferrando SJ: Mood and Substance Use Disorders in Older Adults with HIV/AIDS: Methodological Issues and Preliminary Evidence, AIDS 2004; 18 Suppl 1: S43-8.
25. Robinson FP: Measurement of Quality of Life in HIV Disease, *J Assoc Nurses AIDS Care* 2004;15 Suppl 5:14S-19S.
26. Rubinstein ML, Selwyn PA: High Prevalence of Insomnia in An Outpatient Population with HIV Infection, J Acquir Immune Defic Syndr Hum Retrovirol, 1998 Nov 1; 19(3); 260-5.
27. Russell CK, Bunting SM, Graney M, Hartig MT, Kisner P, Brown B: Factors that Influence the Medication Decision Making of Persons with HIV/AIDS: A Taxonomic Exploration, *J Assoc Nurses AIDS Care* 2003; 14(4): 46-60.
28. Sewell MC, Goggin K J, Rabkin JG, Ferrando SJ, McElhiney MC, Evans S: Anxiety Syndromes and Symptoms Among Men with AIDS: A Longitudinal Controlled Study, *Psychosomatics*. 2000 Jul-Aug, 41 (4): 294-300.
29. Starace F, Bartoli L, Aloisi MS, Antinori A, Narciso P, Ippolito G, Ravasio L, Moioli MC, Vangi D, Gennero L, Coronado OV, Giacometti A, Nappa S, Perulli ML, Montesarchio V,

La Gala A, Ricci F, Cristiano L, De Marco M, Izzo C, Pezzotti P, D'Arminio Monforte A: Cognitive and Affective Disorders Associated to HIV Infection in the HAART era; Findings from the Neurol CONA Study. Cognitive Impairment and Depression in HIV/AIDS. The Neurol CONA Study, *Acta Psychiatr Scand*, 2002; 106(1) : 20-6.

30. World Health Organization, International Classification of Diseases, 10th Ed. (ICD-10), WHO, Geneva, 1992.

31. World Health Organization, Report of Second Consultation on the Neuropsychiatric Aspects of HIV-1 Infection, Global Programme on AIDS, Geneva, Annex 3. WHO/GPA/MNH, 90.1.1990; World Health Organization, Geneva.

CHAPTER

12 Medico-legal Aspects of Sexually Transmitted Diseases and HIV/AIDS

S.K. Verma

Intimate physical relation is among one of the few most pleasurable moments in the life of all creatures and that's why most of them practice it regularly. But, it is also a hard fact that the sexual contacts entail the risk of diseases. All such diseases that are transmitted through sexual contact are grouped as sexually transmitted diseases (STDs). As a group STDs constitutes one of the most common communicable diseases among sex workers. The number of infected people are continuously on its increase despite the progress in diagnosis and treatment of these illnesses. Some of the factors responsible for the continuous increase in STDs include changes in sexual behaviour, emergence of resistant strains, promiscuity in the society and ignorance amongst the general population and even some of the health professionals.[1] Sexual assault is the criminal sexual violence that broadly can be defined as an act of sexual intimacy performed without the consent of the victim through use of threat or force, or when the victim is unable to give consent because of physical or mental disability.[2] In Indian literature terms like rape, sodomy and incest are used to describe different types of sexual assaults.

Sexually transmitted diseases (STDs) and sexual assault (SA) are significant contributor of morbidity and mortality worldwide. The exact incidence of STDs is very difficult to find because all STDs are not reported and even reportable diseases are generally under reported in most of the countries, specially like ours. Thus data from different parts of the world is sketchy. However, as per the WHO estimates of 1995, at least 333 million new cases of curable STDs (Syphills, gonorrhea, Chlamydia and Trichomoniasis) were reported globally in 15 to 49 years of age. These estimates also suggest that 90 per cent of STDs are in developing countries.[3] The annual incidence of STDs in India is estimated around 5 percent or approximately 40 million infections occurring in the country annually.[4]

The situation regarding HIV/AIDS is for more complex and alarming. The joint United Nations Programme on HIV/AIDS (UNAIDS) and the WHO report states that since HIV/

AIDS epidemic begin, almost 58 million people throught that world have been infected with HIV and almost 22 million people have died. HIV continues to spread causing 15,000 new infections every day and 95% of them in low and middle income country.[5] India has more than 4 million HIV infected individuals with 29,007 cases of AIDS upto October 2001.[6] India, in fact is the second largest country in the world of having such a large number of HIV infected persons. Moreover, the infection is percolating from high risk groups to general population. Globally, about 70% of all HIV infections are caused by hetro-sexual transmission and about 5-10% of all HIV cases are due to sexual transmission between men who have sex with other men. In India, more than three-fourth of all HIV transmission are caused by the hetrosexual mode of transmission.[7]

The exact incidence and prevalence of (SA) is not easy to estimate as the majority of the incidences go unreported. Incidence of sexual assault in USA has increased from 17 to 80 per lac population in a period of 2 decades from 1970-1990.[8] Nine to twenty four percent of women in US are assaulted sexually at least once in their life time.[9] Indian annual national figures reported for rape are as given in Table-1.

Table 1. *Indian Figures for Rape*

Year	*No. of cases*
1988	9099
1998	15031

(Source : Crime in India, 1998, NCRB[10])

The number of victims of rape have increased by over 65% during the period from 1988 to 1998. Amongst the states, the highest number of cases reported in 1998 was from Madhya Pradesh (3354), followed by Uttar Pradesh (1605) and Bihar (1421) cases, Mizoram has the maximum crime rate for rape being 9.3 crimes per 100,000 population followed by Madhya Pradesh (4.3) and Delhi (3.4) per 100,000 population.[10]

Medico-legal Aspects

The medico-legal aspects of the STDs and SA are peculiar and multifaceted due to:

(a) High incidence and prevalence rate;

(b) Transmission by intimate physical contact;

(c) Present incurable status of HIV/AIDS, and

(d) Social stigma attached to these diseases and assault;

Medico legally and ethically STDs and SA can be related to issues such as:

A. Consent

B. Confidentiality and privilege communication

C. National/International laws

D. Human Rights

E. Other issues related to STDs and SA

A. Consent

Every adult human being with a sound mind has a right to determine what should be done with his body and before performing any act on the body of any person, his consent is required. Consent is an essential ingredient of even the doctor patient relationship, as per Section 13 of the Indian Contract Act. Ordinarily the term consent means a free and voluntary. agreement, approval or permission for compliance of some act.[11] Globally, none of the issues regarding consent had lead to such a controversy as testing for HIV. Presently, testing for HIV is more than a mere biological test and hence involves ethical, human and legal dimensions. The topic has been debated at different forums and comprehensively included in the draft of National AIDS Policy. As per the National Guidelines for HIV Testing[12], the testing for HIV should be carried out on a voluntary basis with appropriate pre and post test counseling. The objectives of the HIV testing in India are:

1. Surveillance;
2. Transfusion safely;
3. Identification of asymptomatic with HIV infections for diagnosis or for voluntary testing purposes; and
4. Research.

Most of the time these separate objectives can not be met by a single strategy hence the different strategies adopted for different purposes are:

(a) Unlinked and Anonymous – for surveillance purposes;
(b) Voluntary and confidential – for asymptomatic or AIDS cases and research; and
(c) Mandatory – for transfusion safety purposes

There is persistent demand from health professionals for mandatory HIV testing of all patients at the time of hospital admission, based on the fear of needle stick and other sharp instrument injury. But, the National HIV testing policy reiterates that no individual should be made to undergo a mandatory testing for HIV. Further, the mandatory testing is definitely not an alternative to the Universal Safety Precautions that needs to be practiced irrespective of the HIV status of the patient. It is argued that testing without explicit consent of the patient has proved to be counter productive in the long run in control of the HIV epidemic. Such testing, it is feared, will drive the target people underground, making the interventions even more difficult.

The UNAIDS and Human Rights International Guidelines also stress that, "Apart from surveillance testing and other unlinked testing done for epidemiological purposes, public health legislation should ensure that HIV testing of individuals should only be performed with the specific informed consent. Exceptions to voluntary testing would need specific judicial authorization granted only after due evaluation of the important considerations involved in terms of privacy and liberty.[13]"

B. Confidentiality and Priviledged Communication

Confidentiality is an integral part of medical practice. The Hippocratic Oath itself states, "Whatever in connection with my professional practice or not in connection with it, I see or hear, in my life, which ought not to be spoken of abroad, I will not divulge as reckoning that all should be kept secret.[11]" Although medical confidentiality is necessary to be observed by every medical practitioner, it is much more important for the doctor dealing with STDs and AIDS/HIV because of the stigma, taboo and fear surrounding these illnesses specially HIV/AIDS. The United Nation HIV/AIDS and Human Rights International Guidelines recommend, "Public health legislation should ensure that HIV/AIDS cases reported to public health authorities for epidemiological purposes are subject of strict rules of data protection and confidentiallty.[13]

However, the information about a patient can be divulged under following situations:

(a) with the consent of the patient;

(b) by order of a court or a person authorized by law to examine witnesses called absolute privilege communication;

(c) to a person who is involved in providing care to, or treatment or counseling of, the other person if such information is required in connection with treatment, providing such care and counseling;

(d) to the concerned person or authority by virtue of his duty to protect the interest of the community or the society called qualified privilege communication;

(e) in the best interest of the patient to the close relative about the exact state of the patient's illness; and

(f) in the self-defence by the medical practitioner, when a charge of medical negligence is brought against him or to realize his professional dues.

Qualified privileged communication is very important while dealing with cases of STDs and HIV. In such cases first of all the patient should be counseled to adopt safer sex practices and avoid marriage till they are cured. But, if the patient does not listen to doctor's advise, then the doctor can inform the person whom he is planning to marry about his illness. Similarly, a patient with ulcerative lesions of STD should avoid using public swimming pools. If he still insist on using public pools, the caretaker of the pool can be informed about his illness in order to protect the society. The common saying in his regard is, "The protective privilege ends where the public peril begins."

The relevance of the medical secrets to HIV/AIDS is clear: should physicians warn current or post sexual partners of an HIV positive patient not taking proper precautions and whose lives may be at risk due to an unknowing exposure? In the USA, many states have adopted "privilege to disclose" legislation, that provide physicians an option of warning without imposing on them a legal duty to do so.[14] The term partner notification encompasses two separate approaches:

(a) Patient referral (also known as self referral), whereby the patient themselves are encouraged to notify partners at risk; and

(b) Provider referral, wherein health care workers assist in notifying the partner's at risk.[15]

A considerable amount of public opinion, both for and against has been marshaled, primarily directed at the use of partner notification in HIV control. Confusion between both approaches has led many to mischaracterize processes that are fundamentally voluntary.[16] However, it might discourage patients from seeking to know their HIV status, which may be a net loss from the perspective of public health. So, an alternative to partner notification is contact tracing. In contact tracing the threat to the breach of confidentiality is not that challenging. Here, the index case is asked to provide the names of all those who might have been exposed. Then all such contacts are warned about the risk but they are not informed about the identity of the index case. Thus, the privacy of the index patient is maintained.

C. International/National Laws

Due to specific nature of HIV/AIDS and different interconnected medico legal issues, the disease forced various international and national agencies to think about a separate law dealing with this disease. The Interdisciplinary International Conference of AIDS: Law and Humanity in 1995, adopted a declaration called, " The New Delhi Declaration and Action plan on HIV/AIDS."[17] The paragraph 5 of the declaration deals with the basic principles for developing any law related to HIV/AIDS and the same are enumerated below:

1. All laws and policies on HIV/AIDS should be based upon sound and scientific data. They should rest upon this foundation and not upon pre-supposition, prejudice and strereotypes;
2. In combating HIV/AIDS, it is essential and urgent as rarely before, to adopt a global approach. This includes a model global AIDS law which supports action at the local, national and international level;
3. The approach, which is adopted, should respect and protect the human rights of all persons at risk of HIV/AIDS and against discrimination on the ground of HIV/AIDS. It is recognized that one of the most effective strategies for changing behaviours and ensuring against spread of HIV infection lies in the protection of the rights of those at risk;
4. Laws should be made for prevention of HIV and for protection of persons affected by HIV/AIDS which are effective and enforceable;
5. Law makers who have a special responsibility in responding to HIV/AIDS, must work in an interdisciplinary way with health care workers, government and non-government organizations, representatives of vulnerable groups, people living with HIV/AIDS and citizens in general, who must be well informed about how HIV/AIDS is transmitted and how the infection from the same can be prevented;

6. The importance of moral, spiritual and religious values in response to the HIV/ AIDS epidemic should be emphasized.

Law can be an effective device in the prevention of STDs to the extent that it is wielded as one tool in comprehensive prevention, diagnosis, treatment and management strategy. Many traditions of public health and legal precedents are valuable standards against which responses to new conditions such as HIV infection must be measured.[18]

STDs and HIV are not notifiable diseases as per WHO. For many years in the US, physicians are required to report infected individuals for suspected STD as a part of STD prevention. But, it is not legally binding on a physician. In India, all AIDS cases are supposed to be reported to National AIDS Control Organisation (NACO), preserving confidentiality about that data related to identity of the patient. The use of quarantine and confinements, seems to have little practical value in cases of STDs and HIV/AIDS. However, Cuba has sought to quarantine all individuals with HIV infection.[19] But, fierce opposition has surfaced to all efforts to being AIDS within the scope of state quarantine statutes.[16]

Marriage is the sacred union, legally permissible, of two healthy bodies of opposite sexes. Mental and physical health is of prime importance in any marriage. That is why in every system of matrimonial law, it has been provided that if a person was found to be suffering from any disease, including STDs in a communicable and incurable form, it will be open to the other partner to seek divorce. The law has offered this remedy to avoid spouses from contacting a contagious disease, which may prove ruinous for the other spouse. Further, if a person suffering from a dreadful disease like HIV, knowingly marries and thereby transmits infection to the spouse, he she would be guilty of "negligent act likely to spread infection or disease dangerous to life" (Section 269 IPC) and of, "malignant act likely to spread infection of disease dangerous to life" (Section 270 IPC). This means that the right of marriage of a HIV positive individual gets suspended, as long as he/she is HIV positive, with a HIV–ve person. However, there is an alternative for two HIV positive individuals of opposite sex can marry but they should be counseled avoid having a child. As the chances of child born after such a wedlock being HIV positive are quite high (The risk for vertical transmission danger from 25 to 45 percent in developing countries [20]).

D. Human Rights in STDs & HIV/AIDS

Human rights are generally defined as the rights, which every human being is entitled to enjoy and have protected. All societies and cultures even in the past have developed some conception of rights and principles that should be honoured and respected.[21] The conception of the rights which every human being is entitled to enjoy by virtue of being a member of the human species have not developed in a short period but has a long history. The global manifestations of the international human rights movement really gathered pace after the terrible suffering and revolution that followed the Second World War. The Universal Declaration of Human Rights 1948 and the International Convention of Human Rights 1966 incorporate fundamental principles, which are now part of international law.[22] Apart from the international laws, Article 21 of our constitution guarantees that, "No person shall be deprived of his life and personal liberty except according to the procedure established by law." These rights cannot be taken away even if a person is suffering from a dreadful disease like HIV. Some of the internationally accepted rights of human beings includes:

- Right to healthcare
- Right to privacy
- Right to shelter and housing
- Right to employment without discrimination
- Right to protection against oppressive laws and policies of the state

Right to healthcare is enshrined as a human right. But still the healthcare facilities and attitude of the health care providers is appalling with the neglect and denial in relation to HIV/AIDS. There are instances where the patients have been thrown out of the hospital when their blood test for HIV was found positive. These people living with HIV/AIDS have been segregated, isolated terminated from these jobs, denied work and formal education, deprived of social status and even denied the right to marry.[23, 24] In many countries including India, the association between HIV and promiscuous sexual behaviour has created a belief that people who are infected with HIV somehow deserve their fate. This attitude needs change. The government has already issued general guidelines for not refusing to admit and treat any case of HIV/AIDS in the government sector. As far as the legal position is concerned, municipal and state aided hospitals fall within the definition of 'state' in Article 12 of the Constitution as expansively to respect and observe the fundamental rights guaranteed in Part-III of our Constitution. Refusal to accept HIV cases as a matter of policy would be discriminatory and thus, contravene Article 14 of the Constitution which guarantees equality of treatment and freedom from discrimination. Further, avoiding treatment to AIDS victims may well deprive them of their life, that is clearly violative of Article 21 of the Constitution, which guarantees protection against deprivation of life by a procedure which is arbitrary and unfair. The crux of the matter is that risk of infection is an occupational hazard which is not unique with HIV but is also present in other infectious diseases as well. In most instances, the risk of contracting HIV does not exceed if requisite precautions are adhered to. In the struggle against HIV/AIDS, we need to learn again the lessons that were taught nearly a century ago, when syphills presented a major challenge to the public health, in the same way that now presents with HIV.

It is not that only the patient's rights are jeopardized due to HIV/AIDS but the rights of health care workers (HCWs) are equally affected once it is known that a health care worker is HIV positive. They are discriminated against, not allowed to see patents and even lose their jobs. Respect for human rights is at the heart of the debate about HIV. In accordance with the principle of 'do no harm', some people are of the opinion that this debate is biased in favour of patients, and infected health care workers (HIV) have received little support from the profession and the media.[23] In 1991, the centers for Disease Control and prevention (CDC) recommended that the health status of health care workers infected with HIV or HBV should be reviewed by an expert panel and they should inform patients of their serologic status before engaging in exposure prone procedures.[25] Health Care Workers HCWs living with HIV/AIDS face loss of their livelihood, professional status and self image. They have been forced to resign, reassigned, denied rotations, or not permitted to continue their education.[26] Due to the fear of discrimination, many HCWs do not seek their HIV status as they have greater legal protection if they are unaware of their serologic status. The current CDC guidelines are under review because existing policies have imposed human rights burdens, driven out qualified HCWs from the medical profession and posed unfair liability risks. These guidelines are also argued inappropriate due to the extremely low risk of HIV transmission from HCWs to the patients.[23] Thus, a new policy focused on management of the work place environment and injury prevention, can achieve high levels of patient safety without discrimination and invasion of the HCW's privacy.[27]

E. Other Issues Related to STDs and Sexual Assault

Other issues pertaining to the victims of sexual assault (SA) can be grouped into:

A. Medical;

B. Legal; and

C. Social.

A. Medical

The role of health care workers incases of sexual assault start as soon as such a case in reported. The duties of a health care workers can be enumerated as;

i. Care of physical and psychological trauma;
ii. Performing a proper medico legal examination;
iii. Prevention of STDs, and AIDS;
iv. Prevention of pregnancy and medical termination of pregnancy; and
v. Long term follow up.[28]

In the coming paragraphs, emphasis is laid on the medical issue of STDs and sexual assault. Managing the cases of STDs, in victims of sexual assault is different from STDs, in other sexual relationships, often the assailant in SA is a stranger or a casual acquaintance and that's why his health status is not known. However, habitual offenders have a high prevalence of STDs and HIV.[29, 30] Further, the infectivity of various organisms causing STDs after a single episode of SA is not very well known as it depends upon multiple factors such as amount and site of trauma to genitals during assault, stage of disease in the assailant, age and health of the victim, infectivity and virulience of the strain of the organism, number of assailants etc. Different studies have reported variable figures for some of the diseases in this regard as shown in Table 2.

Table 2

Disease	*Incidence after single episode of intercourse*
1. Chlamydia[31]	45-80 percent
2. Gonorrhoea[32]	22-25 percent
3. HIV[33]	3.2-5.6 percent

The various STDs encountered in the victims of sexual assault are: gonorrhoea, chlamydia, Trichomonas vaginalis, bacterial vaginosis, condyloma acuminata, syphilis, genital herpes and HIV. These incidences have been reported from a low percentage of 0.8 for HIV to a high percentage of 38.3 per cent for bacterial vaginosis and all other disease in between this range.[34, 35]

Management of STDs in victims of sexual assault includes diagnosis and prophylaxis. After a thorough examination conducted with consent of the victim or victim's guardian (if the age of the victim is less than 12 years, Section 89 of Indian penal code), samples for diagnosis of common STDs can be obtained. Before collecting the sample for HIV, pre-test counseling should be done and an informed expressed consent should be obtained. The diagnostic test as recommended by CDC for common STDs are given below in Table 3:

Table 3

	Disease	*Diagnostic Test*
1.	Gonorrhoea	Culture from site
2.	Lymphogranuloma Venereum	Culture/Presumptive non-culture tests
3.	Vaginitis (Trichomonas, Giardia Entamoeba)	Wet mount and vaginal swab culture
4.	Bacterial Vaginitis	Vaginal swab culture
5.	Syphills	Serum (VDRL)
6.	Hepatitis B	Serum (HbsAg)
7.	HIV	Serum (ELISA & WB)

Source: CDC Guidelines[36]

Repeated follow up is usually required at 2, 6, 12 and 24 weeks in victims of a sexual assault in order to detect new infections; to complete hepatitis B immunization (it indicated); to complete counseling and treatment of injuries, STDs and HIV; and for rehabilitation purposes. As per the CDC guidelines, for prophylaxis of the victims of sexual assaults, the regimes consisting of Ceftriaxone 125 mg 1/m plus Metronidazole 2 gm orally in a single dose plus Azithromycin 1 gm orally in a single dose or Doxycycline 100 mg BD × 7 days can be used.

In cases, where the assailant is a known HIV positive and the assault history is suggestive of a potential risk of transmission such as: non condom use; ejaculation; anal intercourse; and vaginal tear/bleeding, and the victim is examined within 24-36 hours after assault.

Anti-retroviral post exposure prophylaxis should be considered, along with information about the limited knowledge on efficacy and known toxicities of anti-retrovirals in this situation.[35] Similarly, if the assailant is hepatitis B positive than the victim should be immunized using hepatitis B vaccine. The management of sexual assault victims is a team effort consisting of the members of different disciplines of medicine and STD along with, law enforcing agencies and rehabilitation centers. The emphasis in such cases should be an immediate attention to the medical condition of the patients a proper medicolegal examination with collection of trace evidence and the prevention of medical and psychological sequalae.

B. Legal

A person who is suffering from STD/HIV and is fully aware of his condition and infectivity, and even after knowing these facts, it he/she willfully or negligently spreads the infection he/she can be under section 269, section 270, section 304A or even under section 302 IPC depending upon the magnitude of the sufferings of the victim and other circumstances of the case. A Georgian man in USA who inflicted a police officer with HIV after a bite was convicted for attempted murder in 1990.[37] Number of such cases of international spread by HIV positive patients have been reported and prosecuted in the west. However, the first person to be successfully prosecuted for sexual transmission of HIV pertains to Stephan Kelly, who has been convicted by the High Court of Glasgow in Feb, 2001. Stephan Kelly has been sentenced to five years imprisonment for the offence of recklessly causing injury to another (his former girl friend).[38] It is a point of discussion that criminally the case of AIDS is whether a direct consequence of HIV or it was latent in the individual that has surfaced once the option of longevity of life is closed.[39] Such a person also owns civil responsibilities for which he can be used for damages suffered by the victim. Recently in England a person has been jailed under Scottish common law for causing HIV infection to his lover (reported in the Times of India, May 22, 2001). Fortunately, no similar case where HIV has been caused by a deliberate set has been reported from India till now.

Evidential Value of STDs in Sexual Assault

STDs are of significant evidential value in sexual assaults as a proof of sexual contact specially when the victim is a child or a young adolescent and both the assailant and victim suffer from the same disease. When STD is found in the victim and is thought to be the result of sexual contact with the accused, positive cultures or blood tests for antibodies from the defendant can be helpful as corroborative evidence.[40] For some organisms such as Herpes simplex virus, Hepatitis B Virus, or HIV, highly specific serological tests exist to detect seroconversion in the victim which may indicate whether or not the infection was recently acquired. But, ordinarily a defendant can not be forced to be examined and give blood or other samples for investigation, without his consent. However, an accused under section 53(1) of the Criminal Procedure Code of India can be examined even without consent and by using reasonable force, when requested by the police and there is reasonable grounds to believe that such an examination will afford evidence, as to the commission of the offence.

Once the positive cultures are obtained from both victim and accused, matching of the strains can be done by molecular and other techniques. However, a negative culture obtained from the accused does not necessarily prove his innocence as the accused may or may not become infected after a single act of intercourse as evident from Table –2.

C. Social

Social stigma exists about STDs and especially about HIV. The attitude and behaviour of relatives and even family members changes drastically always towards an HIV patient. This mind set needs to be changed as any attempt of segregation/isolation is bound to generate negative thinking in the patient. However, practice of abstinence, single partner and use of condoms should be advocated to reduce the prevalence of HIV and STDs.

Liability for Failure to Diagnose AIDS

Two cases have been reported upto 1994, (this number must have been increased significantly now) where patients have sued their doctors for falling to diagnose AIDS resulting in a delay for providing treatment.[41] A legal duty is established by way of the doctor patient relationship, to manage the patient with reasonable skill and care. A proper diagnosis of the patient's disease is required as failure to diagnose can lead to improper treatment and even no treatment. This can be a reason for medical negligence case against the doctor, if the patient suffers. In light of the potential legal repercussions of failing to diagnose HIV/AIDS, doctors should take proper care, while taking history of patients and be on the look out for the clinical features indicating to be of HIV/AIDS, specially among high risk patients.

Concluding Remarks

In nutshell, behaviour modifications are hard to achieve. They are even harder to sustain where people's pleasures are involved and that is the reason STDs and HIV are difficult to curtail. The increasing sphere of STDs and HIV is bound to affect the social, medical, legal and ethical panorama of life. The problems which were unthinkable in olden times are posing threats and creating medico legal and ethical issues. One must be aware of these issues and plan out strategies to address them effectively.

References

1. Herbst MC: AIDS—A right to be informed, Med Law 1991; 10: 83-93.
2. Roadabaugh BJ, Austin M: Sexual Assault, New York, Gariand STPM Press 1981: 6 –10.
3. Gerbace AC *et al.*: Global Prevalence and Incidence Estimate of Selected Curable STDs, Sex *Trans Infect* 1998; 74 (Supple) : S15.
4. Rathore AS, Ramesh V: Sexually Transmitted Diseases, in Ghai OP, Gupta P (edS). Essential Preventive Medicine, New Delhi, Vikas Publishing House Pvt. Ltd., 1999 : 428-38.
5. The 10/90 Report on Health Research 2001-2002, Global Forum for Health Research C/o WHO, Switzerland, WHO, 2002 : 146-149.
6. AIDS update 2002; 7(1) : 1.
7. Indian Council of Medical Research Bulletin, ICMR, New Delhi, Dec. 2000; 138.
8. U S Bureau of the Census: Statistical Abstracts of the United States, 1996, 106th Ed. Govt. Printing Office, Washington DC, 1996: 166.
9. Koss MP: Detecting the Scope of Rape—A review of prevalence research methods, *J Interpersonal Violence* 1993; 8: 198.
10. Crime in India 1998, National Crime Records Bureau, Min of Home Affairs, Govt. of India, New Delhi, 1999; 56-123.
11. Verma SK: Medico Legal Issues in Clinical Practice, In: Ghai OP, Gupta P (Eds), Essential Preventive Medicine, New Delhi, Vikas Publishing House Pvt. Ltd., 1999 : 907-920.
12. Specialist's Training and Reference Module, National AIDS Control Organisation, Delhi, Delhi State AIDS Control Society 2001 : 67-69.
13. HIV / AIDS and Human Rights—International Guidelines, United Nations, New York and Geneva, 1998.
14. Bayer R: Ethical Issues In : Holmes KK, *et al* (Eds), Sexually Transmitted Diseases 3rd ed. New York, McGraw Hill, 1999: 1449-54.
15. Toomey KE, Gates W: Partner Notification for the Prevention of HIV Infection, AIDS 1989; 3(Supple); 557-562.
16. Rothenberg RB, Potterat JJ: Partner Notification for Sexually Transmitted Diseases and HIV Infection. In : Holmes KK, Sparling PF *et al* (Eds), Sexually Transmitted Diseases, 3rd Ed. New York, McGraw Hill 1999: 745-752.
17. Jayasuriya DC: Interdisciplinary International Conference of AIDS—Law and Humanity (New Delhi, 6-10 December, 1995). Int. Digest of Health Legislation 1996; 47(3) : 396-400.
18. Richards EP, Bross DC: Legal and Political Aspects of STD Prevention : Public Duties and Private Rights. In : Holmes K K *et al* (Eds), Sexually Transmitted Diseases, 3rd Ed, New York McGraw Hill 1999 : 1441-54.

19. Bayer R, *et al*.: Controlling AIDS in Cuba : The Logic of Quarantine, *N Engl J Med* 1989; 83: 1022.
20. Ton ML: Mother to Child Transmission AIDS Action 1999; 45: 8-9.
21. Dev A, Dev SA, Das S (Eds): Human Rights – A source book. New Delhi, NCERT, 1996; 1-10.
22. Kirby M: Human Rights and the HIV Paradox, Lancet 1996; 348: 1217-18.
23. Erridge P: The Rights of HIV Infected Health Care Workers, *B M J* 1996; 312 : 1625-26.
24. Verma SK: Supreme Court Curtails Right of PLWHA in India, *J Forensic Med Toxicol* 1999; 16(2) : 61-62.
25. Recommendations for Preventing Transmission of Human Immuno-deficiency Virus and Hepatitis B Virus to Patients during Exposure Prone Invasive Procedures. MMWR Mort Mortal Wkly Rep 1991; 40(RR-8); 1-9.
26. Schatz B: Supporting and Advocating for HIV Positive Health-care Workers. Bull New York *Acad Med*, 1995 : 263-272.
27. Gastin LO: A Proposed National Policy on Health-care Workers living with HIV / AIDS and Other Blood for Pathogens, *JAMA* 2000; 284 (15) : 1965.
28. Verma SK, Agarwal BBL: Medical Aspects of Rape Victim—Indian Perspective, *Int. J Med Toxicol Leg Med* 1999; 1(2) : 23-26.
29. Heimberger TS *et al*.: High Prevalence of Syphilis Detected through Jail Screening Program—A Potential Measure to address the Syphilis Epidemic, *Arch Intern Med* 1993; 153 : 1799.
30. National Commission on AIDS. HIV Disease in Correctional Facilities. National Commission on AIDS, Washington DC, 1999; 10.
31. McCutchan JA: Epidemiology of Veneral Urethritis—Comparison of Gonorrhea and Non-gonococcal Urethritis, *Rev Infect Dis* 1984; 6 : 669.
32. Holmes KK, *et al*.: An Estimate of the Risk of Men Acquiring Gonorrhea by Sexual Contact with Infected Females. *Am J Epidemiol* 1970; 91: 170.
33. Royce RA *et al*.: Sexual Transmission of HIV, *N Engl J Med*, 1997; 336: 1072.
34. Jenny C *et al*.: Sexually Transmitted Diseases in Victims of Rape, *N Engl J Med*, 1990; 322 : 713.
35. Glaser JB *et al*.: Sexually Transmitted Diseases in Postpubertal Female Rape Victims, *J Infect Dis*, 1991; 164 : 726.
36. Centre for Disease Control and Prevention, 1998 Guidelines for Treatment of Sexually Transmitted Diseases, MMWR 1998; 47: 108.
37. Wecht ND, Wecht CH: Scaipe and Quill, Pittsburg's Institute of Legal Medicine, In : Update of AIDS : Medical, Legal and Social Concern 1991; 35 : 8-9.
38. Chalmers J: The Criminalization of HIV-transmission, *J Med Ethics* 2002; 28 : 160-163.
39. Husain M, Usmani JA: AIDS and Criminality—A New Legal Perspective, *J Forensic Med Toxicol* 2000; 17(2) : 10-12.
40. Beck-Saque CM, Jenny C: Sexual Assault and STD, In : Holmes KK, *et al* (Eds). Sexually Transmitted Diseases 3rd Ed. New York, McGraw Hill, 1999 : 1433-39.
41. Hirsch D: Liability for Failure to Diagnose HIV Infection and AIDS, In : Stewart G (Ed) could it be HIV, 2nd Ed. North Sydney, Australasian Medical Publishing Company Ltd., 1994 : 72-73.

CHAPTER

13 HIV Counseling in Adolescents

Manju Mehta and *R Sadhu*

INTRODUCTION

Counselling is the process of interaction in which the counselor builds rapport with the client/patient and helps him/her to clarify his/her current life situation and helps him/her to decide about the future plan of action. Grossly speaking the term counseling embraces functions such as information giving, guidance, helping activities etc. and now a days it is applied in treatment of medical and psychiatric disorders.

For a counselor, the skills of listening, encouraging, acknowledging, summarizing, connecting, reflecting, challenging, checking understanding, motivating etc. along with unconditional positive regard expressed through genuineness, empathy, non-possessive warmth and congruence in the therapeutic relationship are important assets.

A patient who has been newly diagnosed as HIV infected can show psychological reactions like grief, surprise, indifference, denial, family concern, loss, suicidal ideation etc. which can influence his decision making capacity and actions. Counselling sessions help him/her to take correct, realistic decisions in such a context.

The slow progressive and fatal course of HIV infection and limitations of our current pharmacological treatments, produces a huge psychological burden not only for the HIV infected, but also for their partners, family members, office colleagues, employers (classmates, teachers in case of children and adolescents). Hence psychological treatments are used regularly as a tool for overall management of HIV infection. Educational measures in the form of simple conversation between the child and the parent on the use of condoms or the communication between the government and the young population through the media can help in prevention as well as bring great changes in high risk behaviour and attitude. The counseling is required with persons at high risk and is individually given to persons having problems.

Who does the Counseling?

HIV/AIDS counselling is usually given by a person trained in various aspects of counseling and specifically related to AIDS/HIV. Various professionals/social groups like social workers, doctors, nurses, psychologists, laboratory technicians, teachers, health educators, religious leaders, community leaders etc. can also be trained in counseling if they possess the motivation and dedication.

Who are to be Counseled?

All those persons who get directly or indirectly affected by the HIV infection, those persons exhibiting high risk behaviour and also those persons want to undergo HIV testing can be given the benefit of counseling. They can be divided into the following groups (Futterman et al., 2000; Maj. et al., 1991):

1. People who are worried that they might be infected with HIV
2. People want to undergo HIV testing
3. People having previous history of high risk sexual behaviour who want/do not want to undergo HIV testing
4. People with AIDS/other diseases related to their HIV infection
5. Men who have sex with men
6. Current or previous sexual partner are/were HIV positive
7. People having high risk injecting drug practices
8. Partners and family members of HIV infected
9. School authority in cases of children and adolescents (in cases where the authority has come to know about the disease of the student)
10. Office colleagues and employers (where they have come to know about the disease of the employee).

The Centers for Disease Control and Prevention (CDC) recommends (Rothman, 2004; Gallant, 2004) that in patients aged between 18 to 54 years coming to the emergency department from places where the HIV prevalence is greater or equal to 1%, in all pregnant women, in all patients with possible acute occupational exposure to HIV and in all patients with known sexual or needle sharing exposure to an HIV infected person, routine HIV testing should be done, and the time consuming prevention counseling may be offered to those who have a positive test result and to those having high risk for HIV as identified through screening. CDC recommends target testing and prevention counseling to patients coming from places where the HIV prevalence is less than 1% and presenting to the emergency department, who reported high risk behaviour and showed clinical signs and symptoms suggestive of opportunistic infections.

Aims of the Counseling

Counseling in such a situation can have multiple purposes depending upon the problem, mental development and the serostatus of the client, the time gap between the knowledge of the seropositivity and the current counseling session. The objective of such counseling can be as follows:

1. Prevent and control the spread of HIV/AIDS infections.
2. Provide emotional and psychosocial support to those already having the disease, their partners and family members.
3. Helping the patients to accept the information, understand its consequences and assist them in decision making.
4. Helping the patients in adherence to the combination anti-retroviral therapy.
5. Helping the school authority and office colleagues to gain knowledge about HIV/AIDS, reduce misconceptions and to be supportive to the patients.

Prevention and control of HIV infection can be achieved through assessment of high risk sexual behaviour, high risk intravenous drug use behaviour etc; working with the patient in making him/her understand the risk involved in them, the patients potential to change his/her behaviour and helping him/her to achieve and sustain such behaviour change. Patients who just came to know about their HIV seropositivity should be counseled in stages in which patients should be given adequate time for adjustment between the information about the meaning of HIV seropositivity and the information about the course of HIV infection, the usual life span with the disease etc.

Special Issues in Counseling of Adolescents

The adolescent age group is a risk group because of its characteristic tendencies of striving for independence, experimentation getting influenced more by the peer group as compared to the guardians and newly achieved sexuality. The counselor should keep in mind the following things while counseling an adolescent:

1. Depending on the level of cognitive maturity, the presence of concrete thinking and unclear concepts about death and dying can be expected.
2. Issue like disclosure to parents about homosexuality, drug use can be threatening.
3. Relaying on adults because of illness can go against the developmental need for establishment of independence.
4. Disclosure about HIV seropositivity to sexual partners can disrupt the small social world of adolescents.

Studies on HIV counseling of adolescents (like that by Rawitscher et al., 1995) had shown that adolescents had difficulty in initiating discussion on sex, safe sex, condom, homosexuality etc. Though adolescent boys preferred female physicians and physicians with whom they had previously spoken about sex to teachers or family members, adolescent girls choe family members and friends for discussion on these topics and getting HIV related information, thereby emphasizing the suitability of techniques like peer counseling, family education, school outreach programmes for them.

In the same study it had been found that adolescents preferred getting tested for HIV by people they did not know.

Context of Counseling

The ways to counsel people can vary depending upon the contexts and the needs. It can take any of the forms as described below:

1. ***Pre-test HIV counseling:*** It is conducted on subjects described previously before they undergo serological test for HIV as a part of taking their informed consent for the test. It usually consists of the following components:
   (a) Discussing the meaning of the positive results and negative results, clarification of distortions, concept of window period of HIV infection.
   (b) Discuss why the test is necessary i.e., the medical advantages of knowing the HIV status and treatment options.
   (c) Assess the high risk sexual behaviours, high risk injectable drug use behaviour, discuss about the potential routes of transmission of HIV, such that the client is able to comprehend his/her risk and encourage safer practices.
   (d) Explore the past reactions of the client to severe stress and also explore the potential reactions of the client to positive result. Take appropriate precautions to intervene a catastrophic reaction, assess coping skills of the patient and support network.
   (e) Discuss about the confidentiality issues, possibility of HIV testing being done completely anonymously (where the result is not made a permanent part of hospital chart), whom to tell about the test and the results, partner notification issues.
   (f) Discuss about the HIV seropositivity hampering the social status.
   (g) Document the discussion in chart and give time for clarifications and answering the client's questions.

2. ***Post-test counseling:*** This is carried out on the subjects who underwent HIV serological testing, after the report of the test is available and it has the following components:
   (a) Interpretation of the test results is conveyed to the client, distortions are clarified (like necessity of repeating HIV serological testing after 3 to 6 months of exposure i.e., the concept of window period is re-emphasized if the test is negative). Questions for assessing the client's level of understanding and his/her emotional reactions to the test result should be asked.
   (b) Recommendations about the reduction of high risk behaviour and promotion of positive health behaviour (i.e., about the use of condoms, stoppage of needle sharing, safer injection practices) should be emphasized.
   (c) Recommendations on the follow-up of sexual partners and needle contacts of the client.

(d) If the client is found to be HIV positive, reconfirmation of the test result on a second serum specimen in a reference laboratory should be done, he/she should be conveyed the information and adequate time gap should be given to him/her before giving him further information about the meaning of the test, the likely course and outcome of the illness; all of these should be conveyed gradually in multiple well spaced sessions. In the initial few sessions overloading the patients with information should be avoided and the emphasis should be on planning about the immediate few days.

(e) Evaluation of the suicide potential, enhancement of the coping skills of the patient, mobilizing support system should be done. Crisis intervention counseling can be done if needed.

(f) Discussion about disadvantages and advantages of informing key people in patients life, the importance of informing partner about patient's seropositivity should be done. Referral to a partner notification programme can be done if needed.

(g) Information on tuberculosis, TB screening, symptoms associated with the spectrum of HIV disease.

(h) Information on pregnancy and perinatal transmission.

(i) Recommendations against donating blood, sperm or organs and against sharing needles, razors etc.

(j) Referrals for appropriate medical and psychological support.

3. ***Counseling for medication adherence (Tuldra et al., 2002; Rawlings et al., 2003):*** This emphasizes the importance of adherence to the combination anti-retroviral therapy, helps the patients to cope with the side effects of medications and the reality of being HIV infected. To improve the medication compliance in adolescents infected with HIV a multilevel compliance initiative — Project TREAT (Treatment Regiments Enhancing Adherence in Teens) has been designed which is based upon Prochaska and Declemente's model of change. Overall it can have the following components:

(a) Information about the drugs and their dosings.

(b) Knowledge about the adverse effects of the drugs, their managements, when and how to seek help.

(c) Understanding of the risk of drug resistance on inadequate adherence.

(d) Discussion on patients knowledge and beliefs about medications.

(e) Use of reminder systems (like Medimom) to combat simple forgetting.

4. ***Crisis intervention counseling:*** An HIV infected person who comes to know about his/her sero status, because of the implications of the infection on his/her survival and the social stigma, can undergo an emotional crisis characterized by

the feelings of helplessness, hopelessness, loss of control and extreme anxiety. Crisis intervention counseling helps in management of such a situation and is characterized by:

(a) Encouragement to express anxiety, fear, sadness, anger and to grieve with the understanding that grief can be a healing process.

(b) Use psychosocial support to dispel self-blame, guilt; providing reassurance; sharing information, experience; reducing feelings of isolation, loneliness.

(c) Offering encouragement, comfort, concern, affection, legal and spiritual assistance through the social network.

(d) Teaching relaxation exercises

5. ***Bereavement counseling:*** This type of counseling deals with the emotions provoked by the loss or impending loss in the family members/partners of the HIV infected and is characterized by review of the lost relationship, encouragement to express the emotions and to undergo a healthy process of mourning along with provision of adequate social support.
6. ***Decision-making counseling:*** This type of counseling helps the patient in taking disturbing but necessary decisions. In the context of an HIV infected patient the following questions may prove to be crucial.

(i) Who will need to be told about the condition?

(ii) How and when will they be told?

(iii) Who will be asked to manage the client's affairs and provide care?

(iv) How will the client continue to attend to certain legal, financial or other matters?

(v) What kinds of change can be made in diet or lifestyle to keep as healthy as possible?

The counsellor helps in suggesting different alternatives, comparing the pros and cons of the alternatives and taking the best possible decision by the client. Usually this type of counseling is done after the initial crisis period is over.

7. ***Problem solving counseling:*** After the resolution of the initial crisis period this type of counseling is used to help the client deal his/her different problems. This type of counseling needs assessment of the client regarding his/her number of sexual partners, use of needles, blood transfusion history etc. alongwith provision of factual information about the problem to the client on which to base the decision. It consists of the following components:

(a) Helping the client to define his/her problem and expressing concern and support for it

(b) Discussing the clients feelings and fears

(c) Discussion on the actions the client has already taken

(d) Discussing the personal and other resources available or needed.
(e) Explaining accurately the protective action the client will need to take.
(f) Helping the client to establish a plan of action.

8. ***Family and relationship counseling (Maj, 1991):*** This should take place only after the consent from the patient and it deals with the partners and family members of HIV infected person. This can be an essential component for the management of unhealthy emotional reactions of the partners and family members towards the HIV infected and it has the following components:
   (a) Information about HIV infection and AIDS, their psychological impact on the infected partner
   (b) Address fears of infectiousness, provide guidelines on sexual behaviour and domestic hygiene
   (c) Encourage open communication between sexual partners about issues related to infections (special sessions can be devoted)
   (d) Taking temporary break when despair becomes overwhelming
   (e) Make plans for bereavement
9. ***Telephone/hotline counseling:*** In some developed and developing countries this method is used for conveying information, temporary management of crisis and for giving support.
10. Another difficult situation is to counsel adolescent, who have hemophilia or other blood related disorders and have acquired HIV (with or without HBV, HCV etc.) through blood transfusion in their early childhood and their relatives (Miller, 1995). Though with modern blood screening techniques this phenomenon has become rare, it can be a very demanding situation to deal with. It has been found that if the parents disclose early to their children about their disease, before they become ill or start making relationship, the situation becomes easier, however early disclosures rarely happen. Ideally speaking, adolescents under age 16 years should not be informed about their HIV seropositivity by the counsellor, without prior parental discussion and consent. Prior discussion with parents is also preferred while informing adolescents aged over 16 years about their seropositivity. Counseling in such a context can be done through
    (i) Family sessions
    (ii) Session with parents alone – when there are secrets about the diagnosis
    (iii) Group sessions – help to learn coping skills from others, and also reduce feelings of isolation.

The goals of such sessions can be as follows:
   (a) Careful use of language to establish rapport and to convey difficult messages
   (b) Focused brief sessions to identify what each family knows, they want to know and what their concerns might be, dealing with them according to the order of priority

(c) Educating adolescents safer sexual practices

(d) Encouraging responsible behaviour choices without diminishing their ability to cope effectively with the threat of disease.

(e) Helping adolescents to maintain hope whilst living within the realities of HIV.

(f) Helping family members to cope with the difficulties.

11. ***Peer counseling:*** Efficacy of peer based HIV prevention education has been established in many studies. In a study conducted in China peer counseling has been found to be an effective measure in the diffusion of sexual health message among Thrishaw pullers (Shugiang et al., 2003).

Some programmes which have been designed to educate the young generation about safe sexual behaviours and HIV also hold promise, for example.

(a) School based and community based programmes — preventive health education, sex education etc. are the important components of this programme.

(b) Outreach programmes – to reach the undetected HIV infected community the "adolescent AIDS programme" has started campaigning on the importance of HIV prevention, testing and care using the youth language and the media. One successful component of the programme was "get tested" week launched at youth led townhall meeting in USA (Futterman et al., 2000).

(c) Prevention of mother to child transmission of HIV services (PMTCT) – It had been found that many mothers had inadequate knowledge on many aspects of HIV transmission for example, in a study conducted in Nigeria 41.7% Nigerian women were not aware about the relation between breast milk and HIV transmission (Ekanem et al., 2004). Hence, PMTC programme has been launched in many countries (for example, Zimbabwe) which consists of recruiting counseling staff and trained health professionals, improving mother child helath (MCH) facilities and conducting information, education and communication activities within the community to address to HIV/AIDS awareness and stigma. MCH service emphasizes uses of voluntary counseling and testing of HIV using rapid testing, nevirapine short regimen to all HIV infected mothers and their newborns alongwith exclusive breast feeding (Perez et al., 2004).

Counseling Using other Modalities

— Internet counseling – internet has been used for this purpose in many countries, for example in Peru "the Perurian Institute for responsible parenthood" administers a questionnaire for keeping track of the age, gender, educational level and geographic location of the user while providing counseling and sexuality information through e-mail (Acevedo et al., 1998).

— Project "Necessaire" on sexual and reproductive health promotion – this technique was used to inform young women and was evaluated in Switzerland. The kit consisted of a brochure, written in the form of a diary of a woman called Rosa, which focused on love, sexuality and prevention of sexually transmitted diseases, along with several other items (like chewing gum, condom, sticker) (Page et al., 2000).

— Considering the popularity of hiphop music among the African Americans, it has been used for HIV/AIDS prevention counseling (Stepens et al., 1998).

Indian Scene

With the HIV epidemic engulfing the Indian population, the HIV/AIDS picture in India has started resembling other affected parts of the world. However, when we think of HIV counseling in such a sociocentric context issue like shared confidentiality come up.

Counselling in such a situation varies where the client becomes more dependent and the counsellors more directive. Counseling using different techniques and modalities is equally applicable in India. One such attempt, the "Rajiv Gandhi Mobile AIDS counselling and Testing Services" a joint venture of Indian Health Organization (IHO) and Rajiv Gandhi Foundation (RGF) was launched in Mumbai in October, 1999. It provides services like information – education – communication; condom distribution; counseling; instant HIV testing, networking with clinics, hospitals and nursing homes for management of STDs, HIV/AIDS, TB and other related disorders. Free of cost counseling and provision of anonymous HIV testing are the exciting features of this service.

Obstacles in HIV counseling – The obstacles to the use of counseling and in the counseling process itself can be grouped as follows:

(a) It has been found that after pretest counseling many patients refuse to undergo serological test for HIV or do not give consent for testing.

(b) The disease process itself can produce cognitive dysfunction thereby resulting in less gain from counseling of patients who presented in the later part of the illness (as is found in adolescents who got infected perinatally).

(c) Sense of immortality, unclear concepts about death and concrete thinking which can be found in adolescents can limit the benefits of the counseling.

(d) The guardedness of the patient in revealing his/her high risk behaviours and the emotional reactions of the relatives to the stigma of the HIV infection of the patient can limit the efficacy of the counselling.

(e) Prolonged asymptomatic period after sero conversion and also associated denial of the patients may act as a barrier to the efficacy of the counseling.

(f) Limitations in terms of time and resources.

(g) Traditional and religious beliefs of the client may be a barrier to the purpose of counseling.

(h) Communication problems.

Efficacy of HIV counseling – Counseling has been proposed to improve the outcome at multiple levels in the management of the HIV infected persons. Some recent studies have proved its overall efficacy in the management (Kamb et al., 1998) though they have also hinted towards the existence of a few groups which are relatively resistant to the counselling interventions for example, females, adolescents, previously HIV tested and counseled, persons who have STD. However another study (project –RESPECT) conducted by Bolu et al., (2004) have found brief counseling to be equally effective in these groups also. A study conducted by Richardson et al., (2004) which compared two brief safer sex counseling techniques in the forms of gain frame approach (i.e., positive consequences of safer sex) and loss frame approach to be more effective in reducing high risk sexual behaviours in HIV positive persons (mainly males who have sex with > or = 2 male partners). Unfortunately, efficacy studies on many aspects of HIV counseling are still lacking as it is a topic which came to focus only recently.

To conclude it can be asserted that till today, HIV infection is one of those many conditions which reminds doctors of their limitations and in such a setting we should not forget to show our love and respect for humanity and should remember the golden words "Prevention is better than cure."

REFERENCES

1. Acevedi E, Delgado G, Segil E: INPPARES uses internet to provide Peruvians with Sexuality Information and Counselling, SIECUS Rep 1998; 26(5): 14.
2. Bolu, OO, Lindsey C, Kamb ML, Kent C, Zenilman J, *et al*.: Is HIV/Sexually Transmitted Disease Prevention Counselling Effective Among Vulnerable Populations? Sexually Transmitted Diseases, 2004; 31:469-474.
3. D'Angelo L J: Adolescents and HIV Infection—A clinician's perspective, *Acta Paediatr Suppl.* 1994 Aug; 400: 88-94.
4. Ekanem EE, Gbadegesin A: Voluntary Counselling and Testing (VCT) for Human Immunodeficiency Virus: A study on acceptability by Nigerian women attending antenatal clinics, *Afr Reprod Health* 2004; 8(2): 91-100.
5. Futterman D, Chabon B, Hoffman ND: HIV and AIDS in Adolescents. *Pediatr Clin North Am* 2000; 47:171-188.
6. Gallant JE: HIV Counselling Testing and Referral, *Am. Fam Physician*, 2004; 70: 295-302.
7. Gelder MG, Lopez-Ibor Jr JJ, Andreasen NC: New Oxford Textbook of Psychiatry, Oxford University Press, Oxford, 2000.
8. Kamb ML, Fishbein M, Doughas JM *et al*.: Efficacy of Risk Reduction Counselling to Prevent Human Immunodeficiency Virus and Sexually Transmitted Diseases: A randomized controlled trial. *JAMA* 1998; 280: 1161-167.
9. Koblin B, Chesney M *et al*.: Effects of a Behavioural Intervention to reduce Acquisition of HIV Infection Among Men who have Sex with Men: The Explore Randomized Controlled Study. Lancet 2004; 364 (9428) : 41-50.
10. Maj M: Psychological Problems of families and Health Workers Dealing with People Infected with Human Immunodeficiency Virus 1, *Acta Psy Scand*, 1991; 83: 161-8.
11. Miller R: Guidelines for Counselling Adolescents with Hemophilia and HIV Infection and Their Families, *AIDS care*, 1995; 7(3): 381-9.

CHAPTER

14 Management of Sexually Transmitted Infections in Indian Adolescents

Shilpa Mehta and *Archana Singal*

Adolescence is a time of great change, when young people take on new roles and responsibilities; renegotiate relationship with adults, peers and the community, and experiments with things symbolic of adult life. These developments are often accompanied by adoption of risk taking behaviour that compromise health. Healthy risk taking is a positive tool in adolescent's life for developing and consolidating his or her own identity. It is the extent to which an adolescent engages in high risk behaviour and the overall impact of these behaviours on personal health and development that are of increasing public health concern. The research suggests that young people who participate in multiple risks taking behaviour increase the chance of damaging their health.[1]

An important and complex area of adolescent behavioural health is sexuality. Issues of experience and activity include the timing of first intercourse, number of sex partners, contraceptive use, pregnancy, and sexually transmitted infections (STIs). Each of these outcomes varies between ages, gender, race, ethnicity, socio-economic status and religious groups.[2,3] Complexity is also reflected in the particular influences associated with adolescent sexual activity. Neighbourhood (socio-economic status, joblessness), peer (sexually active friends), familial (family instability), single parent household, sibling sexual activity and individual characteristics (race/ethicality, gender, age, pubertal status) have all been associated with adolescent sexual outcomes.[2,4]

TRENDS IN ADOLESCENT SEXUAL BEHAVIOUR

High risk behaviour has been defined as 'behaviour that increases the likelihood of adverse physical, social or psychological consequences'.[1] Worldwide, approximately half of 16 year olds are sexually active, which facilitates the spread of STIs.[5] The past four decades have been a period of great change in adolescent's sexual activity and its consequences. Though adolescents are initiating sexual activity at younger ages, the teen pregnancy rates are now declining since their peak in 1991. Important trends in areas of adolescent sexual behaviour include sexual experience and activity, pregnancy and STIs, including human immunodeficiency virus (HIV) and acquired immunodeficiency syndrome (AIDS).[6]

Regarding sexual experience approximately 12.1% of males and 30% of females aged 18 to 21 reportedly have had sexual intercourse, by 12 years of age. For over 20% of these young women, early sexual initiation was not voluntary. The Center for Disease Control and Prevention (CDC) reported that between 1990 and 1997, 15 to 19 years old males and females increased their condom use. However consistent adolescent contraceptive use remains lower than that for adults.[2,3]

Despite the increased proportion of youth practicing protected intercourse adolescents are disproportionately at risk for STIs.[2,5] STI rates have declined among the total population; however the rate of decline among adolescents has not been as great. In the United States, about 25% of sexually active adolescents contract an STI each year and more than half of all new HIV infection occur among persons under age 25 representing about 20,000 new HIV cases each year.[5]

Common STIs in adolescence can manifest as:

1. Urethral Discharge
2. Genital Ulcer
3. Vaginal Discharge
4. Lower Abdominal Pain

1. Urethral Discharge: Urethritis is probably the most common STI in adolescent men in developing countries with an incidence varying from 7-10%. Although *Chlamydia trachomatis* and *Ureaplasma urealyticum* are the major causes of urethritis in the developed world, *Neisseria gonorrhoea* continues to be the major cause in developing countries.[7] A gram stain of the urethral discharge and/or the first void urine is used for the detection of intracellular gram negative diplococci. The presence of 5 or more polymorphs on high power field of urethral smear is suggestive of urethritis. However gonococeal infection cannot always be excluded by Gram stain, as culture is the true gold standard.

2. Genital Ulcer: Like urethritis, genital ulcers are much more common in developing countries than in industrialized countries. The most common causes of genital ulcers in all the developing countries are chancroid, syphilis and genital herpes. Two rather rare causes of genital ulcers are lymphogranuloma venerum and donovanosis.[8]

Table 1. *Clinical Features of Genital Ulcers*[8]

	Syphilis	*Herpes*	*Chancroid*	*LGV*	*Donovanosis*
Etiological agent	*Treponema pallidum*	*Herpes Simplex Virus (HSV)*	*Hemophilus ducreyi*	*C. trachomatis* $(L_1 - L_3)$	*Calymmatobacterium granulomatis*
Incubation period	9-90 days	2-7 days	1-4 days	3 days-6 weeks	1-4 weeks (upto 6 months)
Primary lesions	Papule	Vesicle	Pustule	Papule, pustule or vesicle	Papule
Number of lesions	Usually one	Multiple, may coalesce	Usually multiple, may coalesce	Usually one	Variable
Diameter	5-15 mm	1-2 mm	Variable	2-10 mm	Variable
Edges	Sharply demarcated, elevated, round or oval	Erythematous	Undetermined ragged, irregular	Elevated, round or oval	Elevated, irregular
Depth	Superficial or deep	Superficial	Excavated	Superficial or deep	Elevated
Base	Smooth, nonpurulent, relatively nonvascular	Serous, erythematous, nonvascular	Purulent, bleeds easily	Variable, non-vascular	Red and velvety, bleeds readily
Induration	Firm	None	Soft	Occasionally firm	Firm
Pain	Uncommon	Frequently tender	Usually very tender	Variable	Uncommon
Lumphadenopathy	Firm, non-tender, bilateral	Firm, tender, often bilateral with initial episode	Tender, may suppurate, loculated, usually unilateral	Tender, may suppurate, loculated, usually unilateral	None, pseudobuboes
Microscopy	Darkfield or direct immuno-fluorescence	Antigen detection	Gram-staining has low sensitivity and specificity	Not available	Giemsa-or Wright stained tissue smears and sections
Culture	Not available	Cell culture	Sensitive, selective media available	McCoy Cell culture	Not available

(Contd...)

Serology	RPR/VDRL FTA-abs, TPHA, MHATP	1gM and 1gG Ab	Experimental	Complement fixation and immuno-fluorescent antibody test	Experimental
Molecular techniques	PCR	PCR	PCR	PCR/LCR	Not available

3. Vaginal Discharge: Abnormal vaginal discharge and dysuria are very common complaint among adolescent women.[9] It is the main symptom of both vaginitis and cervicitis. The underlying cause of cervicitis in women are gonococcal or chlamydial infection which are usually localized to the endocervix and urethra. The presence of a minimum of 30 polymorphs per high power field on endocervical gram stain is suggestive of cervicitis. Gonococcal and chlamydial cultures are commonly performed on modified MacConky's and McCoy cell cultures respectively. The most frequent causes of vaginal discharge are candidiasis, bacterial vaginosis and trichomoniasis.[9]

Table 2. ***Diagnostic Features and Management of Vaginal Infection in Pre-menopausal Adults[9]***

	Normal Vaginal Examination	*Canidial Vaginitis*	*Trichomonal Vaginitis*	*Bacterial Vaginosis **(NSV)***
Etiology	Uninfected; Lactobacillus predominant	*Candida albicans* and other yeasts	*Trichonomas vaginalis*	Associated with *Gordrenella vaginalis,* various anaeroibic bacteria, and mycoplasma
Typical Symptoms	None	vulval itching, burning or irritation	Profuse purulent discharge	Malodorous, slightly increased discharge
Discharge: Amount	Variable, usually scant	Scant to moderate	Profuse	Moderate
Colour	Clear or white	Curdy white	Yellow	Usually white or gray
Consistency	Non-homo-genous, floccular	Clumped, adherent plaques	Homogenous	Homogenous, low viscosity; uniformly coating vaginal walls

(Contd...)

Inflammation of vulvulal or vaginal epithelium	None	Erythema of vaginal epithelium, introitus; vulvar dermatitis common	Erythema of vaginal and vulvar epithelium; colpitis macularis	None
pH of vaginal fluid + Amine ("fishy") odor with 10% KOH	Usually < 4.5 None	Usually < 4.5 None	Often > 5.0 May be present	Usually > 4.5 present
Microscopy	Normal epithelial cells, lactobacilli predominate	Leukocytes, epithelial cells; yeast, mycelia, or pseudomycelia in up to 80%	Leukocytes; motile trichomonads seen in 80 to 90% of symptomatic patients, less often in the absence of symptoms	Clue cells; few leukocytes; lactobacilli out-outnumbered by profuse mixed flora, nearly always including G. vaginalis plus anaerobic species, on Gram stain
Usual treatment	None	Miconazole, clotrimazole, or other imidazoles	Metronidazole or tinidazole 2.0 g orally (single dose)	Metronidazole 500 mg orally twice daily for 7 days
Usual management of sex partners	None	None; topical treatment if candidal dermatitis of penis is present	Examine for STD; treat with metronidazole 2 gm p.o.	Examine for STD; no treatment if normal

4. Lower Abdominal Pain: Pelvic inflammatory disease (PID) is a common complication of untreated cervicitis. The most common symptoms of PID are lower abdominal pain, fever, cervical motion tenderness, palpable mass and vaginal discharge.[7]

The estimated risk of PID is highest among sexually active young adolescents, with a progressive decline with increasing age. The investigators calculated that the risk of developing salpingitis for those with chlamydial infection was approximately 70% greater among women between 15 to 19 years than among women 20 to 24 years old; among those with gonorrhoea, the risk for 15 to 19 years old was about 20% less than among the 20 to 24 years old.[10]

Partner notification and treatment, counselling, HIV and VDRL testing and condom promotion are four keys of comprehensive case management, which should be insured in every case reporting to the STD clinic.

Human papilloma virus

Studies demonstrate that prevalence of human papilloma virus (HPV) is highest among adolescents and young adults.[11]

Identifying Risk and Protective Factors

Sexual behaviour is socially negotiated, heavily affect laden, motivated by individual arousal and subject to moral and socio-cultural standards that vary across religion and in relation to age and gender. Thus sexual behaviour has unique characteristics when social, biological, behavioural and developmental factors all act in concert to increase the likelihood of STD acquisition.[5]

Known risk factors for health risk behaviour of adolescents include[1]:

1. Biological factors
2. Poverty and homelessness
3. Poor academic performance
4. Low self esteem, a sense of hopelessness
5. Family history of mental and physical health problems
6. Intellectual and developmental disabilities
7. Illiteracy
8. Tobacco smoking, alcohol use and illicit drug use.

Risk Factors

Biological Factors

The histology of cervix and vagina undergo dramatic changes from childhood through puberty and into adulthood. Soon after birth, the squamous cells of the vagina are replaced with columnar epithelium. At puberty, estrogen exposure causes the vaginal lining to thicken again with layers of squamous epithelium. Such epithelial changes may be particularly important at the cervix, since the persistence of cervical, columnar epithelium in young women appear to significantly increase their vulnerability to STDs. Although cervical columnar epithelium eventually recedes completely, replacement is a gradual process, continuing well into adulthood. Typically the cervix in adolescence still displays areas of exposed columnar epithelium, a condition often referred to as ectopy. This is significant because both Chlamydia trachomatis and Neisseria gonorrhoea preferentially attach to columnar and not squamous epithelium. In addition, ectopy may contribute to HIV acquisition and HIV shedding. The vasculature found with columnar epithelium associated with ectopy is more superficial and easily traumatized than that of squamous epithelium.[7,12,13,14]

The higher vaginal pH of early adolescence may be associated with lower prevalence of hydrogen peroxide producing organisms. Mucus production is greatly increased in early puberty, but the mucus is thinner than that found in older adolescents or adult women. Thinner mucus may permit organisms to penetrate more easily and to attach mucosal sites or gain access to the upper tract.[7]

Psychological and Cognitive Development

The stages of adolescence have arbitrarily catagorised as "early" (females : 9–13 years and males 11–15 years), "middle" (females 12–16 years and males 14–17 years) and "late" (females > 16 years and males > 17 years).[15]

Cognitive development in each of these stages is strongly influenced by the quality of teaching or role modeling they experience. This is particularly relevant to STD acquisition where adults may use indirect methods of educating or "rely" on scare tactics rather than utilize skills training.[16] Younger adolescent frequently use concrete style or reasoning, focusing on the present time and are unable to conceptualise the long term impact, that current actions may have until they reach middle or late adolescence. Furthermore, adolescents may have difficulty correctly implementing complex tasks (such as condom use) involving a series of steps that must be accomplished in a certain sequence to be effective. Finally many parents, educators and health care workers do not teach about STD risks or even details of pubertal development until long after many adolescents are at risk of STDs. Therefore, these youth do not even have the basic information to make informed choice.[16]

Sexual Behaviour

Socio-cultural and behavioural changes, over the last few decades, have combined with changes in the aspects of developmental physiology of adolescents, to increase the risk of STDs among young adolescents. Biologically, the average age of menarche has decreased and at the same time, societal changes have resulted in increasing the average age at which young men and women marry. Today the interval between maturation and marriage has increased and this fact has expectedly increased the incidence of pre-marital sex.[17,18,19]

Changes in sexual behaviour, have placed adolescents at an increased risk of STDs, with the trend to earlier age at first intercourse occurring worldwide. These trends have occurred despite concern about HIV infection. At each age a greater percentage of males than females have been sexually active and in general, the percentage of males who have had sexual intercourse is equal to that of females 1 year older.[20] In addition the younger age of sexual "debut" is associated with a greater number of sexual partners, an important determinant of STD risk.

Population based data demonstrate that condom use has increased substantially, but the use is not always consistent. Follow up data indicate that as males get older and as the duration of existing relationship increases, condoms are less likely to be used, while other forms of contraception that offer less protection against STDs are more used, particularly oral contraception. This fact may aid in the increased exposure and transmission of organisms such as HSV-2, chlamydia. HPY and HIV, which are associated with chronic and often asymptomatic infection.[21]

Use of condoms is a complex behaviour. Many studies have noted that perceived risk, peer pressure and partner support are important factors in condom use. A major concern, however is the belief that their partners, particularly their steady partners, would view the request to use a condom as indicating lack of trust. Approaches to reconciling these issues are complex and require skillful and practiced communication, as well as intervention suitable for sexually active adolescents who are in the formative phase of social skill developments. Other barriers to condom use that are unique to adolescents include lack of easy availability.[22,23]

Sexuality Among Adolescents with Intellectual and Developmental Disabilities

Sexuality and sexual expression are highly controversial issues among individuals having intellectual and developmental disabilities, with organizational and structural policies existing in school, community and work site setting, leading to unhealthy sexual expression.[24]

Tobacco smoking, alcohol use and illicit drug use is associated with range of health risk behaviour of which unsafe sex and STIs, form an important proportion.[1]

Protective Factors Include[1]

1. An attachment to an adult carer
2. Independence and competency
3. High aspiration with adult support
4. Effective schooling, connectedness with the teachers
5. Good health
6. Motivation to access resources

Issue of Age of Consent and Confidentially[1]

General practitioners (GPs) who treat young people need a good understanding of law relating to the age of consent and confidentiality of medical treatment and the conflicts that can arise between the screening for risk behaviour and legislative reporting requirement.

Knowing that young people under the age of 16 years who show sufficient maturity and understanding can consent to treatment without the knowledge of legal guardians is crucial to GPs treating young women.

Medical and Non-medical Interventions

Effective STD prevention for adolescents requires involvement by numerous individuals and institutions that have contact with young people and it should include activities implemented in different settings.

Psychological Screening for Health Risk Behaviour

A widely used and valuable screening device for exploring psychosocial functioning with adolescents is the "HEADSS" approach. It provides the comprehensive framework for examining the "Four worlds of the adolescents" while weighing upto the balance of health risk and protective factors.[1]

Influences in each of the "Four worlds of adolescents"

Inner World: Temperament, mental and physical health, intelligence, self-esteem and genetic factors.

Non-medical and Medical Interventions

Family World: Family dynamics, history of illness, relationships, culture and spirituality.

Peer World: Friendship, activities, pro or anti social groups

School World: Academic and sporting achievements and ability, relationships with teachers and peers.

Despite the many challenges facing prevention of STIs among adolescents, there are encouraging findings from interventions based in schools or in community, implemented in clinics or via mass media, or resulting from policy discussion.[1]

Counseling

Counseling is defined as confidential dialogue between a client and a care provider aimed at enabling the client to cope with stress and take personal decisions related to HIV/AIDS. The counseling process includes an evaluation of personal risk of HIV transmission and facilitation of preventive measures. This includes information, education and psychosocial support and allows individuals to make decisions that facilitate coping and adopt preventive behaviour.[25]

Indication for HIV Counseling and Testing[25]

- Clinical indications
- Signs and symptoms for HIV (e.g. unexplained weight loss, fever, atypical pneumonia or oral thursh)
- Acute HIV seroconversion symptoms
- Confirmation, if prior reported positive test is not documented.
- Prior risk behaviour
- Multiple sexual partners, sexual partner at risk, prior or recent STD diagnosis, injection drug use and transfusion with blood and its products before screening for HIV was introduced, haemophiliacs who received factor VIII before screening for HIV, men who have sex with men (MSM).
- Pregnant women
- Exposure to HIV
- Occupational
- Sexual or drug abuse
- Persons who request HIV testing

Essential Stages of Counseling[25]

Stage One : Forming rapport and gaining the client's trust
Stage Two : Definition and understanding of roles, boundaries and needs
Stage Three : Process of ongoing, supportive counselling
Stage Four : Closure or ending the counselling relationship

Elements of Counseling[25]

The GATHER approach can be understood as follows:

G : Greet the client politely
A : Ask about their needs, doubts, concerns
T : Tell the client about the facts, side effects and give options
H : Help the client to choose
E : Explain about the different issues
R : Return for follow-up

Different Types of HIV/AIDS Counseling[25]

1. Pre-test counseling: Counseling before the test for HIV
2. Post-test counseling: Counseling after the HIV test is done, whether positive or negative
3. Risk reduction assessment
4. Counselling after a diagnosis of AIDS has been made
5. Family and relationship counseling
6. Bereavement counseling
7. Outreach counseling
8. Crisis counselling
9. Telephone and hotline counseling

Pre-test Counseling[26]

The content of the pre-test counseling visit should be tailored to the individual, taking into account whether the client has been counselled and tested for HIV previously, his or her knowledge about HIV diagnosis and treatment, and the clients level of reported risk. For the clients who are being tested for HIV for the first time the discussion of HIV transmission and natural history may need to be more detailed than for persons who have been counselled previously.

1. Ascertain risk status

   ↓

   Discussion risk reduction plan and referral to other services
   (support groups, drug treatment, needle exchange)
2. Assess understanding of HIV transmission and natural history.
   - difference between HIV (the virus) and AIDS (clinical condition)

- presence of antibody test indicates HIV infection but not the clinical syndrome of AIDS.

3. Test results: can be positive, negative, indeterminate
   - generally positive within 3 months but may take upto 6 months
   - therefore repeat testing after 6 months of exposure, if initial test is negative
4. Psychological support, social support, impact of positive result.
5. Ensure that follow up is available, importance of obtaining test results, post-test counselling.
6. Discuss confidentiality
7. Obtain informed consent

Post-test Counseling[26]

1. Prepare patient for the result
2. Disclose result and its interpretation (positive/negative/indeterminate)

For HIV Seronegative Persons

1. Readdress and reinforce risk reduction plan
2. Discuss need for repeat testing for those with recent (< 6 months) exposure or ongoing risk behaviour

For Indeterminate HIV1 WB (Western Blot)

1. Discuss the prevalence and risk factors of indeterminate test (10% of the reactive results)
   - prevalence of cross reacting autoantibodies as in pregnancy
2. Low risk individuals – reassurance
   Repeat testing at 3-6 months
3. High risk individual, those with P_{24} band
   - possibility of acute HIV infection
   - need for follow up at 1, 3, 6 months
   - safe sexual/drug abuse behaviour
4. Consider supplement assay (e.g. PCR, P_{24} antigen, culture)
   - For early diagnosis of seroconverters
   - Reassure those without HIV infection

For HIV Seropositive Persons

1. Give time to handle potential distress
2. If positive result is unexpected/inconsistent with risk behaviour – repeat testing

3. Differentiate between HIV-infected and having AIDS
   - Review natural history of HIV
   - Degree of immunosuppression
4. Emphasize importance of early clinical intervention to slow disease progression
   - Anti-retroviral therapy
   - Prophylasis against opportunistic infections
5. Ways to avoid transmitting HIV to others and to avoid acquisition of other STDs that theoretically may accelerate HIV disease
6. Provide referrals for medical, psychological or social services.
7. Follow-up visits to
   - Reassess psychological status
   - Discuss partner notification/counselling issues
   - Referral services

School Based Programs

Adolescent Reproductive Health (ARH) programs in school have the potential to reach large number of adolescents especially where school enrollment rates are high. School based programs are able to provide educational message and skill-based programs to a captive audience of youth.[27-30]

HIV/AIDS/STI educational programs: There is evidence that best school based program can be effective in postponing the age of first intercourse and in decreasing the rates of unprotected intercourse, but the curriculum in many schools needs to be strengthened. Contrary to the popular belief, sex education has not increased the percentage of young people becoming sexually active. However, the program needs to be strengthened in terms of proper training in STD prevention and correct use of condom.[7,27]

Mass Media Based Programs

Communication research indicates that media can be an effective strategy for influencing adolescent sexual and contraceptive behaviour. In the recent years, programs efforts directed to adolescents have increasingly emphasized the combination of educational material with entertainment to attract the young audience. This "enter-educate" approach is thought to have considerable potential with young adolescents. These programs usually include a mass media component (radio, television and/or print media), social marketing of condoms and peer educators who sold condoms. Studies conducted in developing countries found that in the intervention group, youth reported greater use of condom and delayed sexual initiation.[7]

Community Based Program[31,32]

Community based programs are operationally defined as programs whose activities are not limited to a particular setting and/or are undertaken in multiple settings concurrently. These programs include:

1. *Youth Development Programs*: These programs usually include nonformal education, family life education, vocational skill training, health education and public awareness creators.
2. *Peer Programs*: Peer programs recruit and train a core group of youth to serve as role models and sources of information for their peers. Moreover, in the same setting, peers have been able to distribute and/or sell certain types of contraception, thus increasing access to non-clinical contraception in a non-threatening environment.
3. *Educational Programs*: These programs have been implemented in Lucknow in India involving sessions that are partly didactic and partly interactive. This project found greater improvements in the intervention community's knowledge of STIs, knowledge of asymptomatic cases of STIs and the knowledge that individuals other than prostitutes can also transmit STIs.

Workplace Based Programs

The first of these was the government of Thailand's 100 percent condom promotion program among visitors to brothels. The second intervention behavioural impact undertaken was an STI/HIV intervention among commercial sex workers and madams in the red light district of Mumbai. This program included motivational and educational videos about HIV, group discussion and visual materials. Both these programs were partly successful, however the sex workers and madams reported that they were concerned that they would lose clients if condoms use were insisted upon.[27]

Health Facility Based Program

"Youth friendly services" and "youth centers" are geared towards making existing reproductive health services more acceptable or less traumatizing to adolescents.[33]

There is a significant number of shortcomings in our current understanding of the efficiency of the ARH intervention. Firstly only a small proportion of ARH intervention undertaken to date have been rigorously evaluated and thus the relative merits of alternative intervention approaches remains unclear. Second the majority of programs that have been rigorously evaluated, have provided small scale evidence on long-term behavioural effects of intervention.

Medical Management of Sexually Transmitted Diseases[34-37]

Syndromic approach is designed to follow a diagnostic logic and provides a readymade tool to health markers.

1. Urethral Discharge

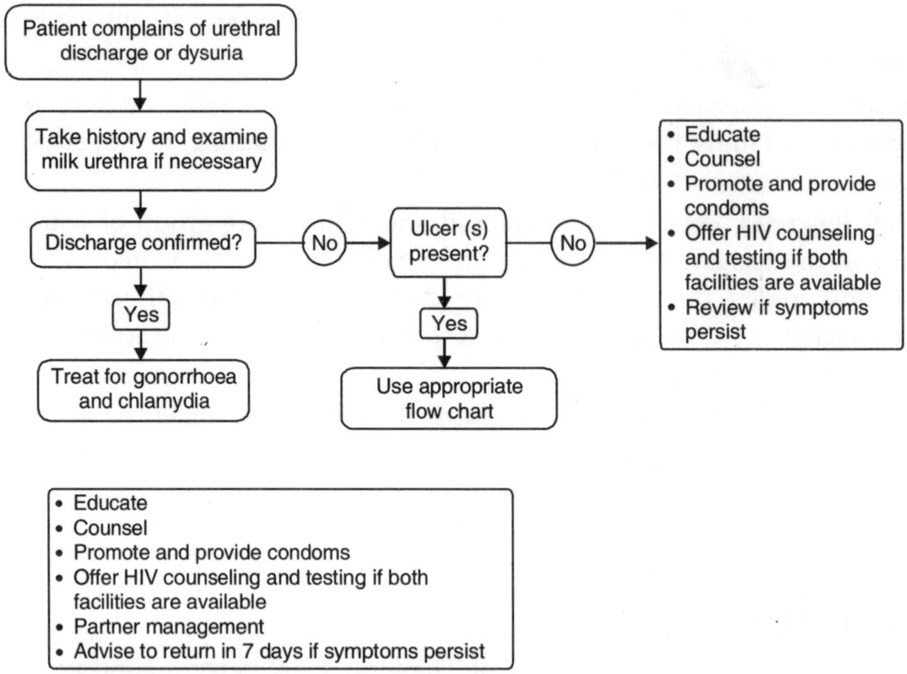
Patient complains of urethral discharge or dysuria
Take history and examine milk urethra if necessary
Discharge confirmed?
No
Ulcer (s) present?
No
• Educate
• Counsel
• Promote and provide condoms
• Offer HIV counseling and testing if both facilities are available
• Review if symptoms persist
Yes
Yes
Treat for gonorrhoea and chlamydia
Use appropriate flow chart
• Educate
• Counsel
• Promote and provide condoms
• Offer HIV counseling and testing if both facilities are available
• Partner management
• Advise to return in 7 days if symptoms persist

2. Uncomplicated Gonococcal Infections

Tab Azithromycin, 2g orally as a single dose (for both gonococcal and chlamydial infections).

or

Inj. Ceftriaxone, 250 mg IM as a single injection

or

Tab. Cefixime, 400 mg orally as a single dose

3. Chlamydial Urethritis or Cervicitis

Tab. Azithromycin 2g orally as a single dose (for both gonococcal and chlamydial infections)

or

Cap. Doxycycline 100 mg orally twice daily for 7 days.

(**Caution**: Doxycycline is contraindicated during pregnancy).

or

Tab. Erythromycin base/erythromycin stearate, 500 mg orally for 7 days.

4. Vaginal Discharge

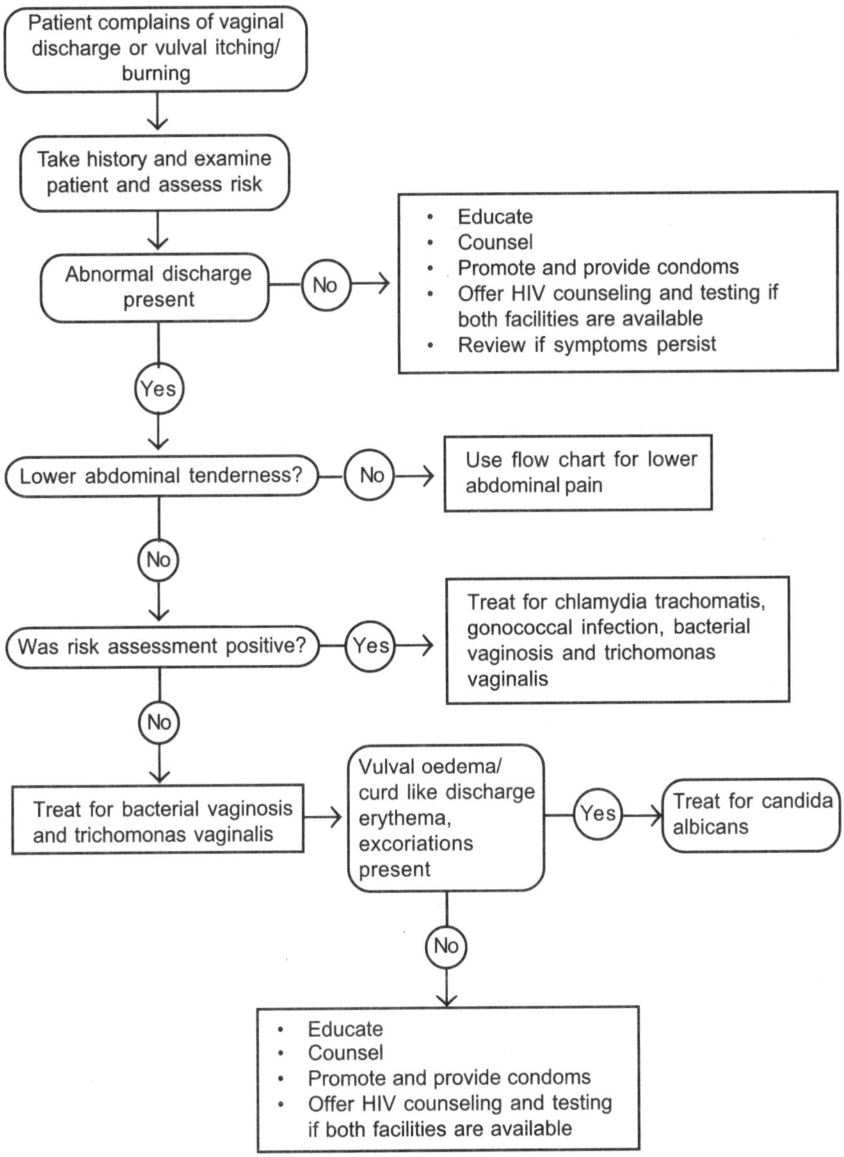

Patient complains of vaginal discharge or vulval itching/ burning
Take history and examine patient and assess risk
Abnormal discharge present
No
• Educate
• Counsel
• Promote and provide condoms
• Offer HIV counseling and testing if both facilities are available
• Review if symptoms persist
Yes
Lower abdominal tenderness?
No
Use flow chart for lower abdominal pain
No
Was risk assessment positive?
Yes
Treat for chlamydia trachomatis, gonococcal infection, bacterial vaginosis and trichomonas vaginalis
No
Treat for bacterial vaginosis and trichomonas vaginalis
Vulval oedema/ curd like discharge erythema, excoriations present
Yes
Treat for candida albicans
No
• Educate
• Counsel
• Promote and provide condoms
• Offer HIV counseling and testing if both facilities are available

For **Gonococcal cervicitis and Chlamydial cervicitis** same as in urethral discharge.

Trichomoniasis

Tab. Metronidazole, 2g orally in a single dose/metronidazole 400 mg orally twice daily for 7 days.

or

Tab. Tinidazole, 2g orally in a single dose.

Bacterial vaginosis

Tab. Metronidazole, 2g orally in a single dose/metronidazole 400 mg orally twice daily for 7 days.

or

Tab. Tinidazole, 2g orally in a single dose.

However, in symptomatic woman, in the first trimester and those intolerant to metronidazole/tinidazole, imidazole pessaries/cream may be given for 7 days.

5. Vaginal Discharge (Speculum and Bimanual)

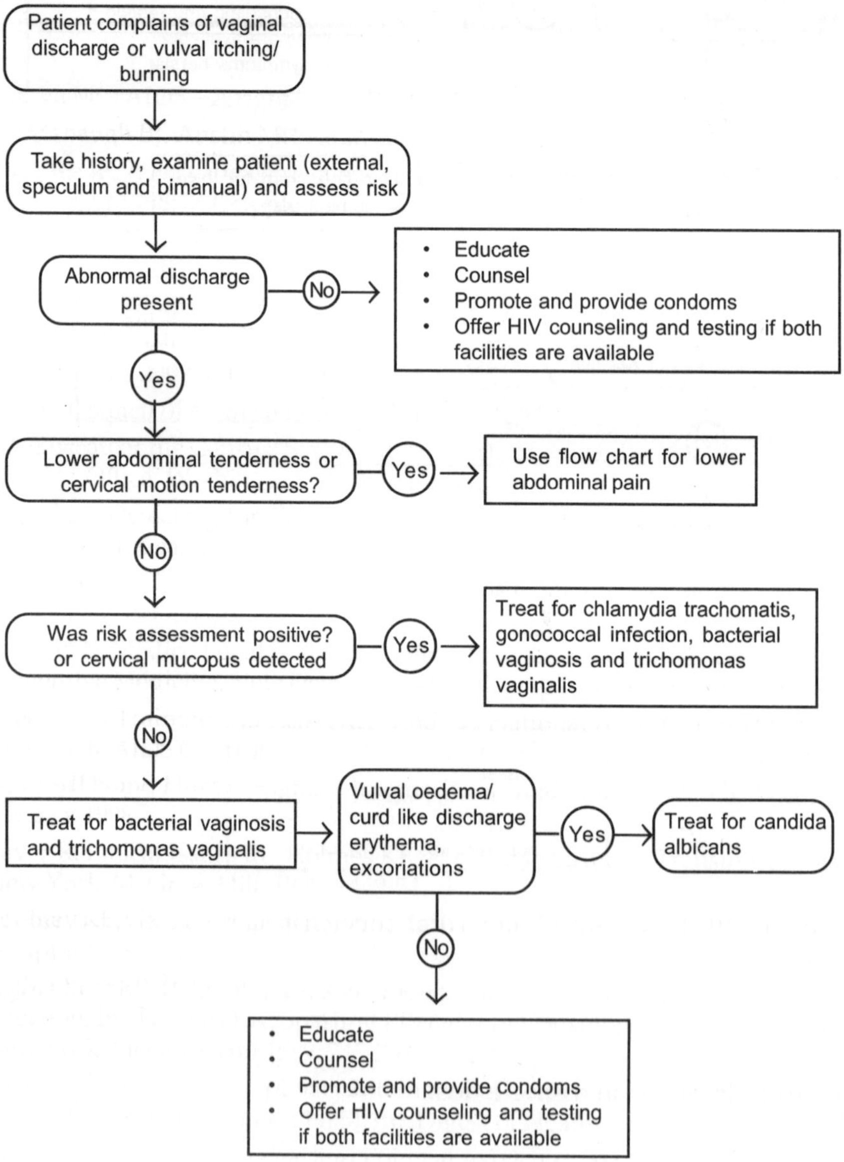
Patient complains of vaginal discharge or vulval itching/ burning
Take history, examine patient (external, speculum and bimanual) and assess risk
Abnormal discharge present
No
• Educate
• Counsel
• Promote and provide condoms
• Offer HIV counseling and testing if both facilities are available
Yes
Lower abdominal tenderness or cervical motion tenderness?
Yes
Use flow chart for lower abdominal pain
No
Was risk assessment positive? or cervical mucopus detected
Yes
Treat for chlamydia trachomatis, gonococcal infection, bacterial vaginosis and trichomonas vaginalis
No
Treat for bacterial vaginosis and trichomonas vaginalis
Vulval oedema/ curd like discharge erythema, excoriations
Yes
Treat for candida albicans
No
• Educate
• Counsel
• Promote and provide condoms
• Offer HIV counseling and testing if both facilities are available

6. *Vaginal Discharge (Speculum and Microscope)*

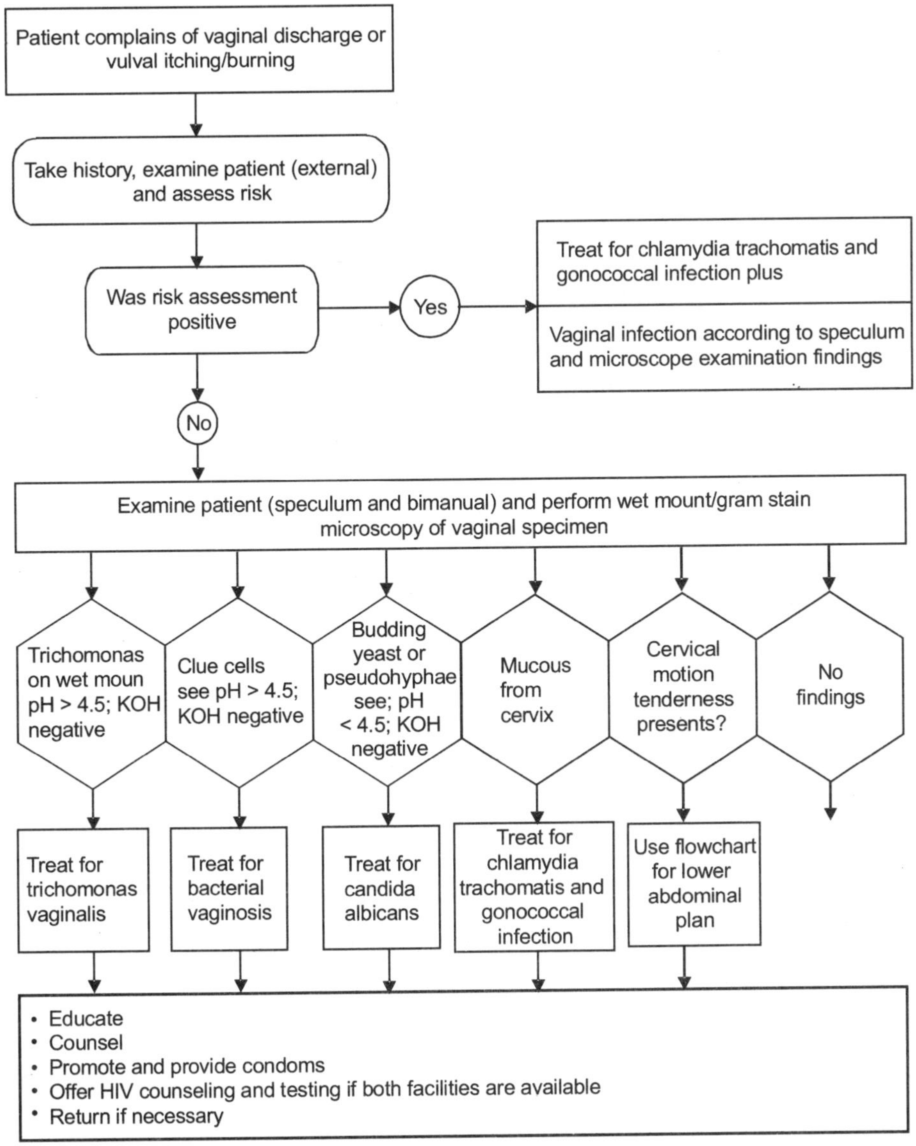
Patient complains of vaginal discharge or vulval itching/burning
Take history, examine patient (external) and assess risk
Was risk assessment positive
Yes
Treat for chlamydia trachomatis and gonococcal infection plus
Vaginal infection according to speculum and microscope examination findings
No
Examine patient (speculum and bimanual) and perform wet mount/gram stain microscopy of vaginal specimen
Trichomonas on wet moun pH > 4.5; KOH negative
Clue cells see pH > 4.5; KOH negative
Budding yeast or pseudohyphae see; pH < 4.5; KOH negative
Mucous from cervix
Cervical motion tenderness presents?
No findings
Treat for trichomonas vaginalis
Treat for bacterial vaginosis
Treat for candida albicans
Treat for chlamydia trachomatis and gonococcal infection
Use flowchart for lower abdominal plan
• Educate
• Counsel
• Promote and provide condoms
• Offer HIV counseling and testing if both facilities are available
• Return if necessary

Notes:
1. KOH test : 1 drop 10% KOH to reveal the amine odour (fishy)
2. Wet mount : smear slide with 1 drop of saline and view at 400x
* Risk factors need adaptation to local social and behavioural epidemiological situation

Risk assessment
Symptomatic partner?
Recent new partner?
Multiple partner?

Spouse returning home after a long stay away?

Vulvo-Vaginal Candidiasis

Cap. Fluconazole 150 mg orally as a single dose.
(**Caution:** safety in pregnancy is not established).
or
Clotimazole 500 mg vaginal pessary intravaginally as a single dose.
or
Micronazole/Clotrimazole 100 mg vaginal pessary intravaginally daily for 6 days.

7. Genital Ulcer

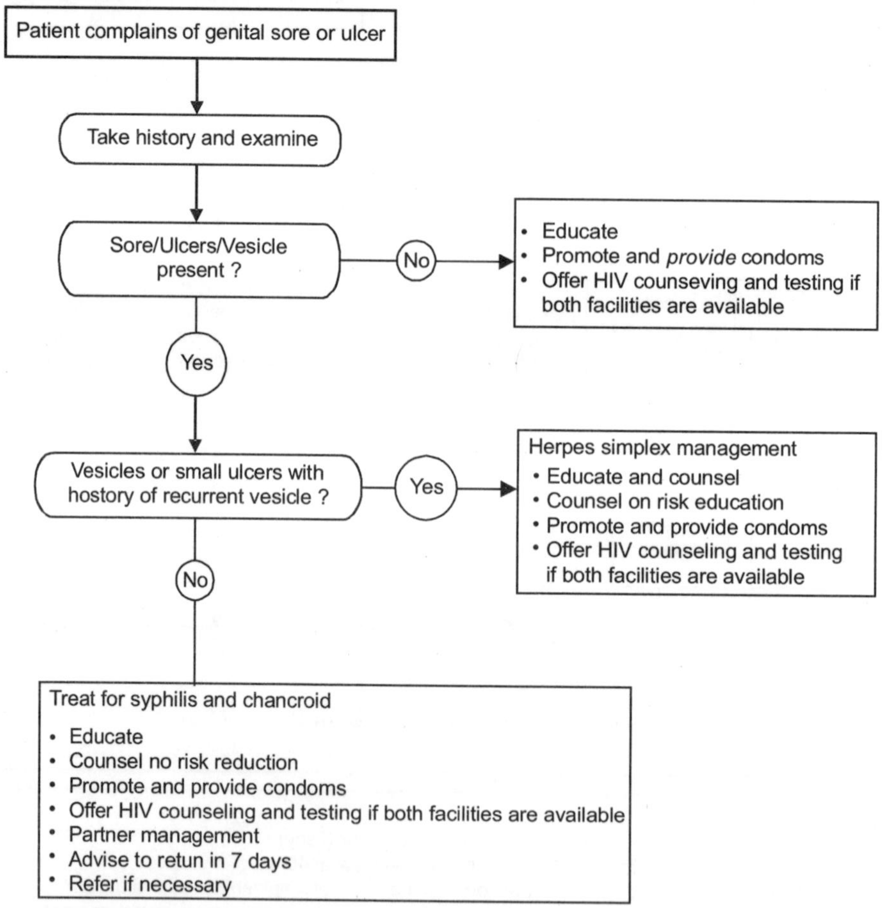

I. Genital Herpes (first clinical episode)

Tab. Acyclovir 200 mg orally five times a day for 7 days or Tab. Acyclovir 400 mg orally 3 times daily for 7 days.

Recurrent Infections

Tab. Acyclovir 200 mg orally 5 times daily for 5 days or Tab. Acyclovir 400 mg orally 3 times daily for 5 days or Tab. Acyclovir 800 mg orally twice daily for 5 days.

Suppressive therapy (in patients with six or more recurrence per year). Tab. Acyclovir 400 mg orally twice a day continuously for at least 6 months to 1 year.

II. Syphilis

Early Syphilis (includes primary, secondary and early latent infection up to 2 years duration).

Inj. Benzathine benzylpenicillin, 2.4 million IU deep IM in a single session (two equally divided doses in each buttock) after intradermal sensitivity test for penicillin.

or

Inj. Procaine benzylpenicillin, 1.2 millions IU (3 vials, each having combination of 1 lakh units of benzylpenicillin or sodium plus 3 lakh units of procaine benzylpenicillin) IM once daily for 10 days.

Alternative regimes for penicillin hypersensitive, non-pregnant patients

Cap. Doxycycline 100 mg orally twice daily for 15 days.

or

Cap. Minocycline 100 mg orally twice daily for 15 days.

or

Tab. Erythromycin (as stearate) 500 mg orally 4 times a day for 15 days

or

Tab. Tetracycline 500 mg orally 4 times a day for 15 days.

III. Chancroid

Tab. Azithromycin 1 g orally as a single dose.

or

Inj. Ceftriaxone, 250 mg IM as a single dose.

or

Tab. Ciprofloxacin, 500 mg orally twice a day for 3-5 days or till clearance of lesions

or

Cap. Doxycycline 100 mg orally twice daily for 7 days.

or

Tab. Trimethoprim (80 mg) + sulphamethoxazole (400 mg), 2 tab orally twice a day for 2 weeks.

8. Inguinal Bubo

LGV (Lymphogranuloma Venereum)

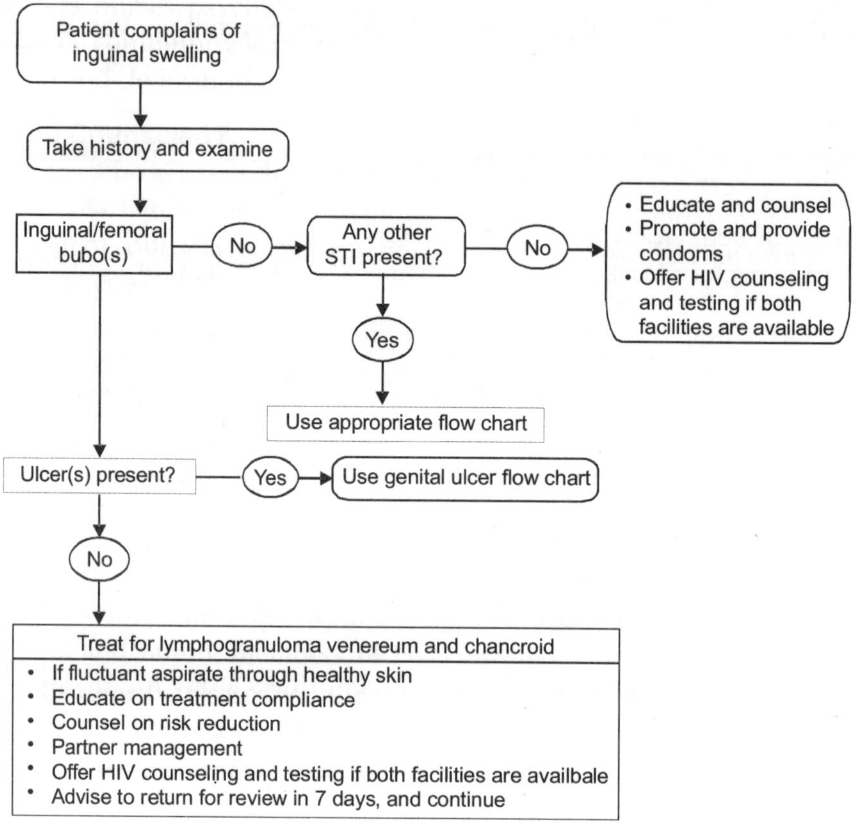

Cap. Doxycycline 100 mg orally twice daily for 21 days.

or

Cap. Tetracycline 500 mg orally 4 times a day for 21 days.

or

Tab. Trimethoprim (80 mg) + suphemathoxazole (400 mg) 2 tablets twice daily for 21 days.

or

Tab. Erythromycin stearate or base 500 mg orally 4 times a day for 2 weeks.

Patient education

- Education and counselling for patients
  - Cure your infection
  - Do not spread STD
  - Help your sexual partner to get treatment

- Come back to make sure you are cured
- Stay cured with condoms
- Keep safety by staying with just one sexual partner
- Protect yourself against AIDS and protect your baby, attend ANC during pregnancy.

9. Scrotal Swelling

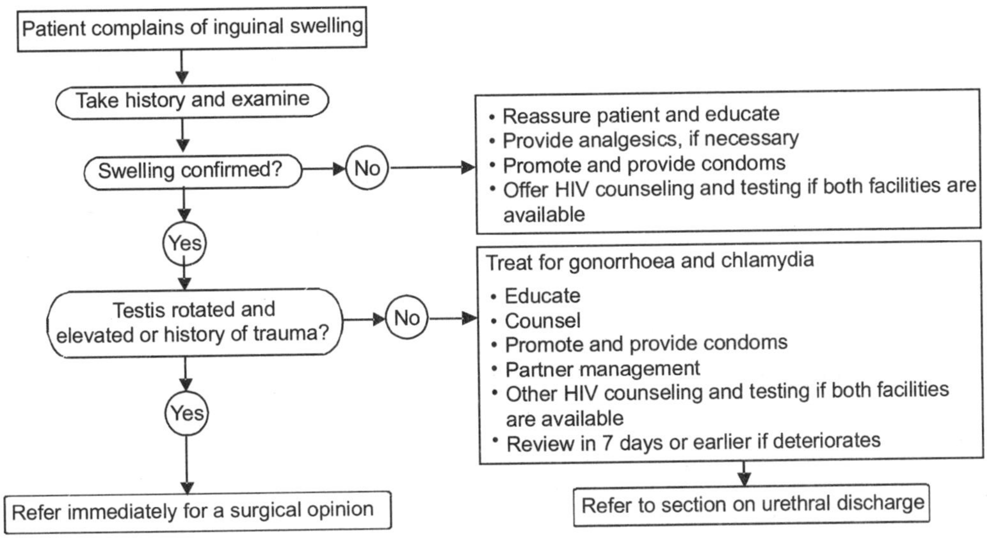
Patient complains of inguinal swelling
Take history and examine
Swelling confirmed?
No
• Reassure patient and educate
• Provide analgesics, if necessary
• Promote and provide condoms
• Offer HIV counseling and testing if both facilities are available
Yes
Testis rotated and elevated or history of trauma?
No
Treat for gonorrhoea and chlamydia
• Educate
• Counsel
• Promote and provide condoms
• Partner management
• Other HIV counseling and testing if both facilities are available
• Review in 7 days or earlier if deteriorates
Yes
Refer immediately for a surgical opinion
Refer to section on urethral discharge

References

1. Gregg MRC, Enderby KC, Grover SR: Risk-taking Behaviour of Young Women in Australia: Screening for Health-risk Behaviours, *Med J Aust*, 2003; 178: 601-5.
2. Meschke LL, Bartholomae S, Zentali SR: Adolescent Sexuality and Parent, adolescent Processes: Promoting Healthy Teen Choices, *J Adolesc Health*, 2002; 31: 264-79.
3. Guttmacher A Institute, Sex and America's Teenagers, New York: Alan Guttmacher Institute, 1994.
4. Child Trends: Facts at a Glance, Washington, DC: Child Trends, Inc., 1997. (2/13)
5. Schaalma HP, Abrahan C, Gillmore MR, Kok G: Sex Education as Health Promotion—What does it take? *Arch Sex Behav*, 2004; 33(3): 259-69.
6. U S Department of Health and Human Services, Healthy People 200: Midcourse review and 1995 revisions, Washington, DC: U.S. Department of Health and Human Services, 1996.
7. Berman SM, Hein K: Adolescents & STDs. In: Holmes KK, Mardh PA, Sparting PF, Lemon SM; Sexually Transmitted Diseases, 3rd edn., New York; McGraw Hill, 1997; 129-142.
8. Ballard RC: Genital Ulcer Adenopathy Syndrome. In: Holmes KK, Mardh PA, Sparting PF, Lemon SM, Sexually Transmitted Diseases. 3rd edn, New York; McGraw Hill, 1997; 887-92.
9. Holmes KK, Stamm WE: Lower Genital Tract Infection in Women. In: Holmes KK, Mardh PA, Sparting PF, Lemon SM, Sexually Transmitted Diseases, 3rd edn., New York; McGraw Hill, 1997; 761-82.
10. Westrom L *et al.*: Chlamydial and Gonococcal Infections in a Defined Population of Women. *Scand J Infec Dis* (suppl) 1982; 32: 157.
11. Burk RD *et al.*: Declining Prevalence of Cervicovaginal Human Papillomavirus Infection with Age is Independent of Other Risk Factors,. *Sex Transm Dis*, 1996; 23:333.
12. Critchlow CW *et al.*: Determinants of Cervical Ectopia and of Cervicitis-age Oral Contraception, Specific Cervical Infection, Smoking and Douching. *Am J Obstetr Gynecol*, 1995; 173:534.
13. Stergachis A, *et al.*: Selective Screening for Chlamydia Trachomatis Infection in a Primary Care Population of Women, *Am J Epidemiol*, 1993; 138: 143.
14. Johnson BA, *et al.*: Derivation and Validation of a Clinical Diagnostic Model for Chlamydial Cervical Infection in University Women, *JAMA*, 1990; 265: 3161.
15. Haffner DW: Facing Facts–Sexual Health for America's Adolescents, Reports of the National Commission on Adolescent Sexual Health, 1995.
16. Gilligan C, Wiggins G: The Origins of Morality in Young Children, Jerome Kagan, Sahron Lamb (eds). Chicago, University of Chiago Press 1987; 277-305.

17. Forrest JD: Timing of Reproductive Life Stages, *Obstetr and Gynecol* 1993; 82: 105.
18. Friedman HL: Changing Patterns of Adolescent Sexual Behaviour: Consequences for Health and Development, *J Adoesc Health*, 1992; 13: 345.
19. Graham CA, AIDS and the Adolescent, Internat, J STD AIDS 1994; 5: 305.
20. Centres for Disease Control and Prevention: Premarital Sexual Experience Among Adolescent Women—United States, 1970-1988. MMWR 1991; 39: 929.
21. Mosher WD, Mc Nally JW: Contraceptive Use at First Premarital Intercourse: United States, 1965-1988, *Fam Plann Perspect*, 1991; 23 : 108.
22. Hingson RW *et al*.: Beliefs about AIDS, Use of Alcohol and Drugs and Unprotected Sex Among Massachusetts Adolescents, *Am J Public Health*, 1990; 80: 295.
23. Donald M: Determinants of Condom Use by Australian Secondary School Students, *J Adolesc Health*, 1994; 15: 503.
24. Ailey SH, Marks BA, Crisp C, Hahn JE: Promoting Sexuality across the Life-span for Individuals with Intellectual and Developmental Disabilities, *Nurs Clin N Am*, 2003; 38: 229-52.
25. Mathur D, Acharya V: Counseling in HIV/AIDS. In : Sharma VK *et al*. Sexually Transmitted Diseases and AIDS. 1st edn, Delhi; Viva Book Pvt. Ltd., 2003; 125-8.
26. Culem C, Buchbinder S: Counseling and testing for HIV Infection. In: Holmes KK, Mardh PA, Sparting PF, Lemon SM, Sexually Transmitted Diseases, 3rd edn., New York; McGraw Hill, 1997; 963-71.
27. Speizer IS, Magnani RJ, Colvin Charlotte: The Effectiveness of Adolescent Reproductive Health Interventions in Developing Countries: A review of the evidence, *J Adolesc Health*, 2003; 33 (5): 324-8.
28. Bongaarts J, Cohen B: Introduction and overview, *Stud Fam Plann*, 1998; 29:105.
29. Kirby D *et al*.: School-based Programs to Reduce Sexual Risk Behaviours: Review of Effectiveness. Public Health Reports 1994; 109: 339.
30. Gallup A: The 19th Annual Gallup Polls of the Public's Attitudes Towards the Public School, Gallup Poll 1997; 69.
31. Howard M, McCabe JB, Helping Teenagers Postpone Sexual Involvement, *Fam Plann Perspect*, 1990; 22: 21.
32. Perry CL: Prevention of Alcohol Use and Abuse in Adolescence—Teacher vs peer-led intervention, (Special Issue: Preventive Interventions in Adolescence) Crisis 1989: 10: 52.
33. Addiss DG *et al*.: History and Features of the Wisconsin Chlamydia Trachomatis Control Program, *Fam Plann Perspect*, 1994; 26: 83.
34. WHO, Guidelines for the Management of Sexually Transmitted Infections 2001. WHO/RHR/01.10.
35. NACO. STD Treatment Recommendations, 2002.
36. Campbell RL, Plumb J: The Syndromic Approach to treatment of Sexually Diseases in Low Income Countries, Issues, Challenges and Future Directions. *J Obstet Gynaecol Can* 2002; 24: 417-424.
37. Sexually Transmitted infections In : Gynaecology. Shaw RW, Soutter WP, Stanton SL (eds). 3rd edition, 2003, Churchill Livingstone, 901-920.

the feelings of helplessness, hopelessness, loss of control and extreme anxiety [illegible] in such a situation and is

[illegible] sadness, anger and to grieve with the [illegible]

CHAPTER

15 Anti-retroviral Therapy in Adolescents—An Overview

Vikas Aggarwal and *S.N. Bhattacharya*

Anti-retroviral therapy is meant for treating HIV/AIDS patients. It is the mainstay in controlling viral load and hence ensure a good immune response.

Goals of Therapy

1. To decrease the viral load (preferably <20 cells/ml - in 3 months) and rate of replication as low as possible and for as long as possible.
2. To increase CD_4 cell counts and hence restore a good immune response.
3. To decrease morbidity associated with HIV infection.
4. To improve the duration and quality of life.

When to Initiate Therapy [1, 2, 3, 4]

Initiation of therapy is somewhat vague and individual decision. There is no universal guidelines. The predictors of HIV disease markers to AIDS progression are:

1. CD_4 count – It is only partially predictive and more efficient in later stages.
2. HIV–I RNA level – It is a better predictor in early stages.
3. Acid associated p^{24} protein level.
4. Neopterin level.
5. Beta-microglobulin level.

But due to availability and cost factor, CD_4 cell count is the mainstay for deciding and managing ART.

If CD_4 count and HIV RNA level testing is available treat if:

(a) Pt. is in WHO clinical stage IV, irrespective of CD_4 cell count/HIV RNA level.
(b) Pt. is in WHO clinical stage III and CD_4 cell count $\leq 350/mm^3$.
(c) Pt. is in WHO clinical stage I and II with CD_4 cell count $< 200\text{-}250/mm^3$.
(d) Pt. is in WHO clinical stage IV and HIV RNA level is > 55,000.

Drugs available:

1. Nucleoside analogue reverse transcriptase inhibitors:
   — Abacavir
   — Didanosine
   — Entricitabine
   — Lamivudine
   — Stavudine
   — Zalcitabine
   — Zidovudine
2. Non-nucleoside reverse transcriptase inhibitors:
   — Delavirdine
   — Efavirenz
   — Nevirapine
3. Prolease inhibitors:
   — Amprenavir
   — Atazanavir
   — Indinavir
   — Liponavir
   — Nelfinavir
   — Ritonavir
   — Saquinavir
4. Nucleotide analogue:
   — Tenofovir
5. Fusion inhibitor:
   — Enfurvirtide
6. Miscellaneous:
   — Hydroxyurea

Characteristics of Nucleoside Reverse Transcriptase Inhibitors

Characteristic	Zidovudine [5,6,7,8] (AZT, ZDV) (Retrovir)	Didanosine [9,10] (ddI) (Videx)	Zalcitabine[11] (ddC)(HIVID)	Stavudine [12,13] (d4T)(Zerit)	Lamivudine [14,15] (3TC) (Epivir)
Dosing recommendations	200 mg tid or 300 mg bid or with 3TC as Combivir, 1 bid	>60kg : 200 mg bid,<60 kg: 125 mg bid	0.75 mg tid	30 mg	150mg bid <50kg : 2mg/kg bid or with ZDV as Combivir: 1 bid
Oral biovailability, %	60	40	85	86	86
Serum half-life, *h*	1.1	1.66	1.2	1.0	3-6
Intracellular half-life, *h*	3	25-40	3	3.5	12
Elimination	Metabolized to AZT Glucuronide (GAZT), Renal excretion of GAZT	Renal excretion 50%	Renal excretion 70%	Renal excretion 50%	Renal excretion unchanged
Adverse events	Bone marrow supression, anaemia and /or neutropenia. Subjective Symptoms: Gastrointestinal introlerance, headache, insomnia, asthenia	Pancreatitis, peripheral neuropathy, Nausea, Diarrhoea	Peripheral neuropathy, Stomatitis	Peripheral neuropathy	Minimal toxicity

Characteristics of Non-nucleoside Reverse Transcriptase Inhibitors

Variable	*Nevirapine* (*Viramune*)[16]	*Delavirdine* (*Descriptor*)[17]	*Efavirenz* (Efferven)
Form	200 - mg tablets	100 - mg tablets	600 mg tablet
Dosing recommendations	200 mg po qd X 14 days, then 200 mg po bid	400 mg po tid (four 100-mg tabs in atleast 3 oz of water to produce slurry)	600 mg 1 HS empty stomach
Bioavailability	>90%	85	> 99% bound to plasma proteins
Serum half life, *h*	25-30	5.8	52-76
Elimination	Metabolized by cytochrome p450; 80% excreted in urine (glucuronidated metabolites, <5% unchanged), 10% excreted in feces	Metabolized by cytochrome p450; 51 % excreted in urine (<5% unchanged), 44% excreted in feces	Metabolised by cytochrome p450 14-34% excreted in urine & 16-61% excreted in feces
Drug interactions	Induces cytochrome p450 enzymes. The following drugs have suspected interactions that require careful monitoring if coadministered with nevira-pine: rifampin, rifabutin, oral contraceptives, protease inhibitors, triazolam, and midazolam	Inhibits cytochrome p450 enzymes not recommended for concurrent use : terfenadine, astemizole, alprazolam, midazolam, cisapride, rifabutin, rifampin, triazolam, ergot derivatives, amphetamines, nifedipine, and anticonvulsants (phenytoin, carbamazepine, phenobarbitol) Delavirdine increases levels of clarithromycin, dapsone, quinidine, warfarin, indinavir, and saquinavir.	Induces cytochrome p450 enzymes resulting in induction of its own metabolism. Effavirenz must not be administered concurrently with terfenadine, astemizole cisapride, midazolam, triazolam, primozide, bepridil or ergot alkaloids.
Adverse Events	Rash Increased amino-transferase levels Hepatitis	Antacids or didanosine: Separate delavirdine administration by < 1 h Rash Headaches	CNS Toxicity

Characteristics of Protease Inhibitors

Characteristics	Indinavir[18] (Crixiun)	Ritonavir[19] (Norvir)	Saquinavir[20] HGC (Invirase)
Form	200, 400 mg tablets	100-mg tablets 600mg/7.5 ml. po solution	200-mg tablets
Dosing recommendations	800 mg q8h Take 1 h before or 2 h after meals; may take with skim milk or low-fat meal	600 mg q12h Take with food if possible	600 mg tid Take with large meal
Oral bioavailability	65%	Not determined	Hard-gel capsule: 40%, erratic
Serum half-life, *h* Route of metabolism	1.5-2 p450 cytochrome	3-5 p450 cytochrome 3 A 4> 2D6	1-2 p450 cytochrome 3A
Adverse effects	Nephrolithiasis Gastrointestinal intolerance, nausea Laboratory: increased indirect bilirubinemia (in-consequential) Miscellaneous : headache, asthenia, blurred vision, dizziness, rash, metallic taste, thrombocytopenia Hyperglycemia	Gastrointestinal intolerance, nausea, vomiting, diarrhoea Parenthesis-circum-oral and extremities Hepatitis, Asthenia Taste perversion Laboratory: triglycerides increase >200%, aminotransferase elevation; elevated creatine phosphokinase and uric acid, Hyperglycemia	Gastrointestinal intolerance, nausea and diarrhoea Headache Elevated aminotransferase enzymes Hyperglycemia

Dose escalation for ritonavir: days 1-2, 300 mg bid; days 3-5, 400 mg bid; days 6-13, 500 mg bid; day 14,600 mg bid. Combination treatment regimen with saquinavir (400-600 mg po bid) plus ritonavir (400-600 mg po bid).

Drug interactions of Nucleoside Reverse Transcriptase Inhibitors [21]

Primary Drug	*Secondary Drug*	*Interaction*
Adefovir	Nephrotoxic agents	May reduce the elimination and increase the level of adefovir
Abacavir	Isonaizid, disulfiram, ethanol	Increased levels of both agents
Didanosine	Antineoplastic Dapsone Delavirdine	Increase neurotoxicity Decrease dapsone efficacy Decrease delavirdine levels as delavirdine requires acidic pH

(Contd...)

	Flouroquinolones Indinavir Itraconazole Ketokonazole Pentamidine Zalcitabine	Decrease level of FQ Decrease indinavir absorption Decrease absorption of both drugs (require acidic pH) Increase risk of pancreatitis Increase neuropathy risk
Stavudine	Antineoplastic & Zalcitabine Zidovudine	Increase neurotoxicity Antagonism
Zidovudine	Myelosuppresive drugs Probnecid Rifampicin	Increased bone marrow toxicity Increase ZDV level Decrease ZDV level

Drug Interactions of Non-Nucleoside Reverse Transcriptase Inhibitors[21]

Secondary Drug	*Delavirdine*	*Efavirenz*	*Nevirapine*
Anticonvulsant	Decrease level of delavirdine	Decrease level of efavirenz	Decrease level of nevirapine
Antihistaminics	Increase antihistaminic level cardiac toxicity	Same	–
Benzodiazipines	Increase level of benzodiazipines	Same	–
Cisapride	Increase level and cardiac risk of cisapride	–	Increase nevaripine level
Ketoconazole	Increase delavirdine level (Fluconazole)	–	Increase nevaripine level
Lovastatin	Increase lovastatin level and increase risk of myopathy	–	–
Rifabutin	Increase rifabutin level (100%) Decrease delavirdine (80%)	Decrease efavirenz AUC	—
Rifampicin	Decrease delavirdine level	Decrease level of efavirenz (28%)	Decrease nevarapine level (37%)
Sildenafil	Increase sildenafil level	–	–
Oral contraceptives	–	Decrease efficacy	Decrease efficacy

Drug Interactions of Protease Inhibitions[21]

Drug	*Indinavi*	*Ritonavir*	*Saquinavir*	*Nelfinavir*
Fluconazole	No dose change	No dose change	No data	No dose change
Ketcoconazole and itraconazole	Decrease dose to 600 mg q8h	Increases ketoconazole > 3-fold; dose adjustment required	Increases saquinavir levels 3-fold; no dose change	No dose change
Rifabutin	Reduced rifabutin to half dose : 150 mg qd	Consider alternative drug or reduce rifabutin dose to one quarter	Not recommended with either Invirase or Fortovase	Reduce rifabutin to half dose : 150 mg qd
Rifampin	Contraindicated	Unknown	Not recommended with either Invirase or Fortovase	Contraindicated
Oral contraceptives	Modest increase in Ortho-Novum levels No dose change	Ethinyl estradiol level decreased; use alternative or additional contraceptive method	No data	Ethinyl estradiol and norethindrone level decreased, use alternative or additional contraceptive method

Rifampin reduces ritonavir level by 35%. Increase ritonavir dose or use of ritonavir in combination therapy is strongly recommended. The effect of ritonavir on rifampin is unknown. Concurrent use may increase liver toxicity. Therefore, patients on ritonavir and rifampin should be monitored closely.

Tenofovir

Tenofovir belongs to the nucleotide reverse transcriptase inhibitor (NtRTI) class of drugs. Like the nucleoside reverse transcriptase inhibitors (NRTIs) NtRTIs inhibits an enzyme called reverse transcriptase, which is essential to the process of viral replication.

Tenofovir is able to reduce the amount of HIV in blood, help to prevent or reverse damage to the immune system and reduce the risk of AIDS related illnesses. It is also an experimental treatment of hepatitis –B. Main advantage of tenofovir is that side effects are less worrying including renal toxicity, nausea, diarrhoea and vomiting.

Tenofovir is also available in a triple drug combination tablet. This tablet which is the first once daily tablet containing a complete anti-HIV regimen, contains 600 mg efavirenz, 200 mg FTC (emtricitabine) and 300 mg tenofovir. It was approved in United States in July 2006.

Standard dose of tenofovir is one 200 mg tab once-daily. Although taking tenofovir with food results in higher blood levels, this doesn't appear to affect the response to treatment.

So in present era, tenofovir is a good answer as second line drug which is cost effective also.

Enfuvirtide (T-20)[22]

— Administered 100 mg twice daily subcutaneously into upper arm, anterior thigh and abdomen.

— Reduction in viral load if given before resistance to other drug develops. Little benefit is added to a failing regime.
— At 24 week-HIV–1RNA decreased by 1.4–1.log_{10} copies/ml.
— FDA approved on 13th March 2003–useful in salvage therapy.
— Greatest benefit in a triplet regime.
— Side effects:
  — Gastrointestinal - diarrhoea, nausea, vomiting
  — General - fatigue, asthenia, pyrexia, fever
  — Skin - dermatitie, pruritus, hypersensitivity and rash
  — CNS - peripheral neuropathy, headache
  — Psychiatric - insomnia, depression
  — Bacterial pneumonia - increased incidence, sepsis, glomerulonephritis, eosinophilia
  — Infection site reaction - painful subcutaneous nodules, erythema induration. Required analgesia but very few of the patients withdrew from the treatment.

Advantage – It is self administered.

Disadvantage – It is very expensive and has a limited availability.

Hydroxyurea

Hydroxyurea is an inhibitor of DNA synthesis. By inhibiting ribonucleotide reductase, hydroxyurea depletes the pool of deoxynucleoside triphosphates, particularly–ATP, available to DNA synthesis. Hydroxyurea may be a candidate to use with nucleoside analogues, particularly didanosine.

It is also possible that during acute HIV infection, hydroxyurea's cytoclastic properties could contribute to the ultimate preservation of normal immunologic function. Hydroxyurea's dosage level is still uncertain, 500mg twice daily has been used most often.

Combination of drugs

1. Preferred Regime: 2 NRTI (column B) + 1 PI (Column A)

Column A (PI)	Column B (NRTI)
Indinavir	Zidovudine + Didonosine
Nelfinavir	Zidovudine + Lamivudine-Preferred
Ritonavir*	Stavudine + Didanosine (+/– Hydroxyurea)
Saquinavir	Zidovudine + zalcitasine

2. Alternative Regime

   2 NRTI (B) + 1 NNRTI (Efavirenz, Nevirapine, delavirdine)
   1 NRTI + 1 NNRTI + PI
   2 NRTI + Hydroxyurea

*[23] Lopinavir/ ritonavir monotherapy appears as effective as combining the agents with 2 NRTIs in maintaining an undetectable HIV load.

Indications for Plasma HIV RNA Testing [21]

Clinical Indication	Information	Use
Syndrome consistent with acute-HIV infection	Establishes diagnosis when HIV antibody test result is negative or indeterminate	Diagnosis
Initial evalution of newly diagnosed HIV infection	Baseline viral load "set point"	Decision to start or defer therapy
Every 3 to 4 months in patients not receiving therapy	Changes in viral load	Decision to start therapy
4 to 8 weeks after initiation of anti-retroviral therapy	Initial assessment of drug efficacy	Decision to continue or change therapy
3 to 4 months after start of therapy	Maximal effect of therapy	Decision to continue or change therapy
Every 3 to 4 months in patients receiving therapy	Durability of antiretroviral effect	Decision to continue or change therapy
Clinical event or significant decline in $CD4^+$ T cells	Association with changing or stable viral load	Decision to continue, initiate, or change therapy

Prognostic Factors

The speed of viral load decline and movement towards undetectable level is affected by:

Baseline CD4 T cell count

Initial Viral load

Potency of the regime

Prior exposure to anti-retroviral agents

Presence of opportunistic infection

With optimal therapy the viral counts should become undetectable within 6 months (<500 copies/ml) if it remains detectable then the RNA level should be rechecked and change in therapy is advocated.

More sensitive viral load detector have now been developed which can detect viral load as low as 50 RNA copies /ml. Data indicate that lowering the HIV RNA level <50 copies/ml is associated with a more complete and durable viral suppression.

When initial decision regarding the start of therapy is made, both CD_4 and viral load should be performed on two occasions to ensure consistency and accuracy. However in patients who present advanced HIV disease, therapy should generally be initiated after the first viral load measurement. A minimally significant change in plasma viremia is considered to be 3 fold or 0.5 log10 increase/decrease. A significant decrease in CD_4 cell count is a decrease of more than 30% from baseline for absolute cell numbers and a decrease of more than 3% from baseline in percentages of cells. Discordance in the CD_4 cell count and viral load assessment can occur and has been found in 14-20% of the patients. Such discordance can complicate decision regarding anti-retroviral therapy and may be due to many factors like acute illness (bacterial pneumonia, tuberculosis, herpes simplex virus infections, pneumocystis jiroveci pneumonia) and immunization. Viral load assessment should not be performed at this stage. However, the discordant response has been associated with a decrease in disease progression. In general trends in viral load are felt to be more informative for decisions regarding anti- retroviral therapy. However, in later stages of infection the predictive value of HIV RNA decreases over time and that of low CD_4 count increases.[21]

Interruption of Anti-retroviral Therapy

i. Temporary
   a. Intolerable side effects
   b. Drug interactions
   c. Pregnancy—1st trimester
   d. Non-availability of drugs

Preferably all the drugs should be discontinued rather than continuing 1 or 2.

Drug Resistance Assessment/Evaluation

1. Genotypic methods : They are used to identify the presence of aminoacid substitutions in HIV protease/reverse transcriptase enzyme. Different types of methods are as follows.
   a. DNA sequencing of the entire strand
   b. DNA sequencing of selective segment by PCR
   c. Determination of point mutation
   d. Probe hybridization
   e. HIV–1 reverse transcriptase– PCR

   500–1000 HIV RNA copies/ml are required for the genotypic methods.
2. Phenotypic methods : It is used to determine the inhibitory concentration of an anti- retroviral agent that reduces the HIV replication by 50% in tissue culture. About 10,000 copies/ml of HIV RNA are required to perform phenotypic testing.

It is important to perform these tests during treatment as resistant mutations quickly disappear from the major plasma viral population.[21]

ART Failure

There are several overlapping definitions of drug failure, including virological failure, immunologic failure and clinical failure. Virological failure generally precedes immunologic failure and immunologic failure generally precedes clinical failure. Prolonged treatment interruption does not restore anti-viral efficacy for heavily pretreated HIV infected patients with multiple resistance mutations[24]. Before changing therapy, it is important to distinguish drug toxicity from drug failure. For drug toxicity, single drug substitutions from the same drug class may be appropriate. For drug failure, most cases require ≥ 2 new drugs or a new drug regimen.

1. **Virologic failure:** Drug failure is confirmed by significant increases in viraemia on repeat testing not caused by a transient stimulus (i.e. acute illnesses, immunization), regardless of CD_4 counts. Criteria for virologic failure:
   (a) Less than a 0.5–0.75 log reduction in plasma HIV RNA by 4 weeks.
   (b) Failure to suppress plasma HIV RNA to undetectable levels within 4-6 months of starting therapy.
   (c) Repeated detection of virus in plasma after initial suppression to undetectable levels.
   (d) Any reproducible significant ($\geq$ 3-fold) increase from the nadir of plasma HIV RNA
2. **Immunologic failure:** 30% decline in CD_4 cell count or 3% decline in CD_4% from baseline, confirmed in repeat testing.
3. **Clinical failure:** HIV disease progression (e.g. constitutional symptoms, opportunistic infections) or death.

The prevalence of anti-retroviral drug resistance among treatment – naive, HIV-infected patients in the United Kingdom is the highest in the world and still climbing, new study results suggest[25].

Potential Benefits of ART[21]

Control of viral replication and mutation; reduction of viral burden
Prevention of progressive immunodeficiency; potential maintenance or reconstitution of a normal immune system.
Delayed progression to AIDS and prolongation of life
Decreased risk for selection of resistant virus
Decreased risk for drug toxicity

Potential Risks of ART[21]

Reduction in quality of life from advance drug effects and inconvenience of current maximally suppressive regimens
Earlier development of drug resistance
Limitation in future choices of anti-retroviral agents due to development of resistance
Unknown long-term toxicity of anti-retroviral drug
Unknown duration of effectiveness of current anti-retroviral therapies

Acute HIV Infection

- Potential candidates for early therapy
- Evidence of short term benefit but no data indicate a definite long term benefit but trails have recommended early institution on therapy

Patient Selection

i. Patients with detectable HIV RNAs in plasma by PCR/bDNA
ii. P24 antigen positivity
iii. A confirmatory test should always be done but it may be negative in the initial stages.
iv. Patients with history of seroconversion in the last 6 months

ART in some special situations:

1. **HIV and T.B. :** HIV/TB co-infection is one of the most common and challenging issue in dealing with PLHA treatment. Patients with TB merit special consideration because co-management of HIV and T.B. is complicated by rifampicin drug interactions with NNRTIs and PIs, pill burden, adherence and drug toxicity.

   If the patient is on refampicin based AKT, preferably Efavirenz based reqimen should be started. ART can be defered till the time patient is able to tolerate AKT which usually is 15 days.
2. **HIV and Hepatitis B & C :** The resultant hepatic disease may increase the risk of lives toxicity and impair the metabolism of some anti-retroviral agents. Use of agents active against both HIV and hepatitis B such as lamivudine and tenofovir may be useful. Few of the anti-retrovirals are known to cause hepatotoxicity e.g. Zidovudine, Didanosine, Stavudine, Abacavir, Lamivudine, Nevirapine and PIs.
3. **ART in Pregnancy :** It should preferably include drugs shown to be effective in reducing mother to child transmission viz. Zidovudine, Lamivudine and Nevirapine. The most successful experience is with Zidovuduine. Thus it should be included in the regimen provided Zedovudine induced anaemia is checked which may prove fatal in pregnancy. Efavirenz should be avoided because of its teratogenic effects. PIs are associated with development of glucose intolerance and diabetes mellitus. Pregnancy is also a risk factor for hyperglycemia.

This should always be accompanied by nevirapine drops to the child to prevent transmission.

If foetal and maternal blood contact can be avoided (may be through C.S.) and mother doesn't breast fed her child (provided topfeeds are available with full nutritional value and doesn't pose any potential risk of infections), risk of HIV transmission can be avoided upto a large extent.

If the HIV infection is diagnosed during pregnancy, the goal of ART is the maintenance of maternal health and this is the basis for the decision to initiated ART any time during pregnancy.

Women who require ART and who are breastfeeding should continue their ongoing anti-retroviral therapeutic regimen. However, the efficacy of potent ART of the mother to prevent postnatal transmission of HIV through breast milk is unknown.

Short course ARTdrug regimens that do not fully suppress viral replication that are used to prevant mother to child transmission of HIV may be associated with development of ART drug resistance especially where single point mutation can confer drug resistance as with nevirapine and lamivudine.

Prophylaxis for HIV Opportunistic Infection

Infection	*Indication*	*Prophylaxis*	*Criteria for Stopping*
1. Pneumocystis Carnii Pneumonia (PCP)	CD_4 count< 200/cmm^3, oral thrush, constitutional symptoms, past history of PCP	Tab. Septran 1 DS OD in morning or Tab. Dapsone 100mg 1 OD	If repeat CD_4 after 3 months is >200/cmm^3
2. Mycobacterium Complex	CD_4 count <50/cmm^3	Tab. Azithromycin 1200mg once a week	If repeat CD_4 after 3 months >100/cmm^3
3. Candidiasis (Oropharyngeal or vaginal) frequent, severe and recurrent.	CD_4 count <100/cmm^3, +ve past history	Tab. Fluconazol 150mg weekly	If repeat CD_4 after 3 months is > 100/cmm^3
4. Cryptococcal meningitis	CD_4 count <100/cmm^3 +ve past history	Tab. Fluconazol 200mg 1 OD	If repeat CD_4 after 3 months is > 100/cmm^3
5. Toxoplasmosis	If CD_4 is <200/cmm^3 with +ve IgG Serology OR If CD_4 count is < 200/cmm^3	Tab. Septran 1 DS 1 OD OR Tab Dapsone 50mg 1 OD Tab. Pyrimethamine 50 mg 1 weekly Tab. Folinic Acid 25mg1 weekly	If repeat CD_4 after 3 months is >200/cmm^3
6. Pneumococcal Pneumonia	If CD_4 count is <200/cmm^3	Pneumococcal Polysacc. (23 valent) vaccine. Reimmunise after 5 yrs.	
7. Influenza	All Pts	Influenza vaccine given annually in winter. No vaccine if CD_4 is > 100mm^3	
8. Recurrent Herpes simplex		Tab. Acyclovir 200mg TDS OR Tab. Acyclovir 400mg BD OR Tab. Velacyclovir 500mg BD	
9. Salmonella species' Non-typhi		Tab. Ciprofloxacin 500mg BD	

POST-HIV EXPOSURE MANAGEMENT

Immediate Measures

- wash with soap and water
- no added advantage with antiseptic/bleach

Next Step

- prompt reporting
- post-exposure treatment should begin as soon as possible
- preferably within two hours
- not recommended after seventy-two hours
- late PEP may be given.
- PEP is not required for all type of exposures

Post Exposure Prophylaxis (PEP): Source Code (SC)

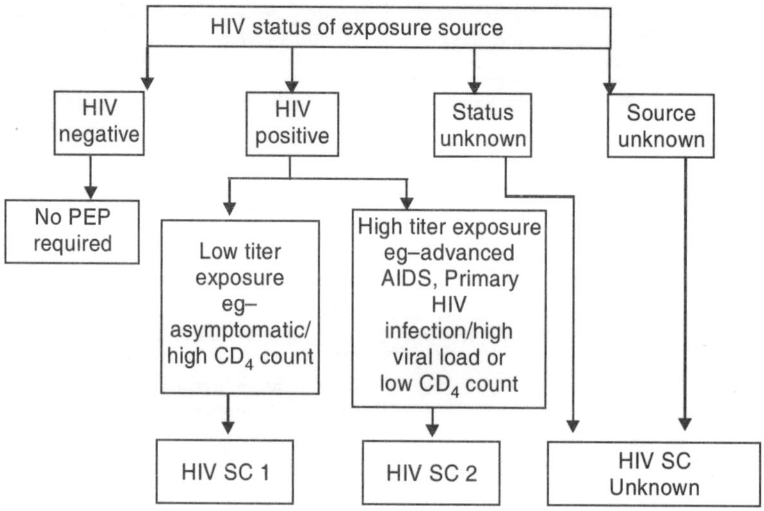

Post Exposure Prophylaxix (PEP): NACO Recommendations

EC	*HIV SC*	*PEP*
1	1	Not warranted
1	2	Consider basic regimen
2	1	Recommended basic regimen
2	2	Recommended expanded regimen
3	1 or 2	Recommended expanded regimen
2/3	unknown	Consider basic regimen if setting suggests possible risk

Post Exposure Prophylaxis (PEP): NACO Recommendations

Basic Regimen

Zidovudine (AZT) — 600 mg in divided doses

(300mg bd or 200 mg tds for 4 weeks + Lamivudine (3TC)

—150 mg bd for 4 weeks

Expanded Regimen

Basic regimen (+ Indinavir — 800 mg tds, or any other protease Inhibitor) for 4 weeks.

Timing and Duration

Started, as early as possible (preferably 2 hours), after an exposure. PEP started after 72 hours of exposure is of no use and hence preferably is not recommended. Optimal duration not known, but probably 4 weeks.

REFERENCES

1. Stein D, Korvick J, Vermund S; CD_4 lymphocyte cell enumeration for prediction of clinical course of human immunodeficiency virus disease: a review. J Infect Dis. 1992; 165:352-63.
2. Carpenter C, Fischl M, Hammer S, et al. Updated recommendations of the International AIDS Society Panel-USA panel. JAMA. 1997; 227: 1962-9.
3. Rabond J, Montaner J, Conway B, *et al*: Variation in plasma RNA levels, CD4 cell counts and p. 24 antigen levels in clinically stable men with human immunodeficiency virus infection. J Infect Dis. 1996; 174: 191-4.
4. Mellors J, Munoz A, Giorgi J, *et al*, Plasma viral load and CD_4 lymphocytes as prognostic markers of HIV-1 infection. Ann Intern Med. 1997; 126: 946-54.
5. Volberding P, Lagakos S, Koch M, *et al*: Zidovudine in asymptomatic human immunodeficiency virus infection: a controlled trial in persons with fewer than 500 CD_4-positive cells per cubic millimeter. N Engl J Med. 1990; 322:941-9.
6. Volberding P, Lagakos S, grimes J *et al*: The duration of Zidovudine benefit in persons with asymptomatic HIV infection: prolonged evaluation of protocol 019 of the AIDS Clinical Trial Group. JAMA 1994; 272: 437-42.
7. Strecher BN, *et al*: Pharmacokinetics of zidovudine phosphorylation in peripheral blood mononuclear cells from patients infected with human immunodeficiency virus. Antimicrob Agents Chemother 1994; 38:1541-47.
8. Richman DD, *et al*: The toxicity of AZT in the treatment of patients with AIDS and AIDS-related complex: A double-blind, placebo-controlled trials. N Engl J Med 1987; 317: 192-97.
9. Lambert JS, *et al*: 2'3'- dideoxyinosine (ddi) in patients with the acquired immunodeficiency syndrome or AIDS-related complex: A phase 1 trial. N Engl J Med 1990; 322:1333-40.
10. Cooley TP, *et al*: Once-daily administration of 2', 3'- dideoxyinosine (ddl) in patients with the acquired immunodeficiency syndrome or AIDS-related complex. N Eng l J Med 1990; 332: 1340-45.
11. Klecker R Jr, *et al*: Pharmacokinetics of 2', 3'- dideoxycytidine in patients with AIDS and related disorders. J Clin Pharmacol 1988; 28: 837-42.
12. Zhu Z, *et al*: Cellular pharmacology of 2', 3'- didehydro-2', 3'- dideoxythymidine (D4T) in human peripheral blood mononuclear cells. Biochem Pharmacol 1990; 39: R15-19.
13. Dudley MN, *et al*: Clinical pharmacokinetics of nucleoside anti-retroviral agents. (Review.) J Infect Dis 1995; 171: S99-112.

14. Van Leeuwen R, *et al*: Evaluation of safety and efficacy of 3TC (lamivudine) in patients with asymptomatic or mildly symptomatic human immunodeficiency virus infection: A phase I/II study. J Infect Dis 1995; 171: 1166-71.

15. Pluda JM, *et al*: A phase I/II study of 2-deoxy-3- thiacytidine (lamivudine) in patients with advanced human immuno deficiency virus infection. J Infect Dis 1995; 171: 1438-47.

16. Havlir D, *et al*: High-dose nevirapine: Safety, pharmacokinetics, and anti-viral effect in patients with human immuno deficiency virus infection. J Infect Dis 1995; 171: 537-45.

17. Para M, *et al*: Randomised phase I/II concentration-controlled trial of the anti-HIV activity of delavirdine. Paper presented at the 3rd Conference on Retroviruses and Opportunistic Infection, Washington DC, January 28-February 1, 1996.

18. Stein DS, *et al*: A24-week open-label I/II evaluation of the HIV protease inhibitor MK-639 (indinavir). AIDS 1996; 10: 485-92.

19. Danner SA, *et al*: for the European —Australian Collaborative Ritonavir Study Group: A short term study of the safety, pharmacokinetics, and efficacy of ritonavir, an inhibitor of HIV-1 protease. N Engl J Med 1994; 333: 1528-33.

20. Schapiro JM, *et al*: The effect of high-dose saquinavir on viral load and CD4+ T cells counts in HIV-infected patients. Ann Intern med 1996; 124: 1039-50.

21. Hommes KK, Mardh PA, Sparling PF, Lemon SM et al.: Appendix B: Guidelines for use of anti-retroviral agents in HIV infected adults and adolescents. In: Hommes KK, Mardh PA, Sparling PF, Lemon SM et al., eds. Sexually Transmitted diseases, 3rd edition. New York; McGraw-Hill, 1999; B1-B18.

22. Tashima KT, Carpenter CCJ, Fusion inhibition - A major but costly step forward in the treatment of HIV-1. N Eng J med 2003; 22: 2249-2250.

23. J Acquir immune Defic syndr- Lopinavir/Ritonavir maintains HIV suppression 2005; 40: 280-287.

24. AIDS Treatment interruption no benefit to HIV patients with many resistance mutations 2005; 19: 1643-1647

25. BMJ online first, primary resistance to HIV drugs high in U.K., 2005.

CHAPTER

16 How to Help Caregivers of Patients with HIV/AIDS?

R.K. Chadda and *Amerdeep Kumar*

INTRODUCTION

Human Immunodeficiency Virus (HIV) infection and Acquired Immuno Deficiency Syndrome (AIDS) are the one of the major public health problems, which the medical scientists, health planners and the community are facing in the last two decades. The illness continues to be difficult to manage, and is associated with a number of physical and psychosocial problems, as it progresses to a fatal end. There have been attempts at improving the quality of life of the patients and the caregivers with some success, but much needs to be achieved. Because of absence of a satisfactory treatment, sexual mode of transmission and frequently a terminal nature, HIV infection carries a lot of stigma. The patient as well as the family, and the caregivers often face considerable burden. A lot of work has been done in the area of the affected patients, and strategies developed at helping them, but the caregivers have often remained a neglected lot. This paper discusses about some of the strategies, which would be helpful to the professionals working with the caregivers of HIV patients.

HIV/AIDS is a chronic illness with a long-term, incapacitating, terminal and stigmatizing character. It has a devastating effect on the affected families as also seen with other terminal illnesses such as cancer. Treatments costs, physical disability, need for long term care and loss of employment due to physical disability in the patients have a devastating effect on the family, and also contribute to the caregiver burden. Changes in family roles and relationships drain on the family economy, and deprivation, emotional distress and caregiver burden are the frequently observed outcome. It is not the patient alone, but the whole family is affected by the illness (Seelay et al., 1994).

The caregivers are often in dilemma with their own psychosocial needs because of their caring role in such a major problem, besides having to act as service providers, and are always in need of advice and information to manage ongoing care. Frequently, they also face extra demands from their ward, which they may found difficult to meet, and themelves need support. Further, since the pandemic has struck mainly young adults, care giving engenders role reversals that represent major upheavals for families with the elderly parents and dependent, young children often end up performing the caregiving role, sometimes unsuited for their age. Thus the carcgiving experience for HIV/AIDS patients is a complex one, different from the usual one seen in other chronic conditions. The role of the family in the provision of care in HIV/AIDS is considered to be much more stressful than it is in other diseases.

Situation in India

The HIV/AIDS epidemic in India has reached alarming proportions and it is believed that if current transmission rates continue, India will soon have the largest concentration of AIDS affected individuals in the world (Verma & Roy, 2002). The National AIDS Control Organization (NACO), Ministry of Health and Family Welfare, Government of India updates the HIV estimates for the country every year since 1998 for monitoring the trends and pattern of HIV/AIDS in the country. The number of cases with HIV infection in the country has grown steadily from 3.5 million in 1998 to 5.1 million in 2004. While the rural residence accounts for approximately 60 percent of cases, the urban residence accounts for the rest 40 percent of cases. The bulk of the cases are contributed by the adult population aged 15-49 years which is the most productive age-group placing the burden of care to already vulnerable populations such as the elderly, the children and the non-earning family members. In India, due to limited number of beds and specialized treatment facilities, the families are mostly responsible for the care and support of their seropositive members. This is often a stressful experience for almost all the members of the family. Within the family, caregivers, who have a greater degree of involvement in the care giving process, are subject to more adverse outcomes. These also have detrimental effects on physical and mental health. Thus, caring of caregivers becomes very important for optimal care of cases with HIV/AIDS (D'Cruz, 2002).

Burdens of Caregiving

The term caregiver burden is used to describe the physical, emotional, financial, and social problems associated with caregiving. Burden can be assessed in terms of its objective or subjective impact. Objective burden assesses the extent to which caregiving disrupts daily routines and social relationships, and negatively affects resources. This may include changes in household routines, missed days of work, family frictions, reduced social contacts, loss of income, and reduced energy due to being involved in care of the patient. Subjective burden refers to the caregiver's perceptions and reactions to caregiving demands. Caregivers with high levels of subjective burden may report "feeling trapped", or feeling nervous or depressed due to the additional responsibility of the caregiving, even when their objective burden is relatively low (Pakenham & Dadds, 1995: Sisk, 2000). In addition to the family members who often face the brunt of caring their HIV patient, there is a group of professional caregivers involved in caring the HIV patients in health care settings and institutions.

Role of Caregivers in HIV Cases

The caregivers of HIV patients may include family members, relatives, spouses, and friends who provide in-home care, usually on an unpaid basis. They may differ in the type of tasks performed, the amount of time devoted to caregiving, and living arrangements (i.e., same or separate household). They help their family member or friend with HIV/AIDS adhere to treatment regimens, avoid unnecessary hospital admissions, reduce reliance on formal caregivers, remain at home longer and maintain quality of life.

Important functions taken by them include-

- Emotional support (e.g. reassuring, comforting, sympathizing, empathizing, and providing encouragement).
- Help with activities of daily living (e.g., feeding, bathing, dressing, and toileting)
- Help in household and other responsibilities (e.g., cleaning the house, shopping for household, providing transportation).
- Management of finances, house maintenance, etc.,
- Health and social care (e.g. taking the patient to the formal and informal services, communicating with health professionals, procuring and administering medications, catheter care, etc.).

Causes of Burden in Caregivers of HIV Patients

There are a number of factors which contribute to the burden in the persons, who are caring for HIV/AIDS patients.

- Caregiving usually comes as an unexpected role, one for which people are often unprepared. Caregivers need to restructure preexisting role obligations and social activities and the ways in which they relate to the care recipient. Interpersonal strains may intensify as the caregiver and care recipient attempt to resolve issues of autonomy and reciprocity within the context of an increasingly asymmetrical relationship. Gradually increasing involvement of the caregiver over the course of illness may require further adjustments in family, work, and social commitments, increasing the stress further (Pearlin et al., 1997).
- The physical demands of informal caregiving also contribute to burden. Unlike formal caregivers, the relatives and friends providing in-home care often are "on call" 24 hours a day. While working this 24-hour shift, caregivers may be required to perform multiple, and sometimes conflicting roles. Those who have never cared for a seriously ill person must need to learn basic nursing skills, often under extremely stressful circumstances. They also need to find ways to oversee complex medication schedules while meeting their own home and work obligations.
- A constant fear of contacting disease also adds up to the burden.
- The emotional issues surrounding caregiving are another source of burden. Because HIV is most prevalent among people under age 40, the caregivers also

tend to be relatively young. The experience of caring for someone with a terminal illness can be a major source of stress for the young adults. Of course, for people of all ages, HIV/AIDS caregiving creates the emotional strain of dealing with an unpredictable and currently incurable disease. Some caregivers may be burdened by fears of contracting HIV even when they know there is little basis for concern. Those who are already infected may worry that no one will be around to care for them when they become ill (Mullan, 1998).

- The financial impact of caregiving is also a major source of burden. Many families suffer severe economic hardships when a key wage earner is forced to reduce or stop working due to illness or to care for a sick partner or relative.
- Stigma surrounding HIV disease also adds to the caregiver burden. Community rejection of HIV positive individuals because of their disease or the mode of transmission often extends to the relatives and friends who provide care. Rather than facing stigmatization, some caregivers try to conceal their caregiving activities by withdrawing from the social relationships.
- HIV-positive parents face additional challenges that increase their sense of burden, which include arranging for guardianship of the children, balancing the needs of "sick" and "healthy" family members, and helping their children cope with the disease and possible discrimination. If a child is also HIV-positive, the mother's guilt about transmitting the virus can be overwhelming (Schable et al., 1995).

Consequences of Caregiver Burden

Caring for an individual with a chronic disease, such as HIV/AIDS, leaves little time or energy for self-care and thus affecting the health of the caregiver. The multiple tasks performed by caregivers may cause them to neglect nutrition, exercise, socialization, and sleep. High levels of physical health problems and affective disorders have been reported in caregivers caring for their family members with HIV/AIDS (LeBlanc et al., 1997)

Caregiver burden often produces high levels of chronic stress due to the multiple factors. Caregivers may exhibit a wide range of signs and symptoms as given below:

1. **Physical symptoms:** Backache, change in eating patterns, diarrohoea, elevated blood pressure, fatigue, gastrointestinal problems, headache, insomnia, muscle tension, weight loss, etc.
2. **Psychological symptoms**: Anger and frustration, loss of self-confidence and self-esteem, loss of interest and commitment to work, feeling of inadequacy, helplessness and guilt, feelings of restlessness, depression, sense of being overwhelmed or overloaded, mood swings, sense of failure, anxiety about the future, etc.
3. **Behavioural symptoms**: Emotional outbursts, withdrawal from friends and family, loss of punctuality and neglect of duty, decrease in judgmental ability, inability to focus on tasks, tearfulness, increased use of alcohol or other drugs, difficulty getting along with people, impaired work performance, resistance to change, etc.

The extent to which caregivers experience these symptoms depends on their personality, belief systems, health and energy levels, and coping skills, severity of the care recipient's illness, duration of caregiving, and accessibility of social support and financial resources.

Formal Caregivers

There is another group of persons involved in caring for the HIV and AIDS cases as a part of their professional role. These include health professionals, counsellors, and social workers who are trained and compensated for their caregiving activities. This group has also been called formal caregivers. The trained volunteers and spiritual counsellors working in various agencies associated with care and rehabilitation of HIV and AIDS patients also fall in this category.

Causes of Burden for Formal Caregivers: A number of factors may be responsible for burden in formal caregivers. These include:

- Fear of exposure.
- Formal caregivers may also experience a lack of support from their families and professional colleagues due to concerns about contagion or "stigma".
- They may also feel emotionally distressed about not being able to "cure" the disease.
- The unpredictable course of HIV disease and the wide range of potential complications can create significant burden, particularly for clinicians with limited HIV management experience. While attempting to control chronic symptoms and conditions, clinicians also must be prepared to treat episodes of acute illness and therapy-related side effects.
- Repeated exposure to the death of young patients further adds up to the emotional stress.
- Formal caregivers also may be burdened by workplace-related stressors, such as work overload, unrealistic expectations of what can be accomplished, lack of decision making, autonomy, communication problems and role conflicts, and inadequate medical resources and referral arrangements (Gueritault-Chalvin et al., 2000; Kalichman, et al., 2000).

Rewards of Caregiving

Caregiving is not only associated with increased burden, but may also have a feeling of personal accomplishment, which may be a rewarding experience. Some of the positive emotions associated with the caregiving experience are outlined below:

- Bring a mission and purpose to one's life
- Develop empathy and self-knowledge
- Gain a sense of personal effectiveness by demonstrating competence under very difficult circumstances
- Experience the positive feelings associated with loving, caring, and helping

Caregiver Burnout

The term "burnout" in caregiving is used to describe the process in which everyday stressors, that are not addressed, start gradually affecting the caregiver's mental and physical health. Burnout has three components: emotional exhaustion, depersonalization, and reduced personal accomplishment. Emotional exhaustion is characterized by feeling fatigued and lacking enough energy to face another day. Depersonalization refers to the interpersonal dimension of burnout. One may start feeling emotionally detached and interact with others in a negative and callous manner. Reduced personal accomplishment is the self-evaluation dimension of burnout and is characterized by a growing sense of inadequacy (Ross et al., 1999).

Factors Contributing to Caregiver Burnout: Factors contributing to caregiver burnout can be grouped under individual and situational factors. The situational factors are more strongly predictive of burnout than the individual characteristics. Caregivers experiencing work overload and interpersonal conflict over an extended period of time are particularly vulnerable to burnout (Ross et al., 1999). The situational and individual are summarized as below:

1. **Situational Factors**
   - High expectations of oneself and others
   - High levels of commitment, dedication and idealism
   - Need to work hard
   - Need to prove oneself
   - Strong goal orientation
   - Difficulty saying no
   - Difficulty delegating responsibility to others
2. **Individual Factors**
   - Role ambiguity and conflict between role demands
   - Work overload
   - Job tensions
   - Interpersonal conflict with care recipient, family members, colleagues or supervisors
   - Inadequate preparation for caregiving
   - Insufficient resources to meet the demands of caregiving
   - Inadequate social support
   - Lack of recognition for the caregiving functions performed
   - Workplace-related factors (e.g. unrealistic work targets, lack of decision-making autonomy, inadequate referral arrangements)

Impact of Caregiver Burnout: Caregiver burnout has serious consequences for the caregiver, care recipient, and the health care systems. It is important to identify the burnout at the earliest stage so that effective steps can be taken. Early warning signs may include losing motivation, putting in more hours with poorer results, and/or voicing complaints about the caregiving role. In the later stages, caregivers may develop various physical, psychological, and behavioural problems as described earlier. Gradually, the quality of care provided by the caregiver suffering burnout starts coming down.

Such caregivers often become less sensitive to the care recipient's feelings and needs. The care recipient may be neglected; treated in a detached, mechanical fashion; or even subjected to mental/physical abuse. Burnout symptoms, such as decreased judgmental ability and difficulty focusing on tasks, make it more difficult for caregivers to competently perform clinical roles. As these changes occur, care recipients may be at increased risk for disrupted care or placement in a long-term care facility (Parks & Novielli, 2000).

Preventing and Managing Burnout in Informal Caregivers: It is important to have a regular periodic contact with the caregivers to assess the burden experienced by them and to provide them support and guidance, and clarify their concerns about caregiving, if any. A regular contact helps in identifying the early signs of burnout and taking early steps to prevent its further development.

Counseling Caregivers

Counseling of the informal caregivers can be conducted along with medical reviews during the follow up visits of the patients. Problems faced by the caregivers in their caring role can be discussed when they are accompanying the patients for review. Practical suggestions can be offered for eliminating or better managing stressors. These also can help caregivers recognize and build on aspects of their lives that contribute to physical, psychological, and social well-being. Caregivers experiencing significant anxiety or depression and high levels of burden may need to be referred to mental health professionals for assessment and counseling (Parks & Novielli, 2000).

Health professionals sometimes overlook the importance of extending counseling during the bereavement period. If the relatives and friends providing care had a close relationship with the care recipient, grief may extend for two or more years after death. Bereavement counseling can help caregivers mourn appropriately, cope with the changes resulting from their loss, and plan for the future.

Helping the caregivers define the meaningful and valued aspects of their roles and highlighting the positive emotions associated with caregiving enhances both physical and psychological well-being.

Strategies for Counteracting Burnout and Promoting Self-care

Strategies for preventing and managing burnout focus on ways of managing the caregiving situation rather than on eliminating or reducing stressors in the caregiving environment. Caregivers are advised to reevaluate their caregiving demands and resources, clarify values and priorities, and adopt coping strategies that match the nature of the stressors. The strategies are described as under:

1. **Problem-focused Strategies to Cope with Stress**

   Problem-focused strategies are generally more effective in coping with the caregiver stress than the emotion-focused strategies. Problem-focused strategies include gathering information, planning, and taking direct action. Emotion-focused strategies include efforts to escape or avoid problems, emotional outbursts, and self-accusation.

The following strategies usually encourage the use of problem focused strategies:

- Educating about the patient's condition. Helping understanding the disease process and caregiving issues make it easier for the caregiver to deal with day-to-day problems.
- Encourage questions from the caregivers, when accompanying the patient for a medical appointment.
- Ask the caregiver to keep a daily record of the events that cause stress in life. After several weeks, he/she would be better prepared to identify problems, evaluate the criticality of the situation, and weigh possible solutions.
- Discussing problems in caregiver groups also helps in reducing the associated stress. In addition to learning how others deal with similar problems, one may be able to help them manage stress.
- One should not hesitate in seeking professional help from a counsellor or mental health professional, if finding it difficult to manage oneself.

2. Change Caregiving Patterns

Informal caregivers sometimes get so involved with the caregiving work that they lose all their personal interests and hobbies, and thus burn out quickly. This can be avoided by helping caregivers establish realistic goals based on an honest assessment of what they can and cannot do. Once goals are established, caregiving patterns can be changed by:

- Breaking down tasks into small acts of care
- Taking help from others in caregiving tasks
- Encouraging the care recipient to help with tasks and continue self-care as long as possible

Caregivers with high levels of subjective burden should be reminded that no one expects them to be perfect.

3. Relaxation Techniques

Many caregivers use relaxation techniques to manage stress and prevent burnout. These techniques should fit with the individual caregiver's interests, time, and resources. Some caregivers may wish to learn yoga or meditation, while others may prefer to take a walk, listen to music, or visit a temple or other religious places depending on their religious practices. Other relaxation techniques which can reduce stress include deep-breathing exercises, massage therapy, gardening, exercising, reading, and socializing with friends.

4. Strive for Good Health

Healthy lifestyles play an important role in burnout prevention. By eating three balanced meals each day, engaging in regular physical activity, and sleeping

7 to 9 hours each night, caregivers can increase their capacity to manage stress. Exercise programs increase energy and provide a needed outlet for pent-up emotions. These may involve vigorous workouts, or just walking 20 to 30 minutes each day, depending on personal preferences.

Some caregivers may react to stress by indulging in unhealthy behaviours such as smoking, drinking, and drug misuse. This may increase the problems further and needs to be discouraged. Caregivers should be informed of the harmful effects of these behaviours and encouraged to participate in counselling and/or treatment programs.

5. **Maintain a Life outside the Caregiving Role**

Caregivers often respond to stress by becoming over-involved with caregiving duties. The constant demands of the job may cause caregivers to neglect friends, interests, and activities that once gave them pleasure. Health professionals should encourage caregivers to take regular breaks and to keep up with their interests and hobbies as best they can. For some caregivers, outside employment may provide relief from everyday tensions. Others may simply need to get away for a few hours. Health professionals can help caregivers "jump-start" the self-renewal process by linking them with social support resources.

6. **Build a Support Network**

Caregivers with higher levels of social support are less likely to experience negative outcomes. Social resources can provide emotional comfort and practical support; reduce social isolation; and offer humor, recognition, and encouragement. They can also be a valuable source of new information and insights.

Social support resources should be explored if the caregiver's answers to screening questions suggest a need for outside assistance. Help from NGOs working in the area can also be explored. Informal sources of social support include family members, other relatives, friends and volunteers.

Caregiver Support Groups

Support groups bring caregivers together to share feelings and experiences and to learn from one another. In contrast to group therapy, their purpose is not to change participants' behaviours but to enhance decision-making capacity and coping effectiveness. One of the major benefits of support groups is to provide an outlet for emotions that cannot be expressed in the home. Support groups can significantly reduce caregiver stress; however, they cannot substitute for professional counselling or therapy when these services are needed (Parks & Novielli, 2000).

Some other benefits of support groups include:

- Opportunities to be better informed about HIV/AIDS, new treatments and community resources
- Share problems and brainstorm solutions

- Establish social contacts
- Lessen the sense of stigma associated with HIV care
- Obtain recognition for caregiving efforts

However, stigma associated with HIV often prevents some caregivers to associate with professionals and such groups. Relatives and friends of HIV-positive individuals need to divulge their caregiving status. They also must find the time to attend support group meetings and also locate someone who can provide care in their absence, and make arrangements for transportation. Telephone support groups are another option for caregivers who wish to maintain anonymity or who cannot attend meetings.

Educating Caregivers

Ignorance, lack of information or misconceptions often contributes to the stress as well as burnout. Therefore, it is important for the health professionals working with the caregivers to provide sufficient information and correct the misconceptions of the caregivers. It is important to assess the caregiver's level of knowledge about HIV/AIDS and the types of tasks performed by them, so that relevant information can be given to them. Some important areas of such information may include:

- What is HIV and AIDS?
- Modes of HIV transmission
- Effects and side effects of medications
- Drug-taking schedules and strategies for improving adherence
- Basic information on nutrition
- Symptoms and problems to expect as the disease progresses

Informal caregivers may also be provided information about infection control, pain and symptom management, and simple nursing techniques (e.g., administering injections, cleaning and dressing ulcers). As new treatments are discovered and standards of care change, informal caregivers need to be updated. Audio-visual aids and print materials should be developed for the caregivers.

Preventing and Managing Burnout in Formal Caregivers

Formal caregivers may require somewhat different approach when they develop burnout. In addition to helping individual caregivers develop more effective coping strategies, interventions should target policies and practices in the workplace that create or exacerbate stress. Formal caregivers can benefit from coping effectiveness training.

Some strategies found to be effective to prevent burnout in the formal caregivers include:

- Establishing clear job descriptions and good referral mechanisms
- Setting realistic work targets
- Restructuring jobs to make workloads more manageable
- Providing training on HIV management, new approaches to pain and symptom management, and effective ways of communicating with patients and family members

- Offering on-site health promotion programs
- Encouraging staff to participate in policy decisions that affect their work
- Providing regular time off and appropriate rewards
- Regular forums for case discussion
- Having support groups for the formal caregivers

(Kalichman et al., 2000)

Conclusion

Till now, we don't have satisfactory and effective treatments available for HIV infection and the illness tends to end terminally after running a long course complicated by opportunistic infections and associated disabilities. In this background, the caregivers have a very important role to play. The caregivers face a number of major stresses and strains and may also burn out. Regular support mechanisms addressing the problems faced by the caregivers of HIV and AIDS cases are required and are helpful in reducing stress and burnout in them.

REFERENCES

1. D'Cruz, P, (2002): Engulfing Darkness—The impact of HIVAIDS on the family, Families in Society, 83, 416-430.
2. Gueritault-Chalvin V, Demi A, Peterson JL, Kalichman SC, Work-related Stress and Occupational Burnout in AIDS Caregivers: Test of a Coping Model with Nurses providing AIDS care. AIDS Care 12: 149-61, 2000.
3. Kalichman SC, Gueritault-Chalvin V, Demi A: Sources of Occupational Stress and Coping Strategies Among Nurses working in AIDS care, *J Assoc Nurses AIDS Care*, 11: 31-7, 2000.
4. LeBlanc AJ, London A, Aneshensel CS: The Physical Costs of AIDS caregiving, *Soc Sci Med* 45: 915-23, 1997.
5. Mullan JT: Aging and Informal Caregiving to People with HIV/AIDS. Res Aging 20: 712-38, 1998.
6. Pakenham KL, Dadds MR: Carers' Burden and Adjustment to HIV, AIDS Care 7: 189-203, 1995.
7. Parks SM, Novielli KD: A practical guide to caring for caregivers, *Am Fam Physician*, 62: 2613-22, 2000.
8. Pearlin LI, Aneshensel CS, LeBlanc AJ: The forms and mechanisms of stress proliferation: the case of AIDS caregivers, *J Health Soc Behav*, 38: 223-36, 1997.
9. Ross MW, Greenfield SA, Bennett L: Predictors of Dropout and Burnout in AIDS Volunteers: A longitudinal shidy, AIDS Care II, 723–31, 1999.
10. Schable B, Diaz T, Chu SY, Caldwell MB, Conti L, Alston OM, *et al*.: Who are the primary caretakers of children born to HIV-infected mothers? Results from a multistate surveillance project. *Pediatrics* 95: 511-5, 1995.
11. Seelay J, Kajura E, Bachengana C, Okongo M, Wagner U, & Mulder D, (1994): The Extended Family and Support for People with AIDS in a Rural Population in South West Uganda: A safety net with holes? In R.Bor & J.Elford (Eds.), The Family and HIV (pp. 141-150), London: Cassell.
12. Sisk R J: Caregiver burden and Health Promotion. *Int J Nurs Stud* 37(1): 37-43, 2000.
13. Verma R K & Roy T K, (2002): HIV Risk Behaviour and Socio-cultural environment. In S.Panda, A Chatterjee, & A S Abdul-Quader (Eds.): Living with the AIDS Virus (pp. 77-90). New Delhi, Sage.
14. Wight RG, Le Blanc AJ, Aneshensel C: AIDS Caregiving and Health among Midlife and Older Women. *Health Psychol* 17: 130-7, 1998.

CHAPTER

17 Surveillance of STIs and HIV/AIDS

Parvathy Nair and Vijay Grover

National HIV sero-surveillance was initiated in India in 1985 with a view to find out the magnitude and dimension of HIV infection long before AIDS cases were reported in the country.

The surveillance system for HIV/AIDS includes:

(a) HIV Sentinel Surveillance

(b) AIDS Case Surveillance

(c) Behavioural Surveillance

(d) STI Surveillance

(a) HIV Sentinel Surveillance: Since 1998, Government of India has been conducting nationwide sentinel surveillance, covering all States and Union Territories, in order to assess the spread of the HIV infection in the country. The sentinel sites included both high risk groups of population like STD clinic attendees, injecting drug users, commercial sex workers and men who have sex with men, and low risk population i.e., women attending antenatal clinics.

HIV sentinel surveillance means carrying out cross-sectional studies (also known as prevalence surveys) of HIV prevalence rates at regular intervals among selected groups in the population known as sentinel groups. It can either be community based or/clinic/health facility based. The later being more convenient and therefore preferred.

The procedures for planning and implementation of HIV sentinel surveillance and for analysis of data so obtained includes

Planning

1. Selection of the Sentinel Population:

Groups with high risk behaviour: Those with sexually transmitted diseases sexual intercourse with multiple partners, sharing unsterilized needles.

Groups with low risk of transmission: Pregnant women. In addition blood donors in most countries and military recruits in some are screened to determine the prevalence of HIV infection in low risk groups. Tuberculosis patients have been included as sentinel groups in a few surveillance systems but the data is difficult to interpret due to the complex interrelationship between mycobacterium tuberculosis infection and HIV infection.

Criterion for Establishment of Sentinel Site

A. STD: Annual attendance should be greater than 500 without any clustering
B. IDUs: One in each bigger state and north eastern state
C. ANC: One in each state (Low Prevalent) with representation from both urban and rural population.

The Ratio of High Risk to Low Risk is as follows

- Areas with High Prevalence: 1:2
- Areas with Moderate Prevalence: 2:1
- Areas with Low Prevalence: 3:1

Sampling

NACO advised collection of consecutive samples over a 12 week period from 1st August to 31st October.

Sample Size

- STD Clinic: 250 (150 from Skin and STD clinic and 100 from Obstetric and Gynaecology Department)
- Injecting Drug Users: 250
- Antenatal Clinic: 400 or moreover a 12 week period.

Frequency of Survey

Sentinel surveillance should be carried out using the sample sizes given above and repeated once every year. The stress is on the quality of the data obtained with the emphasis on having more testing centers than on the increased frequency of tests. Also the methodology and laboratory procedures used must be similar to those previously used to ensure comparable results.

Testing Methodology

The unlinked anonymous method of testing is used as it reduces the participation bias. In this method a sample of blood originally collected for other purposes is tested for HIV after all the information that could identify the source of the sample is eliminated. Blood collected for HIV testing is also subjected to screening for Hepatitis B and C to assess the prevalence and monitor the trends over a period of time.

HIV Testing Strategy

ELISA or Rapid or simple assay with higher sensitivity is used to test the serum first. If the serum is found reactive on the first assay the test is repeated with a second ELIZA or rapid simple assay with higher specificity based on a different antigen preparation along/ or with different test principles. If the serum is non reactive in the second test it is considered antibody negative.

Implementation

The HIV sentinel surveillance programme was initially implemented in high risk areas and later extended to other areas.

Staffing at Sentinel Sites: There would be one in charge of the sentinel site, a nursing attendants, a lab technician.

At the HIV testing laboratory there would be one in charge of HIV testing lab and one lab technician.

Data collection: The method of testing is unlinked anonymous in which all efforts are made to delete information that can identify the source of the sample. The data collection forms should include the following information

- The location of the sentinel site
- The population group
- The month and year of serum collection
- Age group
- HIV laboratory test result

Only a unique code number should link the data collection form with the lab result.

All the sera collected at the sentinel site are tested in the same laboratory at the same time during any one sampling period. Minimum of 0.5 ml of serum is collected in specimen tube, properly labeled and stored in the freezer. Ideally 6-7 ml of blood should be drawn to facilitate Hepatitis B and C testing simultaneously. They are dispatched to the HIV testing laboratory not in batched of less than 50 as if less samples are sent it increases the risk of identification of the source of the sample

External Quality Assurance Programme

All samples detected HIV sero-positive by using Rapid HIV test kits will be retested by using two ELIZA kits with different antigens or principles. Also 5% of all negative samples collected would be sent to reference laboratories for confirmation. In both case the result is communicated to the respective laboratories in 15 days time.

Reporting of Data

Data Collection: 1st August to 31st October

All voluntary counselling and testing centers sent their report to State AIDS Control Societies by 15th November.

Regional meetings with states by 15th December

Preliminary report prepared by NACO should be out by 30th December while final report is released by NIHFW with three months after the preliminary report is submitted.

Analysis of HIV sentinel data

!. HIV prevalence trends in each individual site

HIV prevalence rate = Number positive for HIV/Total number tested × 100

Confidence interval is taken as 90% and calculated as follows CI(90%)

= p + Z/px (100-p)/N

P = prevalence. Z = 1.65 (for CI-90%) and N = Number of samples tested.

HIV Prevalence Rates in Each Risk Group (i.e., ANC & STD Patients)

The average prevalence rate is calculated for each risk group in the following manner:

If there are three or less than three sentinel centers, the arithmetic mean is calculated.

If there are more than three sentinel sites the median is calculated.

Distribution of HIV prevalence according to different documented variables like age, sex, location, migration, literacy and occupational status.

Assumptions

The following assumptions on different parameters for estimation of the size of the risk group populations have been recommended and taken for estimation.

1. The census figures and the projected figures for October will be the basis for calculating:
   (a) Population (in the age group of 15–49 years)
   (b) Urban population and rural population
   (c) Male-Female ratio
2. STD prevalence rates in both urban and rural populations as follows:
   STD prevalence in urban areas will be 10% in high prevalent States, 7% in medium prevalent States and 5% in low prevalent States. It will be the same for both males and females. 5% prevalence in rural populations in all States/UTs, for both males and females.
3. For the purpose of HIV estimation in high-risk population, urban rural differential will be 3:1 in all the States. Similarly, for HIV prevalence in low risk population, the urban-rural differential will be 8:1 in all the States.
4. As there are more infected males than females, the following ratio would be applied:

- In high prevalent States, for every infected female there are 1.2 males,
- In moderate prevalent States, for every infected female there are 2 males
- In low prevalence States, for every infected female there will be 3 males.

Similarly, for every male STD patient from highly prevalent States, it is assumed that there would be 0.83 females, for moderate prevalent States, there will be 0.5 females and for low prevalent States, there would be 0.33 female patients.

5. For estimation of HIV infection among IVDUs, the HIV prevalence rate will be applied to the estimated size of IVDUs population in the State.
6. The States will be categorised as high, moderate or low, based on following definition:
   (i) High Prevalent States: States where HIV prevalence in antenatal women is 1% or more.
   (ii) Moderate Prevalent States: States where the HIV prevalence in antenatal women is less than 1% and prevalence in STD and other high risk groups is 5% or more.
   (iii) Low Prevalent States: States where the HIV prevalence in antenatal women is less than 1% and HIV prevalence among STD and other high-risk group is less than 5%.

Sentinel Surveillance Sites in India

The Annual Round of HIV Sentinel Surveillance, 2003, was conducted in 455 sentinel sites in all the States and UTs. These included:

- 271 sites at antenatal clinics (as proxy for the general population)
- 166 sites in clinics for sexually transmitted diseases
- 13 sites among injecting drug users
- 3 sites for men having sex with men
- 2 sites for commercial sex workers.

2001	*2002*	*2002*	*2003*	*2004*
	320 sites	384 sites	455 sites	670 sites (proposed)

India has an overall prevalence of less than 1% among adult population. During year 2004, annual round would be held in 670 sites, to be started from 1st July 2004. The main features of this round are :

Annual data collection for rural sub-set in 124 ANC sites located in high-prevalence States, to closely track the spread of HIV in rural areas.

84 sentinel sites will be located in the on-going targeted intervention projects in order to have high-risk data representative of all States.

Relocation of 18 STD sites in private sector hospitals in order to ensure participation of private sector STD clinics.

- Establishment of sentinel sites in TB hospitals in high-prevalence States to monitor HIV trends in TB patients across these States.

(b) AIDS Case Surveillance: To assess the incidence of AIDS cases in the country, information will be collected from all hospitals having trained Physicians with standard AIDS case definition in Indian context. But the diagnosis and reporting of AIDS cases is very incomplete. And the cases so reported are just a fraction of the actual numbers. The estimated completeness of AIDS reporting varies from 50% in Hong Kong to less than 5% in most South Asian countries.

(c) Behavioural Surveillance: To assess the changing pattern of behaviour in different risk groups of population behavioural sentinel surveillance will be instituted initially on pilot basis which will be expanded as per the needs of the programme from time to time. The general concept of behavioural surveillance was not formulated since 1993 and it would take some years before it is full integrated with National HIV/AIDS programme.

The behavioural indicators would include:

1. The percentage of respondents who report at least one non regular sex partner in the last 12 months.
2. The percentage of respondents who say they used condom the last time they had sex with a non marital, non cohabitating partner, among those who had sex within the last 12 months.
3. Age at first sex among youth
4. Reported sharing of unclean injecting equipment among drug injectors
5. Reported number of clients in the last one week amongst sex workers.
6. Reported condom use with last client amongst sex workers.
7. Prevalence of genital herpes antibodies in young (15-24 yrs olds) can be used as a surrogate measurements for the first two indicators.

The Responses to the above questions can yield basic information that can help setting specific and reasonable targets that can be achieved over a specific period of time and devise specific means of evaluating the effectiveness of programme interventions with regard to started targets.

HIV-risk Behaviour Surveillance Survey by NACO

The main objectives of BSS is to provide repeated measures on behaviour for observing trends in high risk behaviour among selected population groups. A set of 9 indicators were used to assess information derived from BSS in Tamil Nadu conducted the three waves (1996/1997/1998). Information was also collated from monthly reports collected from participating NGOs from other Indian cities. The BSS indicators are as follows:

1. ***Knowledge Indicators***

   Proportion of respondents who cite 2 acceptable ways of preventing STDs

   Proportion of respondents who know condoms prevent STD.

   Proportion of respondents who cite 2 acceptable ways of preventing HIV/AIDS.

   Proportion of respondents who know that condoms prevent HIV/AIDS.

2. ***Behaviour Indicators***

   Proportion of respondents who report heterosexual intercourse with a non-regular partner in the last year

   Proportion of respondents who report condom use during last sexual intercourse with non-regular sexual partner in the last year

3. ***Urethritis Prevalence***

   Proportion of male respondents who report symptoms of urethritis during last year.

   Proportion of male respondents who sought treatment from qualified medical practitioners for urethritis in the last year

4. ***Appropriate Perception of Risk Indicators***

   Proportion of respondents with risk behaviour who perceive that they are at risk of contracting HIV/AIDS.

STI Surveillance

According to WHO estimates there were approximately 370 million STI patients in Asia Pacific Region which contribute about 46% of the global burden of disease in the region. The two main sources of information on STIs are National case reporting systems and Epidemiological or prevalence assessment surveys. However as many as STI infections are asymptomatic or have non-specific symptomatology and also due to the general stigma attached with the disease, there's an under reporting of STI cases. Epidemiological surveys can be a better method but they are mostly conducted on specific population groups, limiting the usefulness the information for national estimates of total burden of infection in the community.

REFERENCES

1. Sero Surveillance for HIV Infection in India. Reprinted from: ICMR bulletin Vol. 17, No. 12, December, 1987.
2. Understanding HIV/AIDS numbers and public health surveillance of HIV/AIDS. HIV/AIDS in Asia and the Pacific Region 2003. World Health Organization, 92-101.
3. Guidelines for HIV Sentinel Surveillance URL: http://www.nacoonline.org/guidelines/guideline_11.pdf
4. NACO: Programs-Targeted Interventions URL: http://www.nacoonline.org/prg_sche_targetint.htm.
5. Indian Journal of Community Medicine Vol. XXVIII, No. Jan-March 2003.

CHAPTER 18

National AIDS and STI Control Program

Vijay Grover

BACKGROUND

Soon after reporting of the first few HIV/AIDS cases in the country in 1986, the Government of India recognized the seriousness of the problem and took a series of important measures to tackle the epidemic. By this time AIDS had already attained epidemic proportion in the African region and was spreading rapidly in many countries of the world. Government of India without wasting any time initiated steps and started pilot screening of high risk population. A high level National AIDS Committee was immediately constituted and National AIDS Control Program (NACP) was launched in year 1987.

National AIDS Committee

To formulate strategy and plan for implementation of prevention and control of HIV/AIDS in the country, Ministry of Health & Family Welfare constituted National AIDS Committee in year 1986 under the Chairmanship of the Union Ministry of Health and Family Welfare with representatives from various sectors. The committee was formed with a view to bring together various ministries, NGOs, and private institutions for effective coordination in implementing the program.

The committee acts as the highest-level deliberation body to oversee the performance of the program and to provide overall policy directions, and to forge multisectoral collaborations. The 5th meeting of the National AIDS Committee was held on 24th September, 1998 in Vigyan Bhavan presided by the Hon'ble Minister of State for Health & Family Welfare.

In the initial years, the program focused on generation of public awareness through more communication programs, introduction of blood screening for transfusion purpose and conducting surveillance activities in the epicenters of the epidemic.

Medium Term Plan for HIV/AIDS Control

In year 1989, with the support of WHO, a medium term plan for HIV/AIDS control was developed with a US $10 million budget provided from external sources. Project documents for the implementation of this plan were developed and implemented in 5 states and UTs, which were most affected, namely Maharashtra, Tamil Nadu, West Bengal, Manipur and Delhi. Initial activities focused on the reinforcement of program management capacities as well as targeted IEC and surveillance activities. Actual preventive activities like implementation of education and awareness program, blood safety measures, control of hospital infection, condom promotion to prevent HIV/AIDS, strengthening of clinical services for both STD and HIV/AIDS gained momentum only in 1992.

NACP in the States & UTs

(a) **State Level Strengthening:** In order to strengthen the program management at the state level, the state governments have established their own managerial organizations which include State AIDS Control Societies (formerly, State AIDS Cells), technical advisory committees and empowered committees as per the guidelines of the strategic plan. The structure of the State AIDS Societies are shown below progress in the development of state management teams has been satisfactory, although some states have responded effectively than others.

(b) **Empowered Committee:** At the state level, an empowered committee has been constituted by the states either under the chairmanship of chief secretary or additional chief secretary at par with the National AIDS Control Board at central level.

This committee takes the policy decisions for implementation of HIV/AIDS control program in the respective states and approve administrative and financial actions which otherwise would have been approved by the state department of finance.

(c) **State AIDS Control Societies:** State AIDS Cells were created in all the 32 States and UTs of the country for the effective implementation and management of National AIDS Control Program. However, over the period of time it was realized that due to many cumbersome administrative and financial procedures, there was delay in release of financial outlay sanction by Government of India due to which the implementation of the program at different levels suffered. In order to remove the bottlenecks faced by the program implementation at State level, Ministry of Health and Family Welfare advised the State Government/Union Territories to constitute a registered society under the chairmanship of Secretary, Health. The society should be broad based with its members representing from various ministries like social welfare, education, industry, transport, finance etc. and Non-Government Organisations. On an experimental basis Tamil Nadu AIDS Control Society was created which was followed by Pondicherry. Successful functioning of these societies led to the Government of India to advise other states to follow this pattern for implementation of the National AIDS Control Program.

With the spread of AIDS from one country to another, it becomes necessary to initiate a National Control Program.

Brief History of NACP

1985	:	A Task Force was constituted by the Government of India to look into this matter. It began by Pilot Screening Program and High Risk Population.
1986	:	First AIDS case reported.
1986	:	National AIDS Committee constituted by MOHFW, representatives from various sectors.
1987	:	NACP was launched to generate public awareness through IEC, Blood screening for transfusion and surveillance.
1989	:	A Medium Term Plan for HIV/AIDS Control with WHO support was started.
1991	:	'Strategic Plan for Prevention and Control of AIDS in India' was prepared for the year 1992-97.
1992	:	National AIDS Control Organisation (NACO) was set up by the Ministry of Health and Family Welfare as a separate working to implement and closely monitor the various components of the program.
1992-1997	:	National AIDS Control Organisation Phase I.
1999-2004	:	National AIDS Control Organisation Phase II.

NACP Phase I (1992-1997)

The Government of India launched a five year HIV/AIDS Control Program Project from September 1992 to September 1997 as hundred percent centrally sponsored project for all States/UTs. The project was later extended upto March 1999.

Objectives

- Involve all States and UTs HIV/AIDS preventive activities with spiritual focus on major epicenters.
- Attain satisfactory level of public awareness on HIV transmission and prevention.
- Development of Health Program intervention among risk behaviour group.
- Screening of all blood units collected for blood transfusion.
- Decrease practices of professional blood donation.
- Development skills on MRI, HE and counselling.
- Strengthen contract of STDs.

Program Management

- Establishment of National AIDS Committee Board and Organisation at the Centre.
- Decentralization and building up AIDS Cell in collaboration with NGOs.
- Conversion of State AIDS Cell into State AIDS Control Societies.

Achievements

- Higher length of awareness.
- Improvement in Blood Society.
- 504 STD centres strengthened.
- Surveillance capacity developed.

<table>
<tr><td colspan="4">Organisational Structure of the State AIDS Control Program Empowered Committee Chief Secretary or Addl. Chief Secretary or Health Secretary, Directorate of Health Services</td></tr>
<tr><td colspan="2">State AIDS Cell
Addl. Director/Jt. Director/Dy. Director</td><td colspan="2">State Technical Advisory Committee
DHS</td></tr>
<tr><td>Officer
STD</td><td>Officer
Blood Safety</td><td>Officer
IEC</td><td>Officer
Surveillance</td></tr>
<tr><td>Pvt. NGOs
Corporate
Individual
Section</td><td>Medical
College
Hospital
STD Centre</td><td>Rural
Health
Care</td><td>NGO
Nodal
Agency
System</td></tr>
<tr><td>1st Level
Health Care
Institution</td><td colspan="2">Distt. Hospital
Municipal Hospital
Centre</td><td>State Communication
Facilities STD
MCH/FP/ANC</td></tr>
</table>

Organisational Structure of National AIDS Control Program

<table>
<tr><td colspan="3">National AIDS Committee
Chairperson
Ministry of Health and Family Welfare</td></tr>
<tr><td colspan="3">National AIDS Control Board
Secretary (H)</td></tr>
<tr><td>Theme Group
Secretary
UNAIDS
Director</td><td>Additional
Project
National
AIDS Control
Organisation</td><td>Technical
Sub-committee
HCL</td></tr>
<tr><td colspan="2">UNAIDS
Addl. Project Director Tech.</td><td>Social, legal
ethical issues
STD Centre</td></tr>
<tr><td colspan="3">Blood Safety
Surveillance</td></tr>
<tr><td colspan="3">IEC</td></tr>
<tr><td colspan="3">Quality Control</td></tr>
<tr><td colspan="3">Research</td></tr>
<tr><td colspan="3">Clinical Case
Management</td></tr>
</table>

Information, Education, Communication and Social Mobilisation (IEC)

A multipronged strategy was adopted. Multi-media approach in collaboration with Ministry for Information and Broadcasting, NGO, mass media.

- Use of advertising agencies for intensive campaign
- Social education program in 15 States on pilot basis
- Focussing on cross border intervention projects
- Training of counsellors and counseling services

Condom Promotion

Enforcement of policies for good quality control condom compared to international standard, social media approach in collaboration with Ministry of Information and Broadcasting, NGO, Mass Media, Social Marketing to increase the use of affordable quality of condom.

- Use of advertising agencies for intensive campaign
- Social education program in 15 States on pilot basis
- IEC packages for groups practicing high risk behaviour
- Focusing on cross borders intervention projects
- Training of counsellors and counselling services

Blood Safety

Aim is to develop and strengthen the national blood transfusion system and ensure adequate supply of safe blood to all blood banks and health facilities.

- Complete ban on professional blood donation w.e.f. 1st Jan, 1998
- Framing and dissemination of national HIV testing policy procedure, mandatory screening and confidentiality
- Establishment of national and state blood transfusion councils as registered societies to screening and confidentiality
- Licences have been issued to 1233 blood banks and no unlicensed blood banks permitted to provide blood transfusion services
- Provision of 100% exemption of income tax for the donation made to national/state blood transfusion councils
- Revision of drugs and cosmetic rules to make it more stringent in respect of procedure for collection, processing, storage and distribution
- Strengthening of 815 public sectors/voluntary sector blood banks
- Mandatory testing for HIV, hepatitis B, malaria and syphilis of all blood units collected at all blood banks
- Establishment of 154 zonal testing centres
- Establishment of 40 blood components separation units
- Clinical management of AIDS patients with opportunistic infections
- Testing for HIV

NACP Phase II (1999-2004)

1. The Phase II of the National AIDS Control Program has become effective from 9th November, 1999. It was a 100% Centrally sponsored scheme implementation in 32 States, UTs and 3 Municipal Corporations namely Ahmedabad, Chennai, and Mumbai through AIDS Control Societies.
2. Project formulation for Phase II, National AIDS Control Program followed a truly participatory process at the State and Municipal Corporation levels. Between April and June 1998, the Technical Laison Officers (TLOs) of NACO in collaboration with State AIDS Control Program officers, conducted State Level Planning Workshops in all the States and the cities of Mumbai, Chennai and Ahmedabad. Each of these workshops was conducted for 2 days in which sector, medical professionals and district level officials participated in each of these workshops. In addition to serving as a tool preparation, these workshops also turned out to be a major advocacy effort. In the formulation of the state implementation plan, the following steps were taken:

   Step 1: Holding of State level workshop in which from Government departments, NGOs etc. discussed the various issues under several components and came out with recommendations.

   Step 2: Constitution of Core team to finalise the specific programs for AIDS Control Project 11 based on the recommendations made under seven components.

   Step 3: Core team held three sittings in June, 1998, examined the recommendation to identify and select program/activities which needed to be given priority and focus.

   Step 4: The activities suggested were listed and prioritized by the Core Team bases on the recommendations at the workshops.

   Step 5: In the end July, the World Bank prescribed cost codes were received. A special Task Force was constituted and the activities were regrouped under five components as per the revised guidelines from NACO and World Bank.

   Step 6: The various activities were divided into sub-activities, cost codes were assigned for each sub-activity. The implementation plan was prepared indicating the process, sub-process, activities, implementing agency, assessment parameters and risks.

   Step 7: The unit cost and the number of units under each activities were finalized by the special Task Force and outlay was worked out. Discussions were held with officials of USAIDS and VHS-APAC to assess the extent of bilateral involvement in Tamil Nadu.

Step 8: The Technical Liaison Officers, World Bank Consultants and the PDNACo reviewed the draft (Project Implementation Plan PIP) prepared and suggest scaling down of outlay, taking into account the past and current expenditure and the absorptive capacity funds in the future. At this state, the Procurement Plan and the Training Action Plan were prepared simultaneously.

Step 9: The special task force held several sittings to review the no. of interventions and units of various activities. After the southern states PIP workshop at Bangalore in the first week of Sept., 1998. It was decided to restrict the interventions and the no. of other units/activities and the outlay was revised. The procurement plan was finalized after excluding the cost of equipment to be procured and supplied by NACO. The training action plan was also revised.

NACP Phase II is Aimed at:

- Shifting focus from raising awareness to changing behaviour through interventions amongst High Risk Group.
- Supporting decentralization of services deliveries to States and Municipalities and a facilitative role for NACO.
- Protecting human rights by encouraging voluntary counselling and testing and discouraging mandatory testing.
- Supporting structure and evidence based annual reviews and operational research.
- Encouraging management reforms to bring about a sense of ownership of the program among the States.

Challenges Facing the National Program

Challenge 1: The need to rapidly build capacities within States

Challenge 2: Ensuring targeted intervention to achieve impact

- Mere delivery of services or HIV awareness not enough to reach marginalised groups
- Supportive inputs need to be provided
- Increased need to work with "bridge population" such as male clients of CSWs

Challenge 3: Achieving behaviour change beyond high risk

- Address behaviour change in the general reproductive age group

Challenge 4: Need to comfort discrimination and stigma

- Public health and human right issue
- Tackle discrimination in health and other primary services
- Work place discrimination

Challenge 5: Addressing the urgency care and support

The National AIDS Control Project Phase II is aimed at two **key objectives** namely:

1. To reduce the spread of HIV infection in India.
2. To strengthen India's capacity to respond to HIV/AIDS epidemic on long term basis.

Operationally The project interventions would seek to achieve the following by end of the project:

1. To keep HIV prevalence rate below 5% of adult population in Maharashtra Below 3% in Andhra Pradesh, Tamil Nadu, Karnataka and Manipur.
2. Reduce blood bank transmission HIV to 4%.
3. Attain awareness level of not less than 90% among the youth and others in the reproductive age group.
4. To achieve condom use of not less than 90% among high risk categories like CSWs.

Project Targets

The program has the following firm targets to be achieved during project period:

1. To reduce blood-borne transmission of HIV to less than 1% of the total transmission.
2. To introduce Hepatitis C as the 5th mandatory test for blood screening.
3. To set up 10 new modern blood banks in uncovered areas, upgrading of 20 major blood banks, setting up of 80 new district level blood banks in uncovered districts, establishing another 40 blood components separation units, promotion of voluntary blood donation and increase its share in total blood collected to atleast 60%.
4. To attain awareness level of not less than 90% among the youth and those in the reproductive age group.
5. To train up at least 600 NGOs in the country in conducting targeted intervention programs among high risk groups and through them promote condom use of not less than 90% among these groups and control of STDs.
6. To conduct annual Family Health Awareness Campaigns among the general population and provide service delivery in terms of medical advice and provision of drugs for control of STDs and Reproductive Tract Infections (RTIs).
7. Promotion of voluntary testing facilities across the country at the end of project.
8. Awareness campaigns will now be more interactive and use of traditional media such as folk arts and street theatre will be given greater priority in the rural areas.
9. Promotion of organisations of people living with HIV/AIDS and giving them financial support to form self-help groups.

Project Components

The project would adopt a multi-pronged approach that would focus on the most critical intervention to begin limiting HIV transmission.

(a) Deliver cost effective intervention against HIV/AIDS

1. Priority targeted intervention for groups at high risk
   (a) Identify groups at higher risk:
      (i) Participating approaches;
         a. Train PHC provider by syndrome case Management of STIs and counselling in condom use.
         b. Improve referral services for STIs, treatment strengthening STI centre in each district and medical college hospital.
         c. Client program – deliver targeted IEC, condom promotion, STI treatment, and counselling for clients.
2. Preventive intervention for the general community
   - Popular service, maintain confidentiality of cases, help caller, clarify doubts and access personal counselling.

School AIDS Education Program

- Raise awarness levels, help young people, resist peer pressure and develop a safe and responsible life style
- Training of teachers, peer education among students
- Providing voluntary testing and counselling

1. Raise availability and demand for voluntary testing especially joint testing of couples, training grass roots health care workers in HIV/AIDS counselling
2. Provide counselling services through all blood banks and STI clinics, IVCTC for each district 145 functioning
   - Review transmission by blood transfusion and occupational experiment
     1. Setting up 10 new modern blood banks
     2. Upgrading 20 existing and setting up 80 new district level blood banks
     3. Mandatory testing of HEPV for screening
     4. Promoting voluntary donation
     5. Setting up 40 component separation units
     6. Communication among blood bank services
     7. Trained counsellors for blood banks
     8. Training health care workers in universal precaution
3. Low cost AIDS care
   - Provide funding for home based and community based care
   - Increase availability of cost effective intervention for community OIs

- Establish best practice guidelines and providing drugs for treatment, common OIs at district level
- Training at selected state level hospitals for provision of referral services
- Establish small community based hospital, HOSPICE program, drop in centres in collaboration with NGOs and CBOs.

  11 centres – shelter, food, nursing care, recreation, spiritual discoveries, training of families and CBOs.
- Expand and improve nationwide STI/HIV/AIDS sentinel surveillance
- Sentinel surveillance in every state
- STI surveillance through special surveys
- Behaviour surveillance surveys
- AIDS care surveillance
- 320 sentinel centre

Training

HIV/AIDS/STDs prevention and control

Objectives

- Preventing the spread of epidemic
- Strengthening local capacity to respond to the epidemic in future
- Central level activities, generic development curricula, training of trainers
- State level training of a Core group in each medical college/tertiary hospital

Train medical and paramedical staff

- To be carried out in several phases

Building capacity for monitoring and evaluation

- Independent monitoring and evaluation would be selected
- Each area to have a M/E Officer
- Performance and expenditure annual review (PEAR)
- Computerized MIS

Increase Indian capacity for research on HIV/AIDS

- Research Advisory Committee to determine research needs in the country in the field of HIV/AIDS
- Enlist institutional to conduct epidemiological and operational research
- HIV vaccine
- MTCT prevention program to be introduced as operational research

Intersectoral Collaboration

- Focus on leveling from innovation HIV/AIDS programs that exists in other sector
- Sharing work of generating awareness and delivering intervention
  - (ii) MSM
  - (iii) Determine access and demand of high services of these groups
  - (iv) Develop strategy based on outreach, peer education and partnership

(b) Provide integrated peer counseling, condom provision and treatment of STIs for high risk
  - (ii) Train PHC providers by syndromic approach, management of STIs and counselling in condom use.
  - (iii) Improve referral services for STIs, treatment and strengthening of STI centres in each district
  - (iv) Client program – deliver targeted IEC, condom promotion, STI treatment, and counselling for clients

1. Preventive intervention for the general community
2. IEC and awareness campaign activities include conducting mass media campaign at States and Municipal level, local IEC counsel program geared youth and college students
3. Providing voluntary testing and counselling
4. Reduce transmission by blood transfusion and occupational exposure
5. A Training Action Plan has been finalized after convening four regional and one national workshop of various states with twin objectives of:
   - Preventing the spread of epidemic and strengthening local capacity to respond to the epidemic in future and
   - Central level activities, generic development curricula, training of trainers
   - State level training of a Core Group in each medical college/tertiary hospital
   - Train medical and paramedical staff
   - To be carried out in several phases
6. Building capacity for monitoring and evaluation
   - Independent monitoring and evaluation would be selected
   - Each area to have a M & E Officer
   - Performance and expenditure annual review (PEAR)
   - Computerised MIS
7. Increase Indian capacity for Research on HIV/AIDS
   - Research Advisory Committee to determine research needs in the country in the field of HIV/AIDS

- Enlist institutional to conduct epidemiological and operational research
- HIV vaccine
- MTCT prevention program to be introduced as operational research
- Focus on leveling from innovation HIV/AIDS program that exists in other sector
- Sharing work of generating awareness and delivering intervention

People Living with HIV/AIDS

Variety of health and social support needs, policies and guidelines developed for clinical management of these cases:

- All Govt. hospitals to admit HIV/AIDS cases without any discrimination
- To be managed in general ward
- Sputum negative TB cases and patients immunity diminished – to manage in separate room
- Special marking of both to be discouraged
- Discharge certificates will refer to OI
- Only case sheet to contain diagnosis of HIV/AIDS
- Death certificate immediate cause of death of opportunistic infection to be mentioned
- All OIs to be treated properly, drug free of cost to be ensured by SACs TB patients to be treated according to RNTCD
- Infection control guidelines in Govt. hospitals to be strictly follow
- PEP should be monitored strictly
- Policy on Anti-retroviral therapy – NACO meeting efforts to be exempt customs and excise not provide under NACP.

A. Organising family health awareness camps on regular basis to generate awareness and provide service delivery for control of STIs/RTIs:
   - Doordarshan and put satellite channels for telecast of messages on HIV/AIDS prevention and control.
   - AIR – JEEYO or JEENO DO
   - AIR FM – NACO film hit parade medical advice, counselling
   - Rural outreach and press activities, street plays. Songs and dramas
   - AIDS Telephone helpline – Toll free
   - Information and counselling – 1097
   - Popular service, maintain confidentiality of cases, help caller, clarify doubts and access personal counselling.

B. Provide the integrated peer counselling, condom use and treatment of STIs for high risk.

Provide integrated peer counselling on condom use and treatment of STIs for high risk;

- Train PHC provider by syndromic case Management of STIs and counselling in condom use
- Improve referral services for STIs, treatment strengthening STI centre in each district and medical college hospital
- Client program – deliver targeted IEC, condom promotion, STI treatment, and counseling for clients

NACO PROGRAM

Sexually Transmitted Diseases (STDs) Control

Introduction

The growing evidence available from all over the world undoubtedly indicates that the incidence of HIV infection is higher in conditions of presence of sexually transmitted diseases (STD). Our country has a high incidence of STD in urban as well as rural areas. Within a short period in Mumbai alone HIV infection has reached 50 percent among sex workers and 36 per cent among STD patients. Evidence also suggests that concomitant infection with other STDs, particularly those characterized by genital ulcers, increase the chance of HIV infection. Therefore, a person already having STD has the greater risk of acquiring HIV from sexual intercourse if he/she comes in contact with an infected partner.

The importance of treatment and control of STD in relation to HIV infection was recognized by NACO. After taking over the STD control program, NACO made it an integral component of AIDS control policy. Suitable strategies were devised for the control and prevention of STD as a priority in the over all planning to control the spread of the infections.

STD Control Program in India

Program for control of STD among the population of India is present for many decades. Even before the country achieved independence, a National STD Control Program was started in 1946. This program continued to operate till 1991 and with the arrival of/ spread of HIV infection in the country and because of the strong relating with STD, the program was brought under the purview of NACO in the year 1992 this program earlier had only a limited number of specialised facilities for diagnosis and treatment. Therefore, the program emphasized more on health seeking behaviour of the individuals having STDs and on the removal of the social stigma attached to the problem of STDs.

It has been found that a very small proportion (only 5-10%) of people suffering from the disease attend public STDs facilities. The majority choose to seek clinical assistance from various other formal as well as informal sources. Some times even reasoning to self-medication. In the rural areas, STD treatment facilities are generally not available. The only health care facility, which is available easily, is that of family welfare services through Maternal & Child Health (MCH)/Family Welfare (FW) and Ante-natal Care (ANC) clinics. These services apart from their mandatory activities also include treatment of STD in their purview. The total gamut of facilities available for diagnosis and treatment for STD however, were not sufficient considering the need and demand for treatment of STD.

STD as a Co-factor for HIV Transmission

- Increasing evidence suggest that STD significantly enhances the acquisition and transmission of HIV.
- The predominant mode of transmission of both HIV infection and STD is through sexual route, other routes of transmission are both blood and blood products, donated organs and tissues and infected women.
- Many of the measures for preventing the sexual transmission of HIV are the same as for prevention of STDs.
- STD clinical services are important access point for persons at high risk for both HIV and STD, not only for diagnosis and treatment, but also for health education counselling and prevention.
- Trends in STD incidence and prevalence sexual behaviour and are easier to monitor than trends in HIV sero-prevalence and thus valuable for determining the impact of HIV/AIDS control program.

Policy on Control of HIV/STDs

The Ministry of Health and Family Welfare has adopted a policy of integrating HIV/AIDS and STDs control within the existing health care systems, both in the public and private sectors. Special emphasis is being placed on the integration of comprehensive STDs management at the primary health care level to provide non-stigmatized services with greater accessibility and acceptability to the patients while maintaining confidentiality and privacy of the patients. The policy strategy also emphasizes on the cooperation and collaboration with the private sector as well as non-government organization for the control of STD. The STD policy document has been widely circulated. A number of manuals and guidelines have been prepared and also distributed in all states and UTs.

Objectives of the STD Control Program

The STD control component of the National AIDS Control Program has two major objectives:

- Reduce STDs cases and there by control HIV transmission by minimizing the risk factor, and
- Prevent the short term as well as long term morbidity and mortality due to STDs

In order to accomplish these objectives, following strategies have been incorporated in the strategic plan for the prevention and control of AIDS in India.

Strategies

The broad strategies for controlling STD as outlined in strategic plan for the prevention and control of AIDS in India are the following:

- Adequate and effective program management
- Prevention of the transmission of STD/HIV infection through IEC and promotion of safer sexual behaviour by the use of condoms
- Adequate and comprehensive case management including diagnosis, treatment, individual counselling partner notification and screening for other disease
- Increasing access to health care for STD by strengthening existing facilities and structures and creating new facilities wherever necessary
- Early diagnosis and treatment of mostly asymptomatic infections through case finding and screening
- Special emphasis on early detection and prompt treatment of STDs among high risk groups through targeted intervention projects

Actions

The following major actions have been taken along the lines suggested in the strategies:

- Training of health care workers in both public and private sectors in comprehensive STDs case management
- Development of appropriate laboratory services for the diagnosis of STDs
- Conduction of Microbiological, Socio-behavioural and Operation research
- Surveillance to assess the epidemiological situation, and monitor and evaluate the on-going STD control program

The details of other actions related to specific strategies are explained below:

Strategy – 1: Develop adequate and effective program management

- Strengthening existing 504 STD clinics in the country by providing drugs, consumables and laboratory support for diagnosis and treatment
- Appointment of STD Programme Officers in State AIDS Control Societies and identification of district nodal officers in each district to supervise the working of STD clinics

Strategy – 2: Promote IEC activities for the prevention and transmission of STDs and HIV infection

- Within the parameters of National AIDS Control Program, IEC activities have been designed for the prevention of STDs and HIV infection including raising of awareness and promotion of appropriate health care seeking behaviour of the people
- Awareness generation activities are being implemented to educate the people for responsible sexual behaviour, safer sex and condom use

Strategy – 3: Make adequate arrangement for comprehensive case management including diagnosis treatment, individual counselling, partner notification, and screening of other disease

- Two sets of guidelines have been published and distributed for use in all first level health care facilities and for reference for STDs specialists
- Training has already been imparted to medical and paramedical workers and Supervisors by the State AIDS Control Societies
- Since laboratory facilities have been extremely limited in most primary health care setting syndromic approach has been favoured in the management of STDs cases because of its cost effectiveness
- In case of improving secondary and tertiary facilities, the existing 504 STD clinics have been further strengthened in different district and taluk hospitals and medical colleges in the country
- The five regional centers with attached regional STD referral laboratories have already been upgraded to provide necessary training for medical and paramedical staff, conducting research and laboratory tests and to ensure quality control of VDRL results

Strategy – 4: Increasing access to health care for STDs by strengthening existing facilities and structures and creating new facilities wherever necessary

- Efforts are on to strengthen the available STD clinics both in the Government as well as private sectors. The HIV prevention efforts such as IEC and the NGO programs are increasing the demand for quality STD services. New facilities are being upgraded to function as First Referral Units in collaboration with Department of Family Welfare. A list of the STD clinics created/upgraded is presented as an annexure to this report.

Strategy – 5: Creating facilities for diagnosis and treatment of asymptomatic infections

- Efforts are on to train lady medical officers in diagnosis and treatment of asymptomatic reproductive tract infections, including sexually transmitted diseases in MCH clinics
- Sensitisation of community about the problems related to RTI/STD through Family Health awareness campaign for early detection and referral to Primary health centres for treatment

STD and Gender Perspective

- Many sexually transmitted infection in women are asymptomatic. For instance, more than 50 percent of gonorrhoeal infection in women are asymptomatic thus there is no felt need to seek health care.
- Most women have very limited understanding and awareness about reproductive health symptoms relating to reproductive tract infections and reproductive of symptoms, they either frequently ignore them or not associate them with RTI/STDs.
- The taboos surrounding sexuality and STD lead to a situation where people, particular women, seeking health care for STDs are stigmatized. This is specially the case where STD care is provided through easily identifiable specialist STD clinics.

- Women feel uncomfortable being examined by male doctors, but very few female doctors are available in STD clinics, thus even if women attend STD clinics, they are usually not examined properly and the necessary treatment may not be given.

Achievements

STD Facility Survey: A 504 STD clinics facility survey is being conducted all over the country covering all STD clinics. The objectives of the survey is to assess the functioning of STDs clinics in reference to their utilization and to find out the deficiencies which influence their functioning. The results will help in formulating a strategy for better utilization of these STD clinics.

STD Referral, Research and Training Centre: A 2-day workshop was organized for conducting facility survey of the 5 STD regional referral centres. The objective of the workshop was to develop tools and action plan for assessing the performance of these centres. A team of four experts visited each site and submitted their observations in regard to the functioning and shortcomings of these institutions. The recommendations of the teams would be utilized for improving the working of these centres.

Production of Training Material

- Interactive training modules have been published and circulated to all states/ UTs. For different categories of health professionals and peripheral health workers. Prevention and control of STDs is one of the key topic in all modules.
- A reference manual "Laboratory diagnosis of Sexually Transmitted Diseases for laboratory workers working in STD laboratories has been published and distributed.
- A protocol and training module on STD surveillance has been prepared.
- Training materials, "Simplified STD treatment guidelines" and STD treatment recommendations have been revised and published.
- Laboratory services in the five Regional STD referral centers and in the STD clinics in medical colleges and district as well as taluk hospitals have been upgraded.
- Laboratory support is provided for diagnosis of difficult cases management of treatment failures and research and antibiotics susceptibility monitoring
- A proposal has been mooted for strengthening the quality assurance system for STD laboratories in relation to serology testing and diagnosis of syphilis and gonorrhoea.

Syndromic Approach to STDs Treatment

This has been devised to simplify treatment of STDs/STIs. This treatment is based on clinical diagnosis in the absence of laboratory support. (Treatment is described under the chapter of management of STIs in adolescents.)

Research

- Baseline studies on STD prevalence in Tamil Nadu, Kolkata and Jaipur have been completed. Similar studies are being conducted in Andhra Pradesh, Himachal Pradesh and Assam.
- A study on the prevalence of STD in pregnant and non-pregnant women in the family planning and child health clinics in East Delhi has been completed
- Studies to validate the flow charts used in the syndromic approach have been completed
- Activities have been initiated on development of an antibiotic susceptibility-monitoring network for gonorrhoea

Surveillance

- Guidelines on STD surveillance based on syndrome approach as well as etiological diagnosis have been developed for district down to health centres for implementation in a phased manner.

REFERENCES

1. Annual Report, M/o Health & Family Welfare, Govt. of India, Nirman Bhawan, New Delhi, 1999-2000, p. 182-189.
2. National AIDS Control Programme: country Scenario, NACO, M/o Health & Family Welfare, Govt. of India, Nirman Bhawan, New Delhi, 1997-98, p. 1-9.
3. National AIDS Control Programme: Country scenario, NACO, M/s Health & Family Welfare, Govt. of India, Nirman Bhawan, New Delhi, 1998-99.
4. National AIDS Control Programme: Country scenario update, NACO, M/o Health & Family Welfare, Govt. of India, New Delhi, Dec., 1995.
5. Annual Report, M/o Health & Family Welfare, Govt. of India, Nirman Bhawan, New Delhi, 1998-99, p. 164-171.
6. Training Modules on Sentinel Surveillance of HIV Infection, National AIDS Control Organization, M/o Health & Family Welfare, Govt. of India, 1993, Annex, B1-B4.
7. National AIDS Control Programme in Health chapter, Ninth Plan (1997-2002), Vol. 11, Planning Commission, Govt. of India, New Delhi.
8. WHO (1981), Technical Report Series No. 660.
9. Control of Sexually Transmitted Diseases, Annual Report (1998-99), M/o Health & Family Welfare, Govt. of India, New Delhi.